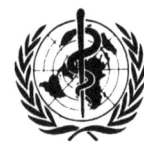 

WORLD HEALTH ORGANIZATION

INTERNATIONAL AGENCY FOR RESEARCH ON CANCER

# IARC MONOGRAPHS
## ON THE
# EVALUATION OF CARCINOGENIC RISKS TO HUMANS

*Some Flame Retardants and Textile Chemicals,
and Exposures in the Textile Manufacturing Industry*

VOLUME 48

This publication represents the views and expert opinions
of an IARC Working Group on the
Evaluation of Carcinogenic Risks to Humans
which met in Lyon,

21–28 February 1989

1990

# IARC MONOGRAPHS

In 1969, the International Agency for Research on Cancer (IARC) initiated a programme on the evaluation of the carcinogenic risk of chemicals to humans involving the production of critically evaluated monographs on individual chemicals. In 1980, the programme was expanded to include the evaluation of the carcinogenic risk associated with exposures to complex mixtures.

The objective of the programme is to elaborate and publish in the form of monographs critical reviews of data on carcinogenicity for chemicals and complex mixtures to which humans are known to be exposed, and on specific occupational exposures, to evaluate these data in terms of human risk with the help of international working groups of experts in chemical carcinogenesis and related fields, and to indicate where additional research efforts are needed.

This project is supported by PHS Grant No. 5-UO1 CA33193-07 awarded by the US National Cancer Institute, Department of Health and Human Services. Additional support has been provided by the Commission of the European Communities since 1986.

©International Agency for Research on Cancer 1990

ISBN 92 832 1248 7

ISSN 0250-9555

All rights reserved. Application for rights of reproduction or translation, in part or *in toto*, should be made to the International Agency for Research on Cancer.

Distributed for the International Agency for Research on Cancer
by the Secretariat of the World Health Organization

PRINTED IN THE UK

# CONTENTS

NOTE TO THE READER ............................................................. 5

LIST OF PARTICIPANTS ............................................................ 7

PREAMBLE

    Background ................................................................. 13
    Objective and Scope ........................................................ 13
    Selection of Topics for Monographs ......................................... 14
    Data for Monographs ........................................................ 15
    The Working Group .......................................................... 15
    Working Procedures ......................................................... 15
    Exposure Data .............................................................. 16
    Biological Data Relevant to the Evaluation of Carcinogenicity to Humans ...... 17
    Evidence for Carcinogenicity in Experimental Animals ........................ 18
    Other Relevant Data in Experimental Systems and Humans ..................... 20
    Evidence for Carcinogenicity in Humans ..................................... 21
    Summary of Data Reported ................................................... 24
    Evaluation ................................................................. 25
    References ................................................................. 29

GENERAL REMARKS ................................................................. 33

THE MONOGRAPHS

    *Flame retardants*
        Chlorendic acid ......................................................... 45
        Chlorinated paraffins ................................................... 55
        Decabromodiphenyl oxide ................................................. 73
        Dimethyl hydrogen phosphite ............................................. 85
        Tetrakis(hydroxymethyl) phosphonium salts ............................... 95
        Tris(2-chloroethyl) phosphate ........................................... 109

    *Textile dyes*
        *para*-Chloro-*ortho*-toluidine and its strong acid salts ................. 123
        Disperse Blue 1 ......................................................... 139

## CONTENTS

Disperse Yellow 3 .................................................. 149
Vat Yellow 4 ....................................................... 161
5-Nitro-*ortho*-toluidine .......................................... 169

*Other textile chemicals*

Nitrilotriacetic acid and its salts ................................ 181

*Industry*

Exposures in the textile manufacturing industry .................... 215

*Glossary* ......................................................... 279

SUMMARY OF FINAL EVALUATIONS ....................................... 281

APPENDIX 1. ACTIVITY PROFILES FOR GENETIC AND RELATED EFFECTS ............................................................. 283

CUMULATIVE INDEX TO THE *MONOGRAPHS* SERIES ........................ 317

## NOTE TO THE READER

The term 'carcinogenic risk' in the *IARC Monographs* series is taken to mean the probability that exposure to an agent will lead to cancer in humans.

Inclusion of an agent in the *Monographs* does not imply that it is a carcinogen, only that the published data have been examined. Equally, the fact that an agent has not yet been evaluated in a monograph does not mean that it is not carcinogenic.

The evaluations of carcinogenic risk are made by international working groups of independent scientists and are qualitative in nature. No recommendation is given for regulation or legislation.

Anyone who is aware of published data that may alter the evaluation of the carcinogenic risk of an agent to humans is encouraged to make this information available to the Unit of Carcinogen Identification and Evaluation, International Agency for Research on Cancer, 150 cours Albert Thomas, 69372 Lyon Cedex 08, France, in order that the agent may be considered for re-evaluation by a future Working Group.

Although every effort is made to prepare the monographs as accurately as possible, mistakes may occur. Readers are requested to communicate any errors to the Unit of Carcinogen Identification and Evaluation, so that corrections can be reported in future volumes.

# IARC WORKING GROUP ON THE EVALUATION OF CARCINOGENIC RISKS TO HUMANS: SOME FLAME RETARDANTS AND TEXTILE CHEMICALS, AND EXPOSURES IN THE TEXTILE MANUFACTURING INDUSTRY

## Lyon, 21-28 February 1989

## LIST OF PARTICIPANTS

**Members**

P. Bannasch, Institute for Experimental Pathology, German Cancer Research Centre, Post Box, 69003 Heidelberg 1, Federal Republic of Germany (*Vice-chairman*)

P.A. Bertazzi, Institute for Occupational Health, Clinica del Lavoro 'Luigi Devoto', University of Milan, via S. Barnaba 8, 20122 Milan, Italy

J.R. Bucher, Carcinogenesis and Toxicology Evaluation Branch, National Institute of Environmental Health Sciences, PO Box 12233, Research Triangle Park, NC 27709, USA

I. Chahoud, Institute for Toxicology and Embryonic Pharmacology of the Free University of Berlin, Garystrasse 1-9, 1000 Berlin 33 (West), Federal Republic of Germany

M.J. Gardner, MRC Environmental Epidemiology Unit, Southampton General Hospital, Southampton SO9 4XY, UK (*Chairman*)

S. Goldfarb, Department of Pathology, The Medical School, University of Wisconsin, 470 North Charter Street, Madison, WI 54706, USA

A.L. Greife, Division of Surveillance, Hazard Evaluations and Field Studies, National Institute for Occupational Safety and Health, R-14, 4676 Columbia Parkway, Cincinnati, OH 45226-1998, USA

A.R. Kinsella, Paterson Laboratories, Christie Hospital and Holt Radium Institute, Manchester M20 9BX, UK

E. Kriek, Division of Chemical Carcinogenesis, The Netherlands Cancer Institute, Antoni van Leeuwenhoekhuis, Plesmanlaan 121, 1066 CX Amsterdam, The Netherlands

Y. Kurokawa, Division of Toxicology, National Institute of Hygienic Sciences, 1-18-1 Kamiyoga, Setagaya-ku, Tokyo 158, Japan

J.A. Merchant, Institute of Agricultural Medicine and Occupational Health, College of Medicine, Oakdale Campus, University of Iowa, Iowa City, IA 52242, USA

Y.D. Parfenov, Laboratory of Carcinogenic Substances, Cancer Research Centre, Kashirskoye Shosse 24, 115478 Moscow, USSR

N.E. Pearce, Wellington Clinical School of Medicine, Department of Community Health, Wellington Hospital, Wellington, New Zealand

E. Priha, Tampere Regional Institute of Occupational Health, PO Box 486, 33101 Tampere, Finland

S. Venitt, Institute of Cancer Research, F Block, Costwold Road, Sutton, Surrey SM2 5NG, UK

**Observers**

*Representative of the National Cancer Institute*

D.G. Longfellow, Chemical and Physical Carcinogenesis Branch, Division of Cancer Etiology, National Cancer Institute, Executive Plaza North, Suite 700, 6130 Executive Boulevard, Bethesda, MD 20892, USA

*Representative of the Commission of the European Communities*

E. Krug, Commission of the European Communities, Health and Safety Directorate, Bâtiment Jean Monnet, Plateau du Kirchberg, BP 1907, 2920 Luxembourg, Grand Duchy of Luxembourg

*Representative of Tracor Technology Resources, Inc.*

S. Olin, Tracor Technology Resources, Inc., 1601 Research Boulevard, Rockville, MD 20850, USA

*Representative of the Chemical Manufacturers Association and Fire Retardant Chemicals Association*

P.A. Martin, Albright & Wilson Ltd, PO Box 3, 210-222 Hagley Road West, Oldbury, Warley, West Midlands B68 0NN, UK

*Representative of the Ecological and Toxicological Association of the Dyestuffs Manufacturing Industry*

R. Jäckh, Toxicology, BASF AG, 6700 Ludwigshafen, Federal Republic of Germany

*Representative of the European Chemical Industry, Ecology and Toxicology Centre*

D. Farrar, Occupational Health, ICI Chemicals & Polymers Ltd, PO Box 13, The Heath, Runcorn, Cheshire WA7 4QD, UK

**Secretariat**

A. Aitio, Unit of Carcinogen Identification and Evaluation

## PARTICIPANTS

H. Bartsch, Unit of Environmental Carcinogenesis and Host Factors

J.R.P. Cabral, Unit of Mechanisms of Carcinogenesis

E. Cardis, Unit of Biostatistics Research and Informatics

J. Cheney, Editorial and Publications Programme

G.J. van Esch, Orange Nassaulaan 65, 3722 JN Bilthoven, The Netherlands, International Programme on Chemical Safety/World Health Organization

J. Estève, Unit of Biostatistics Research and Informatics

M. Friesen, Unit of Environmental Carcinogenesis and Host Factors

E. Heseltine, Lajarthe, Montignac, France

T. Kauppinen, Unit of Carcinogen Identification and Evaluation

M. Kogevinas, Unit of Analytical Epidemiology

K. L'Abbé, Unit of Analytical Epidemiology

D. Mietton, Unit of Carcinogen Identification and Evaluation

R. Montesano, Unit of Mechanisms of Carcinogenesis

I. O'Neill, Unit of Environmental Carcinogenesis and Host Factors

C. Partensky, Unit of Carcinogen Identification and Evaluation

I. Peterschmitt, Unit of Carcinogen Identification and Evaluation, Geneva, Switzerland

A. Sasco, Lyon, France

L. Shuker, Unit of Carcinogen Identification and Evaluation

L. Tomatis, Director

H. Yamasaki, Unit of Mechanisms of Carcinogenesis

*Secretarial assistance*

J. Cazeaux

M. Lézère

S. Reynaud

# PREAMBLE

# IARC MONOGRAPHS PROGRAMME ON THE EVALUATION OF CARCINOGENIC RISKS TO HUMANS[1]

## PREAMBLE

### 1. BACKGROUND

In 1969, the International Agency for Research on Cancer (IARC) initiated a programme to evaluate the carcinogenic risk of chemicals to humans and to produce monographs on individual chemicals. The *Monographs* programme has since been expanded to include consideration of exposures to complex mixtures of chemicals (which occur, for example, in some occupations and as a result of human habits) and of exposures to other agents, such as radiation and viruses. With Supplement 6(1), the title of the series was modified from *IARC Monographs on the Evaluation of the Carcinogenic Risk of Chemicals to Humans* to *IARC Monographs on the Evaluation of Carcinogenic Risks to Humans*, in order to reflect the widened scope of the programme.

The criteria established in 1971 to evaluate carcinogenic risk to humans were adopted by the working groups whose deliberations resulted in the first 16 volumes of the *IARC Monographs* series. Those criteria were subsequently re-evaluated by working groups which met in 1977(2), 1978(3), 1979(4), 1982(5) and 1983(6). The present preamble was prepared by two working groups which met in September 1986 and January 1987, prior to the preparation of Supplement 7(7) to the *Monographs* and was modified by a working group which met in November 1988(8).

### 2. OBJECTIVE AND SCOPE

The objective of the programme is to prepare, with the help of international working groups of experts, and to publish in the form of monographs, critical reviews and evaluations of evidence on the carcinogenicity of a wide range of human exposures. The *Monographs* may also indicate where additional research efforts are needed.

The *Monographs* represent the first step in carcinogenic risk assessment, which involves examination of all relevant information in order to assess the strength of the available evi-

---

[1]This project is supported by PHS Grant No. 5 UO1 CA33193-07 awarded by the US National Cancer Institute, Department of Health and Human Services, and with a subcontract to Tracor Technology Resources, Inc. Since 1986, this programme has also been supported by the Commission of the European Communities.

dence that certain exposures could alter the incidence of cancer in humans. The second step is quantitative risk estimation, which is not usually attempted in the *Monographs*. Detailed, quantitative evaluations of epidemiological data may be made in the *Monographs*, but without extrapolation beyond the range of the data available. Quantitative extrapolation from experimental data to the human situation is not undertaken.

These monographs may assist national and international authorities in making risk assessments and in formulating decisions concerning any necessary preventive measures. The evaluations of IARC working groups are scientific, qualitative judgements about the degree of evidence for carcinogenicity provided by the available data on an agent. These evaluations represent only one part of the body of information on which regulatory measures may be based. Other components of regulatory decisions may vary from one situation to another and from country to country, responding to different socioeconomic and national priorities. *Therefore, no recommendation is given with regard to regulation or legislation, which are the responsibility of individual governments and/or other international organizations.*

The *IARC Monographs* are recognized as an authoritative source of information on the carcinogenicity of chemicals and complex exposures. A users' survey, made in 1988, indicated that the *Monographs* are consulted by various agencies in 57 countries. Each volume is generally printed in 4000 copies for distribution to governments, regulatory bodies and interested scientists. The *Monographs* are also available *via* the Distribution and Sales Service of the World Health Organization.

## 3. SELECTION OF TOPICS FOR MONOGRAPHS

Topics are selected on the basis of two main criteria: (a) that they concern agents and complex exposures for which there is evidence of human exposure, and (b) that there is some evidence or suspicion of carcinogenicity. The term agent is used to include individual chemical compounds, groups of chemical compounds, physical agents (such as radiation) and biological factors (such as viruses) and mixtures of agents such as occur in occupational exposures and as a result of personal and cultural habits (like smoking and dietary practices). Chemical analogues and compounds with biological or physical characteristics similar to those of suspected carcinogens may also be considered, even in the absence of data on carcinogenicity.

The scientific literature is surveyed for published data relevant to an assessment of carcinogenicity; the IARC surveys of chemicals being tested for carcinogenicity(9) and directories of on-going research in cancer epidemiology(10) often indicate those exposures that may be scheduled for future meetings. Ad-hoc working groups convened by IARC in 1984 and 1989 gave recommendations as to which chemicals and exposures to complex mixtures should be evaluated in the *IARC Monographs* series(11,12).

As significant new data on subjects on which monographs have already been prepared become available, re-evaluations are made at subsequent meetings, and revised monographs are published.

## 4. DATA FOR MONOGRAPHS

The *Monographs* do not necessarily cite all the literature concerning the subject of an evaluation. Only those data considered by the Working Group to be relevant to making the evaluation are included.

With regard to biological and epidemiological data, only reports that have been published or accepted for publication in the openly available scientific literature are reviewed by the working groups. In certain instances, government agency reports that have undergone peer review and are widely available are considered. Exceptions may be made on an ad-hoc basis to include unpublished reports that are in their final form and publicly available, if their inclusion is considered pertinent to making a final evaluation (see pp. 25 *et seq.*). In the sections on chemical and physical properties and on production, use, occurrence and analysis, unpublished sources of information may be used.

## 5. THE WORKING GROUP

Reviews and evaluations are formulated by a working group of experts. The tasks of this group are five-fold: (i) to ascertain that all appropriate data have been collected; (ii) to select the data relevant for the evaluation on the basis of scientific merit; (iii) to prepare accurate summaries of the data to enable the reader to follow the reasoning of the Working Group; (iv) to evaluate the results of experimental and epidemiological studies; and (v) to make an overall evaluation of the carcinogenicity of the exposure to humans.

Working Group participants who contributed to the considerations and evaluations within a particular volume are listed, with their addresses, at the beginning of each publication. Each participant who is a member of a working group serves as an individual scientist and not as a representative of any organization, government or industry. In addition, representatives from national and international agencies and industrial associations are invited as observers.

## 6. WORKING PROCEDURES

Approximately one year in advance of a meeting of a working group, the topics of the monographs are announced and participants are selected by IARC staff in consultation with other experts. Subsequently, relevant biological and epidemiological data are collected by IARC from recognized sources of information on carcinogenesis, including data storage and retrieval systems such as CANCERLINE, MEDLINE and TOXLINE — including EMIC and ETIC for data on genetic and related effects and teratogenicity, respectively.

The major collection of data and the preparation of first drafts of the sections on chemical and physical properties, on production and use, on occurrence, and on analysis are carried out under a separate contract funded by the US National Cancer Institute. Efforts are made to supplement this information with data from other national and international sources. Representatives from industrial associations may assist in the preparation of sections on production and use.

Production and trade data are obtained from governmental and trade publications and, in some cases, by direct contact with industries. Separate production data on some agents may not be available because their publication could disclose confidential information. Information on uses is usually obtained from published sources but is often complemented by direct contact with manufacturers.

Six months before the meeting, reference material is sent to experts, or is used by IARC staff, to prepare sections for the first drafts of monographs. The complete first drafts are compiled by IARC staff and sent, prior to the meeting, to all participants of the Working Group for review.

The Working Group meets in Lyon for seven to eight days to discuss and finalize the texts of the monographs and to formulate the evaluations. After the meeting, the master copy of each monograph is verified by consulting the original literature, edited and prepared for publication. The aim is to publish monographs within nine months of the Working Group meeting.

## 7. EXPOSURE DATA

Sections that indicate the extent of past and present human exposure, the sources of exposure, the persons most likely to be exposed and the factors that contribute to exposure to the agent, mixture or exposure circumstance are included at the beginning of each monograph.

Most monographs on individual chemicals or complex mixtures include sections on chemical and physical data, and production, use, occurrence and analysis. In other monographs, for example on physical agents, biological factors, occupational exposures and cultural habits, other sections may be included, such as: historical perspectives, description of an industry or habit, exposures in the work place or chemistry of the complex mixture.

The Chemical Abstracts Services Registry Number, the latest Chemical Abstracts Primary Name and the IUPAC Systematic Name are recorded. Other synonyms and trade names are given, but the list is not necessarily comprehensive. Some of the trade names may be those of mixtures in which the agent being evaluated is only one of the ingredients.

Information on chemical and physical properties and, in particular, data relevant to identification, occurrence and biological activity are included. A separate description of technical products gives relevant specifications and includes available information on composition and impurities.

The dates of first synthesis and of first commercial production of an agent or mixture are provided; for agents which do not occur naturally, this information may allow a reasonable estimate to be made of the date before which no human exposure to the agent could have occurred. The dates of first reported occurrence of an exposure are also provided. In addition, methods of synthesis used in past and present commercial production and different methods of production which may give rise to different impurities are described.

Data on production, foreign trade and uses are obtained for representative regions, which usually include Europe, Japan and the USA. It should not, however, be inferred that those areas or nations are necessarily the sole or major sources or users of the agent being evaluated.

Some identified uses may not be current or major applications, and the coverage is not necessarily comprehensive. In the case of drugs, mention of their therapeutic uses does not necessarily represent current practice nor does it imply judgement as to their clinical efficacy.

Information on the occurrence of an agent or mixture in the environment is obtained from data derived from the monitoring and surveillance of levels in occupational environments, air, water, soil, foods and animal and human tissues. When available, data on the generation, persistence and bioaccumulation are also included. In the case of mixtures, industries, occupations or processes, information is given about all agents present. For processes, industries and occupations, a historical description is also given, noting variations in chemical composition, physical properties or levels of occupational exposure with time.

Statements concerning regulations and guidelines (e.g., pesticide registrations, maximal levels permitted in foods, occupational exposure limits) are included for some countries as indications of potential exposures, but they may not reflect the most recent situation, since such limits are continuously reviewed and modified. The absence of information on regulatory status for a country should not be taken to imply that that country does not have regulations with regard to the exposure.

The purpose of the section on analysis is to give the reader an overview of current methods cited in the literature, with emphasis on those widely used for regulatory purposes. No critical evaluation or recommendation of any of the methods is meant or implied. Methods for monitoring human exposure are also given, when available. The IARC publishes a series of volumes, *Environmental Carcinogens: Methods of Analysis and Exposure Measurement*(13), that describe validated methods for analysing a wide variety of agents and mixtures.

## 8. BIOLOGICAL DATA RELEVANT TO THE EVALUATION OF CARCINOGENICITY TO HUMANS

The term 'carcinogen' is used in these monographs to denote an agent or mixture that is capable of increasing the incidence of malignant neoplasms; the induction of benign neoplasms may in some circumstances (see p. 19) contribute to the judgement that the exposure is carcinogenic. The terms 'neoplasm' and 'tumour' are used interchangeably.

Some epidemiological and experimental studies indicate that different agents may act at different stages in the carcinogenic process, probably by fundamentally different mechanisms. In the present state of knowledge, the aim of the *Monographs* is to evaluate evidence of carcinogenicity at any stage in the carcinogenic process independently of the underlying mechanism involved. There is as yet insufficient information to implement classification according to mechanisms of action(6).

Definitive evidence of carcinogenicity in humans can be provided only by epidemiological studies. Evidence relevant to human carcinogenicity may also be provided by experimental studies of carcinogenicity in animals and by other biological data, particularly those relating to humans.

The available studies are summarized by the Working Group, with particular regard to the qualitative aspects discussed below. In general, numerical findings are indicated as they appear in the original report; units are converted when necessary for easier comparison. The Working Group may conduct additional analyses of the published data and use them in their assessment of the evidence and may include them in their summary of a study; the results of such supplementary analyses are given in square brackets. Any comments are also made in square brackets; however, these are kept to a minimum, being restricted to those instances in which it is felt that an important aspect of a study, directly impinging on its interpretation, should be brought to the attention of the reader.

For experimental studies with mixtures, consideration is given to the possibility of changes in the physicochemical properties of the test substance during collection, storage, extraction, concentration and delivery. Either chemical or toxicological interactions of the components of mixtures may result in nonlinear dose-response relationships.

An assessment is made as to the relevance to human exposure of samples tested in experimental systems, which may involve consideration of: (i) physical and chemical characteristics, (ii) constituent substances that indicate the presence of a class of substances, (iii) tests for genetic and related effects, including genetic activity profiles, (iv) DNA adduct profiles, (v) oncogene expression and mutation; suppressor gene inactivation.

## 9. EVIDENCE FOR CARCINOGENICITY IN EXPERIMENTAL ANIMALS

For several agents (e.g., 4-aminobiphenyl, bis(chloromethyl)ether, diethylstilboestrol, melphalan, 8-methoxypsoralen (methoxsalen) plus ultra-violet radiation, mustard gas and vinyl chloride), evidence of carcinogenicity in experimental animals preceded evidence obtained from epidemiological studies or case reports. Information compiled from the first 41 volumes of the *IARC Monographs*(14) shows that, of the 44 agents and mixtures for which there is *sufficient* or *limited evidence* of carcinogenicity to humans (see p. 25-26), all 37 that have been tested adequately experimentally produce cancer in at least one animal species. Although this association cannot establish that all agents and mixtures that cause cancer in experimental animals also cause cancer in humans, nevertheless, *in the absence of adequate data on humans, it is biologically plausible and prudent to regard agents and mixtures for which there is sufficient evidence* (see pp. 26-27) *of carcinogenicity in experimental animals as if they presented a carcinogenic risk to humans.*

The monographs are not intended to summarize all published studies. Those that are inadequate (e.g., too short a duration, too few animals, poor survival; see below) or are judged irrelevant to the evaluation are generally omitted. They may be mentioned briefly, particularly when the information is considered to be a useful supplement to that of other reports or when they provide the only data available. Their inclusion does not, however, imply acceptance of the adequacy of the experimental design or of the analysis and interpretation of their results. Guidelines for adequate long-term carcinogenicity experiments have been outlined (e.g., 15).

The nature and extent of impurities or contaminants present in the agent or mixture being evaluated are given when available. Mention is made of all routes of exposure that have been adequately studied and of all species in which relevant experiments have been performed. Animal strain, sex, numbers per group, age at start of treatment and survival are reported.

Experiments in which the agent or mixture was administered in conjunction with known carcinogens or factors that modify carcinogenic effects are also reported. Experiments on the carcinogenicity of known metabolites and derivatives may be included.

(a) *Qualitative aspects*

An assessment of carcinogenicity involves several considerations of qualitative importance, including (i) the experimental conditions under which the test was performed, including route and schedule of exposure, species, strain, sex, age, duration of follow-up; (ii) the consistency of the results, for example, across species and target organ(s); (iii) the spectrum of neoplastic response, from benign tumours to malignant neoplasms; and (iv) the possible role of modifying factors.

Considerations of importance to the Working Group in the interpretation and evaluation of a particular study include: (i) how clearly the agent was defined and, in the case of mixtures, how adequately the sample characterization was reported; (ii) whether the dose was adequately monitored, particularly in inhalation experiments; (iii) whether the doses used were appropriate and whether the survival of treated animals was similar to that of controls; (iv) whether there were adequate numbers of animals per group; (v) whether animals of both sexes were used; (vi) whether animals were allocated randomly to groups; (vii) whether the duration of observation was adequate; and (viii) whether the data were adequately reported. If available, recent data on the incidence of specific tumours in historical controls, as well as in concurrent controls, should be taken into account in the evaluation of tumour response.

When benign tumours occur together with and originate from the same cell type in an organ or tissue as malignant tumours in a particular study and appear to represent a stage in the progression to malignancy, it may be valid to combine them in assessing tumour incidence. The occurrence of lesions presumed to be preneoplastic may in certain instances aid in assessing the biological plausibility of any neoplastic response observed.

Of the many agents and mixtures that have been studied extensively, few induced only benign neoplasms. Benign tumours in experimental animals frequently represent a stage in the evolution of a malignant neoplasm, but they may be 'endpoints' that do not readily undergo transition to malignancy. However, if an agent or mixture is found to induce only benign neoplasms, it should be suspected of being a carcinogen and it requires further investigation.

(b) *Quantitative aspects*

The probability that tumours will occur may depend on the species and strain, the dose of the carcinogen and the route and period of exposure. Evidence of an increased incidence of neoplasms with increased level of exposure strengthens the inference of a causal association between the exposure and the development of neoplasms.

The form of the dose-response relationship can vary widely, depending on the particular agent under study and the target organ. Since many chemicals require metabolic activation before being converted into their reactive intermediates, both metabolic and pharmacokinetic aspects are important in determining the dose-response pattern. Saturation of steps such as absorption, activation, inactivation and elimination of the carcinogen may produce nonlinearity in the dose-response relationship, as could saturation of processes such as DNA repair(16,17).

*(c) Statistical analysis of long-term experiments in animals*

Factors considered by the Working Group include the adequacy of the information given for each treatment group: (i) the number of animals studied and the number examined histologically, (ii) the number of animals with a given tumour type and (iii) length of survival. The statistical methods used should be clearly stated and should be the generally accepted techniques refined for this purpose(17,18). When there is no difference in survival between control and treatment groups, the Working Group usually compares the proportions of animals developing each tumour type in each of the groups. Otherwise, consideration is given as to whether or not appropriate adjustments have been made for differences in survival. These adjustments can include: comparisons of the proportions of tumour-bearing animals among the 'effective number' of animals alive at the time the first tumour is discovered, in the case where most differences in survival occur before tumours appear; life-table methods, when tumours are visible or when they may be considered 'fatal' because mortality rapidly follows tumour development; and the Mantel-Haenszel test or logistic regression, when occult tumours do not affect the animals' risk of dying but are 'incidental' findings at autopsy.

In practice, classifying tumours as fatal or incidental may be difficult. Several survival-adjusted methods have been developed that do not require this distinction(17), although they have not been fully evaluated.

## 10. OTHER RELEVANT DATA IN EXPERIMENTAL SYSTEMS AND HUMANS

*(a) Structure-activity considerations*

This section describes structure-activity correlations that are relevant to an evaluation of the carcinogenicity of an agent.

*(b) Absorption, distribution, excretion and metabolism*

Concise information is given on absorption, distribution (including placental transfer) and excretion. Kinetic factors that may affect the dose-reponse relationship, such as saturation of uptake, protein binding, metabolic activation, detoxification and DNA repair processes, are mentioned. Studies that indicate the metabolic fate of the agent in experimental animals and humans are summarized briefly, and comparisons of data from animals and humans are made when possible. Comparative information on the relationship between exposure and the dose that reaches the target site may be of particular importance for extrapolation between species.

*(c) Toxicity*

Data are given on acute and chronic toxic effects (other than cancer), such as organ toxicity, immunotoxicity, endocrine effects and preneoplastic lesions. Effects on reproduction, teratogenicity, feto- and embryotoxicity are also summarized briefly.

*(d) Genetic and related effects*

Tests of genetic and related effects may indicate possible carcinogenic activity. They can also be used in detecting active metabolites of known carcinogens in human or animal body fluids, in detecting active components in complex mixtures and in the elucidation of possible mechanisms of carcinogenesis.

The adequacy of the reporting of sample characterization is considered and, where necessary, commented upon. The available data are interpreted critically by phylogenetic group according to the endpoints detected, which may include DNA damage, gene mutation, sister chromatid exchange, micronuclei, chromosomal aberrations, aneuploidy and cell transformation. The concentrations (doses) employed are given and mention is made of whether an exogenous metabolic system was required. When appropriate, these data may be represented by bar graphs (activity profiles), with corresponding summary tables and listings of test systems, data and references. Detailed information on the preparation of these profiles is given in an appendix to those volumes in which they are used.

Positive results in tests using prokaryotes, lower eukaryotes, plants, insects and cultured mammalian cells suggest that genetic and related effects (and therefore possibly carcinogenic effects) could occur in mammals. Results from such tests may also give information about the types of genetic effect produced and about the involvement of metabolic activation. Some endpoints described are clearly genetic in nature (e.g., gene mutations and chromosomal aberrations), others are to a greater or lesser degree associated with genetic effects (e.g., unscheduled DNA synthesis). In-vitro tests for tumour-promoting activity and for cell transformation may detect changes that are not necessarily the result of genetic alterations but that may have specific relevance to the process of carcinogenesis. A critical appraisal of these tests has been published(15).

Genetic or other activity detected in the systems mentioned above is not always manifest in whole mammals. Positive indications of genetic effects in experimental mammals and in humans are regarded as being of greater relevance than those in other organisms. The demonstration that an agent or mixture can induce gene and chromosomal mutations in whole mammals indicates that it may have the potential for carcinogenic activity, although this activity may not be detectably expressed in any or all species tested. Relative potency in tests for mutagenicity and related effects is not a reliable indicator of carcinogenic potency. Negative results in tests for mutagenicity in selected tissues from animals treated *in vivo* provide less weight, partly because they do not exclude the possibility of an effect in tissues other than those examined. Moreover, negative results in short-term tests with genetic endpoints cannot be considered to provide evidence to rule out carcinogenicity of agents or mixtures that act through other mechanisms. Factors may arise in many tests that could give misleading results; these have been discussed in detail elsewhere(15).

The adequacy of epidemiological studies of reproductive outcomes and genetic and related effects in humans is evaluated by the same criteria as are applied to epidemiological studies of cancer.

## 11. EVIDENCE FOR CARCINOGENICITY IN HUMANS

### (a) *Types of studies considered*

Three types of epidemiological studies of cancer contribute data to the assessment of carcinogenicity in humans — cohort studies, case-control studies and correlation studies.

Rarely, results from randomized trials may be available. Case reports of cancer in humans are also reviewed.

Cohort and case-control studies relate individual exposures under study to the occurrence of cancer in individuals and provide an estimate of relative risk (ratio of incidence in those exposed to incidence in those not exposed) as the main measure of association.

In correlation studies, the units of investigation are usually whole populations (e.g., in particular geographical areas or at particular times), and cancer frequency is related to a summary measure of the exposure of the population to the agent, mixture or exposure circumstance under study. Because individual exposure is not documented, however, a causal relationship is less easy to infer from correlation studies than from cohort and case-control studies.

Case reports generally arise from a suspicion, based on clinical experience, that the concurrence of two events — that is, a particular exposure and occurrence of a cancer — has happened rather more frequently than would be expected by chance. Case reports usually lack complete ascertainment of cases in any population, definition or enumeration of the population at risk and estimation of the expected number of cases in the absence of exposure.

The uncertainties surrounding interpretation of case reports and correlation studies make them inadequate, except in rare instances, to form the sole basis for inferring a causal relationship. When taken together with case-control and cohort studies, however, relevant case reports or correlation studies may add materially to the judgement that a causal relationship is present.

Epidemiological studies of benign neoplasms and presumed preneoplastic lesions are also reviewed by working groups. They may, in some instances, strengthen inferences drawn from studies of cancer itself.

*(b) Quality of studies considered*

It is necessary to take into account the possible roles of bias, confounding and chance in the interpretation of epidemiological studies. By 'bias' is meant the operation of factors in study design or execution that lead erroneously to a stronger or weaker association than in fact exists between disease and an agent, mixture or exposure circumstance. By 'confounding' is meant a situation in which the relationship with disease is made to appear stronger or to appear weaker than it truly is as a result of an association between the apparent causal factor and another factor that is associated with either an increase or decrease in the incidence of the disease. In evaluating the extent to which these factors have been minimized in an individual study, working groups consider a number of aspects of design and analysis as described in the report of the study. Most of these considerations apply equally to case-control, cohort and correlation studies. Lack of clarity of any of these aspects in the reporting of a study can decrease its credibility and its consequent weighting in the final evaluation of the exposure.

Firstly, the study population, disease (or diseases) and exposure should have been well defined by the authors. Cases in the study population should have been identified in a way that was independent of the exposure of interest, and exposure should have been assessed in a way that was not related to disease status.

Secondly, the authors should have taken account in the study design and analysis of other variables that can influence the risk of disease and may have been related to the exposure of interest. Potential confounding by such variables should have been dealt with either in the design of the study, such as by matching, or in the analysis, by statistical adjustment. In cohort studies, comparisons with local rates of disease may be more appropriate than those with national rates. Internal comparisons of disease frequency among individuals at different levels of exposure should also have been made in the study.

Thirdly, the authors should have reported the basic data on which the conclusions are founded, even if sophisticated statistical analyses were employed. At the very least, they should have given the numbers of exposed and unexposed cases and controls in a case-control study and the numbers of cases observed and expected in a cohort study. Further tabulations by time since exposure began and other temporal factors are also important. In a cohort study, data on all cancer sites and all causes of death should have been given, to avoid the possibility of reporting bias. In a case-control study, the effects of investigated factors other than the exposure of interest should have been reported.

Finally, the statistical methods used to obtain estimates of relative risk, absolute cancer rates, confidence intervals and significance tests, and to adjust for confounding should have been clearly stated by the authors. The methods used should preferably have been the generally accepted techniques that have been refined since the mid-1970s. These methods have been reviewed for case-control studies(19) and for cohort studies(20).

*(c) Quantitative considerations*

Detailed analyses of both relative and absolute risks in relation to age at first exposure and to temporal variables, such as time since first exposure, duration of exposure and time since exposure ceased, are reviewed and summarized when available. The analysis of temporal relationships can provide a useful guide in formulating models of carcinogenesis. In particular, such analyses may suggest whether a carcinogen acts early or late in the process of carcinogenesis(6), although such speculative inferences cannot be used to draw firm conclusions concerning the mechanism of action and hence the shape (linear or otherwise) of the dose-response relationship below the range of observation.

*(d) Criteria for causality*

After the quality of individual epidemiological studies has been summarized and assessed, a judgement is made concerning the strength of evidence that the agent, mixture or exposure circumstance in question is carcinogenic for humans. In making their judgement, the Working Group considers several criteria for causality. A strong association (i.e., a large relative risk) is more likely to indicate causality than a weak association, although it is recognized that relative risks of small magnitude do not imply lack of causality and may be important if the disease is common. Associations that are replicated in several studies of the same design or using different epidemiological approaches or under different circumstances of exposure are more likely to represent a causal relationship than isolated observations from single studies. If there are inconsistent results among investigations, possible reasons are sought (such as differences in amount of exposure), and results of studies judged to be of high quality are given more weight than those from studies judged to be methodologically less sound. When suspicion of carcinogenicity arises largely from a single study, these data are not combined with those from later studies in any subsequent reassessment of the strength of the evidence.

If the risk of the disease in question increases with the amount of exposure, this is considered to be a strong indication of causality, although absence of a graded response is not necessarily evidence against a causal relationship. Demonstration of a decline in risk after cessation of or reduction in exposure in individuals or in whole populations also supports a causal interpretation of the findings.

Although a carcinogen may act upon more than one target, the specificity of an association (i.e., an increased occurrence of cancer at one anatomical site or of one morphological type) adds plausibility to a causal relationship, particularly when excess cancer occurrence is limited to one morphological type within the same organ.

Although rarely available, results from randomized trials showing different rates among exposed and unexposed individuals provide particularly strong evidence for causality.

When several epidemiological studies show little or no indication of an association between an exposure and cancer, the judgement may be made that, in the aggregate, they show evidence of lack of carcinogenicity. Such a judgement requires first of all that the studies giving rise to it meet, to a sufficient degree, the standards of design and analysis described above. Specifically, the possibility that bias, confounding or misclassification of exposure or outcome could explain the observed results should be considered and excluded with reasonable certainty. In addition, all studies that are judged to be methodologically sound should be consistent with a relative risk of unity for any observed level of exposure and, when considered together, should provide a pooled estimate of relative risk which is at or near unity and has a narrow confidence interval, due to sufficient population size. Moreover, no individual study nor the pooled results of all the studies should show any consistent tendency for relative risk of cancer to increase with increasing level of exposure. It is important to note that evidence of lack of carcinogenicity obtained in this way from several epidemiological studies can apply only to the type(s) of cancer studied and to dose levels and intervals between first exposure and observation of disease that are the same as or less than those observed in all the studies. Experience with human cancer indicates that, in some cases, the period from first exposure to the development of clinical cancer is seldom less than 20 years; latent periods substantially shorter than 30 years cannot provide evidence for lack of carcinogenicity.

## 12. SUMMARY OF DATA REPORTED

In this section, the relevant experimental and epidemiological data are summarized. Only reports, other than in abstract form, that meet the criteria outlined on p. 15 are considered for evaluating carcinogenicity. Inadequate studies are generally not summarized: such studies are usually identified by a square-bracketed comment in the text.

### (a) Exposures

Human exposure is summarized on the basis of elements such as production, use, occurrence in the environment and determinations in human tissues and body fluids. Quantitative data are given when available.

### (b) Experimental carcinogenicity data

Data relevant to the evaluation of carcinogenicity in animals are summarized. For each animal species and route of administration, it is stated whether an increased incidence of neoplasms was observed, and the tumour sites are indicated. If the agent or mixture produced tumours after prenatal exposure or in single-dose experiments, this is also indicated. Dose-response and other quantitative data may be given when available. Negative findings are also summarized.

### (c) Human carcinogenicity data

Results of epidemiological studies that are considered to be pertinent to an assessment of human carcinogenicity are summarized. When relevant, case reports and correlation studies are also considered.

### (d) Other relevant data

Structure-activity correlations are mentioned when relevant.

Toxicological information and data on kinetics and metabolism in experimental animals are given when considered relevant. The results of tests for genetic and related effects are summarized for whole mammals, cultured mammalian cells and nonmammalian systems.

Data on other biological effects in humans of particular relevance are summarized. These may include kinetic and metabolic considerations and evidence of DNA binding, persistence of DNA lesions or genetic damage in exposed humans.

When available, comparisons of such data for humans and for animals, and particularly animals that have developed cancer, are described.

## 13. EVALUATION

Evaluations of the strength of the evidence for carcinogenicity arising from human and experimental animal data are made, using standard terms.

It is recognized that the criteria for these evaluations, described below, cannot encompass all of the factors that may be relevant to an evaluation of carcinogenicity. In considering all of the relevant data, the Working Group may assign the agent, mixture or exposure circumstance to a higher or lower category than a strict interpretation of these criteria would indicate.

### (a) Degrees of evidence for carcinogenicity in humans and in experimental animals and supporting evidence

It should be noted that these categories refer only to the strength of the evidence that an exposure is carcinogenic and not to the extent of its carcinogenic activity (potency) nor to the mechanism involved. A classification may change as new information becomes available.

An evaluation of degree of evidence, whether for a single substance or a mixture, is limited to the materials tested, and these are chemically and physically defined. When the materials evaluated are considered by the Working Group to be sufficiently closely related, they may be grouped for the purpose of a single evaluation of degree of evidence.

(i) *Human carcinogenicity data*

The applicability of an evaluation of the carcinogenicity of a mixture, process, occupation or industry on the basis of evidence from epidemiological studies depends on the variability over time and place of the mixtures, processes, occupations and industries. The Working Group seeks to identify the specific exposure, process or activity which is considered most likely to be responsible for any excess risk. The evaluation is focused as narrowly as the available data on exposure and other aspects permit.

The evidence relevant to carcinogenicity from studies in humans is classified into one of the following categories:

*Sufficient evidence of carcinogenicity*: The Working Group considers that a causal relationship has been established between exposure to the agent, mixture or exposure circumstance and human cancer. That is, a positive relationship has been observed between the exposure and cancer in studies in which chance, bias and confounding could be ruled out with reasonable confidence.

*Limited evidence of carcinogenicity*: A positive association has been observed between exposure to the agent, mixture or exposure circumstance and cancer for which a causal interpretation is considered by the Working Group to be credible, but chance, bias or confounding could not be ruled out with reasonable confidence.

*Inadequate evidence of carcinogenicity*: The available studies are of insufficient quality, consistency or statistical power to permit a conclusion regarding the presence or absence of a causal association.

*Evidence suggesting lack of carcinogenicity*: There are several adequate studies covering the full range of levels of exposure that human beings are known to encounter, which are mutually consistent in not showing a positive association between exposure to the agent, mixture or exposure circumstance and any studied cancer at any observed level of exposure. A conclusion of 'evidence suggesting lack of carcinogenicity' is inevitably limited to the cancer sites, conditions and levels of exposure and length of observation covered by the available studies. In addition, the possibility of a very small risk at the levels of exposure studied can never be excluded.

In some instances, the above categories may be used to classify the degree of evidence for carcinogenicity for specific organs or tissues.

(ii) *Experimental carcinogenicity data*

The evidence relevant to carcinogenicity in experimental animals is classified into one of the following categories:

*Sufficient evidence of carcinogenicity*: The Working Group considers that a causal relationship has been established between the agent or mixture and an increased incidence of malignant neoplasms or of an appropriate combination of benign and malignant neoplasms (as described on p. 19) in (a) two or more species of animals or (b) in two or more independent studies in one species carried out at different times or in different laboratories or under different protocols.

Exceptionally, a single study in one species might be considered to provide sufficient evidence of carcinogenicity when malignant neoplasms occur to an unusual degree with regard to incidence, site, type of tumour or age at onset.

In the absence of adequate data on humans, it is biologically plausible and prudent to regard agents and mixtures for which there is *sufficient evidence* of carcinogenicity in experimental animals as if they presented a carcinogenic risk to humans.

*Limited evidence of carcinogenicity*: The data suggest a carcinogenic effect but are limited for making a definitive evaluation because, e.g., (a) the evidence of carcinogenicity is restricted to a single experiment; or (b) there are unresolved questions regarding the adequacy of the design, conduct or interpretation of the study; or (c) the agent or mixture increases the incidence only of benign neoplasms or lesions of uncertain neoplastic potential, or of certain neoplasms which may occur spontaneously in high incidences in certain strains.

*Inadequate evidence of carcinogenicity*: The studies cannot be interpreted as showing either the presence or absence of a carcinogenic effect because of major qualitative or quantitative limitations.

*Evidence suggesting lack of carcinogenicity*: Adequate studies involving at least two species are available which show that, within the limits of the tests used, the agent or mixture is not carcinogenic. A conclusion of evidence suggesting lack of carcinogenicity is inevitably limited to the species, tumour sites and levels of exposure studied.

(iii) *Supporting evidence of carcinogenicity*

Other evidence judged to be relevant to an evaluation of carcinogenicity and of sufficient importance to affect the overall evaluation is then described. This may include data on tumour pathology, genetic and related effects, structure-activity relationships, metabolism and pharmacokinetics, physicochemical parameters, chemical composition and possible mechanisms of action. For complex exposures, including occupational and industrial exposures, the potential contribution of carcinogens known to be present as well as the relevance of materials tested are considered by the Working Group in its overall evaluation of human carcinogenicity. The Working Group also determines to what extent the materials tested in experimental systems are relevant to those to which humans are exposed. The available experimental evidence may help to specify more precisely the causal factor(s).

*(b) Overall evaluation*

Finally, the body of evidence is considered as a whole, in order to reach an overall evaluation of the carcinogenicity to humans of an agent, mixture or circumstance of exposure.

An evaluation may be made for a group of chemical compounds that have been evaluated by the Working Group. In addition, when supporting data indicate that other, related compounds for which there is no direct evidence of capacity to induce cancer in animals or in humans may also be carcinogenic, a statement describing the rationale for this conclusion is added to the evaluation narrative; an additional evaluation may be made for this broader group of compounds if the strength of the evidence warrants it.

The agent, mixture or exposure circumstance is described according to the wording of one of the following categories, and the designated group is given. The categorization of an agent, mixture or exposure circumstance is a matter of scientific judgement, reflecting the strength of the evidence derived from studies in humans and in experimental animals and from other relevant data.

*Group 1 — The agent (mixture) is carcinogenic to humans.*
*The exposure circumstance entails exposures that are carcinogenic to humans.*

This category is used only when there is *sufficient evidence* of carcinogenicity in humans.

*Group 2*

This category includes agents, mixtures and exposure circumstances for which, at one extreme, the degree of evidence of carcinogenicity in humans is almost sufficient, as well as those for which, at the other extreme, there are no human data but for which there is experimental evidence of carcinogenicity. Agents, mixtures and exposure circumstances are assigned to either 2A (probably carcinogenic) or 2B (possibly carcinogenic) on the basis of epidemiological, experimental and other relevant data.

*Group 2A — The agent (mixture) is probably carcinogenic to humans.*
*The exposure circumstance entails exposures that are probably carcinogenic to humans.*

This category is used when there is *limited evidence* of carcinogenicity in humans and *sufficient evidence* of carcinogenicity in experimental animals. Exceptionally, an agent, mixture or exposure circumstance may be classified into this category solely on the basis of *limited evidence* of carcinogenicity in humans or of *sufficient evidence* of carcinogenicity in experimental animals strengthened by supporting evidence from other relevant data.

*Group 2B — The agent (mixture) is possibly carcinogenic to humans.*
*The exposure circumstance entails exposures that are possibly carcinogenic to humans.*

This category is generally used for agents, mixtures and exposure circumstances for which there is *limited evidence* of carcinogenicity in humans in the absence of *sufficient evidence* of carcinogenicity in experimental animals. It may also be used when there is *inadequate evidence* of carcinogenicity in humans or when human data are nonexistent but there is *sufficient evidence* of carcinogenicity in experimental animals. In some instances, an agent, mixture or exposure circumstance for which there is *inadequate evidence* of or no data on carcinogenicity in humans but *limited evidence* of carcinogenicity in experimental animals together with supporting evidence from other relevant data may be placed in this group.

*Group 3 — The agent (mixture, exposure circumstance) is not classifiable as to its carcinogenicity to humans.*

Agents, mixtures and exposure circumstances are placed in this category when they do not fall into any other group.

*Group 4 — The agent (mixture, exposure circumstance) is probably not carcinogenic to humans.*

This category is used for agents, mixtures and exposure circumstances for which there is *evidence suggesting lack of carcinogenicity* in humans together with *evidence suggesting lack of carcinogenicity* in experimental animals. In some instances, agents, mixtures or exposure circumstances for which there is *inadequate evidence* of or no data on carcinogenicity in humans but *evidence suggesting lack of carcinogenicity* in experimental animals, consistently and strongly supported by a broad range of other relevant data, may be classified in this group.

## References

1. IARC (1987) *IARC Monographs on the Evaluation of Carcinogenic Risks to Humans*, Supplement 6, *Genetic and Related Effects: An Updating of Selected* IARC Monographs *from Volumes 1 to 42*, Lyon
2. IARC (1977) *IARC Monographs Programme on the Evaluation of the Carcinogenic Risk of Chemicals to Humans. Preamble* (IARC intern. tech. Rep. No. 77/002), Lyon
3. IARC (1978) *Chemicals with* Sufficient Evidence *of Carcinogenicity in Experimental Animals —* IARC Monographs *Volumes 1-17* (IARC intern. tech. Rep. No. 78/003), Lyon
4. IARC (1979) *Criteria to Select Chemicals for* IARC Monographs (IARC intern. tech. Rep. No. 79/003), Lyon
5. IARC (1982) *IARC Monographs on the Evaluation of the Carcinogenic Risk of Chemicals to Humans*, Supplement 4, *Chemicals, Industrial Processes and Industries Associated with Cancer in Humans (IARC Monographs, Volumes 1 to 29)*, Lyon
6. IARC (1983) *Approaches to Classifying Chemical Carcinogens According to* Mechanism of Action (IARC intern. tech. Rep. No. 83/001), Lyon
7. IARC (1987) *IARC Monographs on the Evaluation of Carcinogenic Risks to Humans*, Supplement 7, *Overall Evaluations of Carcinogenicity: An Updating of* IARC Monographs *Volumes 1 to 42*, Lyon
8. IARC (1988) *Report of an IARC Working Group to Review the Approaches and Processes Used to Evaluate the Carcinogenicity of Mixtures and Groups of Chemical* (IARC intern. tech. Rep. No. 88/002), Lyon
9. IARC (1973-1988) *Information Bulletin on the Survey of Chemicals Being Tested for Carcinogenicity*, Numbers 1-13, Lyon
    Number 1 (1973)  52 pages
    Number 2 (1973)  77 pages
    Number 3 (1974)  67 pages
    Number 4 (1974)  97 pages
    Number 5 (1975)  88 pages
    Number 6 (1976) 360 pages
    Number 7 (1978) 460 pages

Number 8 (1979) 604 pages
Number 9 (1981) 294 pages
Number 10 (1983) 326 pages
Number 11 (1984) 370 pages
Number 12 (1986) 385 pages
Number 13 (1988) 404 pages

10. Coleman, M. & Wahrendorf, J., eds (1988) *Directory of On-going Studies in Cancer Epidemiology 1988* (IARC Scientific Publications No. 93), Lyon, IARC [and previous annual volumes]

11. IARC (1984) *Chemicals and Exposures to Complex Mixtures Recommended for Evaluation in* IARC Monographs *and Chemicals and Complex Mixtures Recommended for Long-term Carcinogenicity Testing* (IARC intern. tech. Rep. No. 84/002), Lyon

12. IARC (1989) *Chemicals, Groups of Chemicals, Mixtures and Exposure Circumstances to be Evaluated in Future* IARC Monographs, *Report of an ad-hoc Working Group* (IARC intern. tech. Rep. No. 89/004), Lyon

13. *Environmental Carcinogens. Methods of Analysis and Exposure Measurement*:

   Vol. 1. *Analysis of Volatile Nitrosamines in Food* (IARC Scientific Publications No. 18). Edited by R. Preussmann, M. Castegnaro, E.A. Walker & A.E. Wasserman (1978)

   Vol. 2. *Methods for the Measurement of Vinyl Chloride in Poly(vinyl chloride), Air, Water and Foodstuffs* (IARC Scientific Publications No. 22). Edited by D.C.M. Squirrell & W. Thain (1978)

   Vol. 3. *Analysis of Polycyclic Aromatic Hydrocarbons in Environmental Samples* (IARC Scientific Publications No. 29). Edited by M. Castegnaro, P. Bogovski, H. Kunte & E.A. Walker (1979)

   Vol. 4. *Some Aromatic Amines and Azo Dyes in the General and Industrial Environment* (IARC Scientific Publications No. 40). Edited by L. Fishbein, M. Castegnaro, I.K. O'Neill & H. Bartsch (1981)

   Vol. 5. *Some Mycotoxins* (IARC Scientific Publications No. 44). Edited by L. Stoloff, M. Castegnaro, P. Scott, I.K. O'Neill & H. Bartsch (1983)

   Vol. 6. *N-Nitroso Compounds* (IARC Scientific Publications No. 45). Edited by R. Preussmann, I.K. O'Neill, G. Eisenbrand, B. Spiegelhalder & H. Bartsch (1983)

   Vol. 7. *Some Volatile Halogenated Hydrocarbons* (IARC Scientific Publications No. 68). Edited by L. Fishbein & I.K. O'Neill (1985)

   Vol. 8. *Some Metals: As, Be, Cd, Cr, Ni, Pb, Se, Zn* (IARC Scientific Publications No. 71). Edited by I.K. O'Neill, P. Schuller & L. Fishbein (1986)

   Vol. 9. *Passive Smoking* (IARC Scientific Publications No. 81). Edited by I.K. O'Neill, K.D. Brunnemann, B. Dodet & D. Hoffmann (1987)

   Vol. 10. *Benzene and Alkylated Benzenes* (IARC Scientific Publications No. 85). Edited by L. Fishbein & I.K. O'Neill (1988)

14. Wilbourn, J., Haroun, L., Heseltine, E., Kaldor, J., Partensky, C. & Vainio, H. (1986) Response of experimental animals to human carcinogens: an analysis based upon the IARC Monographs Programme. *Carcinogenesis, 7*, 1853-1863
15. Montesano, R., Bartsch, H., Vainio, H., Wilbourn, J. & Yamasaki, H., eds (1986) *Long-term and Short-term Assays for Carcinogenesis — A Critical Appraisal* (IARC Scientific Publications No. 83), Lyon, IARC
16. Hoel, D.G., Kaplan, N.L. & Anderson, M.W. (1983) Implication of nonlinear kinetics on risk estimation in carcinogenesis. *Science, 219*, 1032-1037
17. Gart, J.J., Krewski, D., Lee, P.N., Tarone, R.E. & Wahrendorf, J. (1986) *Statistical Methods in Cancer Research, Vol.3, The Design and Analysis of Long-term Animal Experiments* (IARC Scientific Publications No. 79), Lyon, IARC
18. Peto, R., Pike, M.C., Day, N.E., Gray, R.G., Lee, P.N., Parish, S., Peto, J., Richards, S. & Wahrendorf, J. (1980) Guidelines for simple, sensitive significance tests for carcinogenic effects in long-term animal experiments. In: *IARC Monographs on the Evaluation of the Carcinogenic Risk of Chemicals to Humans*, Supplement 2, *Long-term and Short-term Screening Assays for Carcinogens: A Critical Appraisal*, Lyon, IARC, pp. 311-426
19. Breslow, N.E. & Day, N.E. (1980) *Statistical Methods in Cancer Research, Vol. 1, The Analysis of Case-control Studies* (IARC Scientific Publications No. 32), Lyon, IARC
20. Breslow, N.E. & Day, N.E. (1987) *Statistical Methods in Cancer Research, Vol. 2, The Design and Analysis of Cohort Studies* (IARC Scientific Publications No. 82), Lyon, IARC

# GENERAL REMARKS

This forty-eighth volume of *IARC Monographs* covers some flame retardants, textile dyes, another textile chemical, as well as occupational exposures in the textile manufacturing industry. It is not the purpose of this volume to consider all of the chemical agents used in textile manufacture. Numerous textile dyes and other agents used in textile processing were evaluated previously by IARC working groups, and these are listed, with the evaluations, in Table 1.

**Table 1. Agents used currently and in the past in the textile manufacturing industry that have been evaluated for carcinogenicity in *IARC Monographs***

| Agent | Evidence for carcinogenicity[a] | | | Use in the textile manufacturing industry[b] |
|---|---|---|---|---|
| | Human | Animal | Group | |
| Acetamide | ND | S | 2B | Cloth plasticizer |
| Acrylic fibres | ND | ND | 3 | Raw material |
| Amaranth | ND | I | 3 | Textile dye |
| Antimony trioxide | I | S | 2B | Flame retardant |
| Auramine (technical grade) | I | S | 2B | Textile dye |
| Asbestos[c] | S | S | 1 | Asbestos textiles |
| Benzidine-based dyes | I | | 2A | Silk dyes |
|   Direct Black 38 (technical grade) | | S | | |
|   Direct Blue 6 (technical grade) | | S | | |
|   Direct Brown 95 (technical grade) | | S | | |
| Benzyl acetate | ND | L | 3 | Solvent |
| Benzyl violet 4B | ND | S | 2B | Textile dye |
| Bis(2-chloroethyl)ether | ND | L | 3 | Scouring agent |
| Blue VRS | ND | L | 3 | Textile dye |
| Brilliant Blue FCF | ND | L | 3 | Textile dye |
| γ-Butyrolactone | ND | I | 3 | Solvent |
| Carmoisine | ND | I | 3 | Wool dye |
| Chlorendic acid[d] | ND | S | 2B | Flame retardant |
| Chlorophenols | L | | 2B | |
|   2,4,6-Trichlorophenol | | S | | Antimildew agent |

**Table 1 (contd)**

| Agent | Evidence for carcinogenicity[a] | | | Use in the textile manufacturing industry[b] |
|---|---|---|---|---|
| | Human | Animal | Group | |
| para-Chloro-ortho-toluidine and its strong acid salts[d] | | | 2A | Dye intermediate |
| para-Chloro-ortho-toluidine | L | | | |
| para-Chloro-ortho-toluidine hydrochloride | | S | | |
| Chromium acetate ($Cr^{+3}$) | I | I | 3 | Textile dye |
| Chromium compounds, hexavalent[c] | S | S | 1 | Textile printing |
| Chromium potassium sulfate ($Cr^{+3}$) | I | I | 3 | Mordant for wool |
| Chromium sulfate ($Cr^{+3}$) | I | I | 3 | Mordant |
| Chrysoidine | I | L | 3 | Textile dye |
| Copper 8-hydroxyquinoline | ND | I | 3 | Textile fungicide |
| Decabromodiphenyl oxide[d] | ND | L | 3 | Flame retardant |
| ortho-Dichlorobenzene | I | I | 3 | Carrier agent |
| para-Dichlorobenzene | I | S | 2B | Carrier agent |
| Dichloromethane | I | S | 2B | Solvent |
| Dieldrin | I | L | 3 | Moth-proofing agent |
| Diepoxybutane | ND | S | 2B | Cross-linking agent |
| Di(2-ethylhexyl)adipate | ND | L | 3 | Cellulose-nylon plasticizer |
| Di(2-ethylhexyl)phthalate | ND | S | 2B | Plasticizer in PVC-coated fabrics |
| 3,3'-Dimethoxybenzidine (ortho-Dianisidine) | I | S | 2B | Acetate rayon dye |
| Dimethyl hydrogen phosphite[d] | ND | L | 3 | Flame retardant |
| Dimethyl formamide | L | I | 2B | Solvent |
| 1,4-Dioxane | I | S | 2B | Solvent |
| Disperse Blue 1[d] | ND | S | 2B | Textile dye |
| Disperse Yellow 3[d] | ND | L | 3 | Textile dye |
| Ethyl acrylate | ND | S | 2B | Back coating agent |
| Evans blue | ND | S | 3 | Textile dye |
| Formaldehyde | L | S | 2A | Finishing agent |
| Glycidaldehyde | ND | S | 2B | Cross-linking agent (wool) |
| Guinea green B | ND | L | 3 | Textile dye |
| Hexachloroethane | ND | L | 3 | Moth repellent |
| Hexamethylphosphoramide | ND | S | 2B | Solvent |
| Hydrogen peroxide | ND | L | 3 | Bleaching agent |
| Isopropyl alcohol | I | I | 3 | Solvent |
| Light green SF | ND | L | 3 | Textile dye |

**Table 1 (contd)**

| Agent | Evidence for carcinogenicity[a] | | | Use in the textile manufacturing industry[b] |
|---|---|---|---|---|
| | Human | Animal | Group | |
| Magenta | I | I | 3 | Textile dye |
| Methyl methacrylate | ND | I | 3 | Back coating agents |
| Mineral oils[c] | | | | Yarn lubricants |
|   Untreated and mildly-treated oils | S | S | 1 | |
|   Highly-refined oils | I | I | 3 | |
| Mirex | ND | S | 2B | Textile insecticide |
| Modacrylic fibres | ND | ND | 3 | Raw material |
| Nitrilotriacetic acid and its salts[d] | ND | | 2B | Chelating agents |
|   Nitrilotriacetic acid and its sodium salts | | S | | |
| 5-Nitro-*ortho*-toluidine[d] | ND | L | 3 | Textile dye |
| Nylon 6 | ND | I | 3 | Raw material |
| Orange I | ND | I | 3 | Textile dye |
| Orange G | ND | I | 3 | Wool dye |
| Phenol | I | I | 3 | Textile printing agent |
| *para*-Phenylenediamine | ND | I | 3 | Textile dye developer |
| *ortho*-Phenylphenol | ND | I | 3 | Carrier agent |
| Polyacrylic acid | ND | ND | 3 | Textile warp sizing agent |
| Polybrominated biphenyls | I | S | 2B | Flame retardants |
| Polyvinyl acetate | ND | I | 3 | Finishing agent |
| Polyvinyl alcohol | ND | I | 3 | Textile warp sizing agent |
| Polyvinyl pyrrolidone | ND | L | 3 | Stripping and colour lightening agent |
| Ponceaux MX | ND | S | 2B | Textile dye |
| Ponceaux 3R | ND | S | 2B | Wool dye |
| Potassium chromate ($Cr^{+6}$) | S | S | 1 | Mordant, dye |
| Potassium dichromate ($Cr^{+6}$) | S | S | 1 | Wool preservative |
| Rhodamine B | ND | L | 3 | Textile dye |
| Rhodamine 6G | ND | L | 3 | Textile dye |
| Styrene-butadiene copolymers | ND | ND | 3 | Carpet and upholstery backcoating agents |
| Tannic acid and tannins | ND | L | 3 | Nylon finishing agents |
| 1,1,2,2-Tetrachloroethane | I | L | 3 | Moth repellent |
| Tetrachloroethylene | I | S | 2B | Solvent |
| Tetrakis(hydroxymethyl) phosphonium salts[d] | ND | I | 3 | Flame retardant |
| Thioacetamide | ND | S | 2B | Solvent |
| Thiourea | ND | S | 2B | Flame retardant |

**Table 1 (contd)**

| Agent | Evidence for carcinogenicity[a] | | | Use in the textile manufacturing industry[b] |
|---|---|---|---|---|
| | Human | Animal | Group | |
| Toluene | I | I | 3 | Solvent |
| 1,1,1-Trichloroethane | ND | I | 3 | Solvent |
| Trichloroethylene | I | L | 3 | Solvent |
| Tris(1-aziridinyl)phosphine oxide | ND | I | 3 | Flame retardant |
| 2,4,6-Tris(1-aziridinyl)-s-triazine | ND | L | 3 | Finishing agent |
| Tris(2-chloroethyl) phosphate[d] | ND | I | 3 | Flame retardant |
| Tris(2,3-dibromopropyl)phosphate | I | S | 2A | Flame retardant |
| Tris(2-methyl-1-aziridinyl)phosphine oxide | ND | I | 3 | Cross-linking agent |
| Trypan blue | ND | S | 2B | Textile dye |
| Vat Yellow 4[d] | ND | L | 3 | Textile dye |
| Xylene | I | I | 3 | Solvent |

[a]From Supplement 7 (IARC, 1987) or *IARC Monographs* volume 47 (IARC, 1990); I, inadequate evidence; L, limited evidence; ND, no adequate data; S, sufficient evidence; 1, Group 1 — the agent is carcinogenic to humans; 2A, Group 2A — the agent is probably carcinogenic to humans; 2B, Group 2B — the agent is possibly carcinogenic to humans; 3, Group 3 — the agent is not classifiable as to its carcinogenicity to humans
[b]From *IARC Monographs* volumes 1-47 and Priha *et al.* (1988)
[c]Excluded from consideration in this volume
[d]In this volume

The main criterion for selecting agents to be evaluated in this volume was the availability of data on carcinogenicity and on human exposure. Originally, data were also collected for three other agents: two groups of flame retardants, bis(2,3-dibromopropyl)phosphate and its salts and tris(dichloropropyl)phosphates, and sodium(2-ethylhexyl)sulfate. Some bis(2,3-dibromopropyl)phosphate salts have been reported to be nephrotoxic to rats and mutagenic to bacteria (Nakamura *et al.*, 1979; Elliott *et al.*, 1982; Lynn *et al.*, 1982; Søderlund *et al.*, 1982; Nakamura *et al.*, 1983). Tris(dichloropropyl)phosphates have induced chromosomal aberrations in animal cells and exerted mutagenic effects in bacteria (Gold *et al.*, 1978; Nakamura *et al.*, 1979; Brusick *et al.*, 1980; Kawachi *et al.*, 1980a,b; Ulsamer *et al.*, 1980; Ishidate *et al.*, 1981; Søderlund *et al.*, 1985; Mortelmans *et al.*, 1986). However, studies on the carcinogenicity of these chemicals had not been published in peer-reviewed journals by the time of the meeting and these compounds were therefore not considered by the Working Group. Sodium(2-ethylhexyl)sulfate is a surfactant used in bleaching and mercerizing textiles, in metal cleaning and in some other applications. This compound was reported to have nephrotoxic effects in mice and rats (Smyth *et al.*, 1941, 1970; National Toxicology Program, 1984; Kluwe *et al.*, 1985). It was not mutagenic to several strains of *Salmonella typhimurium* in the presence or absence of an exogenous metabolic system (National Toxicology Program, 1984; Zeiger *et al.*, 1985). The only carcinogenicity study available on this compound has been retracted (National Toxicology Program, 1984).

Flame retardants are used in a wide variety of products, including carpets, home furnishings, fabrics, plastics, paints, adhesives and construction materials. Tetrakis(hydroxymethyl) phosphonium salts, sulfate and chloride, are flame retardants used in cotton and rayon fabrics. Decabromodiphenyl oxide (used in polyester/cotton blends and nylon) and tris(2-chloroethyl)phosphate (used in carpet backings) are also widely used as flame retardants in the textile industry (Ulsamer *et al.*, 1980), but their main use is in plastics. Similarly, chlorendic acid and dimethyl hydrogen phosphite have some specific uses in textile manufacture, but their major applications are not related to textiles. Chlorinated paraffins are saturated hydrocarbons with usual chain lengths of 10-30 carbon atoms and chlorination grades of 40-70%. They are used mainly as high-pressure lubricant additives in the metal industry but may be added as plasticizers and flame retardants to a variety of products, including plastics, rubber and paints. Chlorinated paraffins are used with decabromodiphenyl oxide and antimony trioxide in polyester fabrics for tents (Priha *et al.*, 1988). Some other chemicals that are used as flame retardants were evaluated previously by IARC working groups. These include tris(2,3-dibromopropyl)phosphate (IARC, 1979, 1987), polybrominated biphenyls (IARC, 1986, 1987) and antimony trioxide (IARC, 1989).

Hundreds of dyes are used in the textile industry in large quantities. In the USA, more than two-thirds of the annual production of dyes is used in textiles (Anon., 1988). Several compounds considered in this volume are used as dyes, dye components or intermediates in the textile industry. The aromatic amines, 4-chloro-*ortho*-toluidine and 5-nitro-*ortho*-toluidine, have two major applications: as intermediates in the manufacture of dyes and some other chemicals and as components of naphthol dyes for fabrics and yarns. Dyeing with naphthol dyes takes places in two phases: the textile is first immersed in a solution of azoic coupling component (naphthol) and then allowed to react with an azoic diazonium component, which is an aromatic amine converted to an azo derivative. An anthraquinone compound, Disperse Blue 1, is a hair colourant which is also used to dye synthetic textiles. Disperse Yellow 3 is a monoazo pigment dye used mainly for synthetic materials. Vat Yellow 4 is a diketone derivative of dibenzo[*a,h*]pyrene which may be applied to a variety of natural and synthetic textile materials. A number of textile dyes were evaluated previously, mainly in *IARC Monographs* volumes 8 and 16 (IARC, 1975, 1978) and in Supplement 7 (IARC, 1987). The evaluations of two of the dyes included in this volume — 4-chloro-*ortho*-toluidine and Disperse Yellow 3 — have been brought up to date on the basis of new data on carcinogenicity that have become available. The previous evaluation of the carcinogenicity of Disperse Yellow 3 was based on a study in mice by Boyland *et al.* (1964). It has since been brought to the attention of the IARC that the compound tested in that study was in fact an isomer of Disperse Yellow 3.

Nitrilotriacetic acid and its sodium salts are chelating agents used, for example, to remove interfering metal ions from textile processing solutions. More than 50% of the 70 000 tonnes of this product that are made annually, however, is used as the basis for laundry detergents. Data on solutions of nitrilotriacetic acid and its sodium salts and metal salts were also included because metal complexes may be formed *in vivo* and because some solutions, e.g., of nitrilotriacetic acid disodium salt and iron nitrate, have been tested for carcinogenicity in animals. Several other solvents, carrier agents, plasticizers, sizing agents, fungicides and other textile chemicals including, e.g., formaldehyde, were evaluated previously by IARC working groups (see Table 1).

The last monograph of this volume covers occupational exposures in the textile manufacturing industry. These exposures include the manufacture of fabrics, yarns, carpets, knitwear, linen, curtains and some other industrial and domestic textiles. The main raw material used in the textile industry is cotton. Other widely used materials include wool and synthetic materials, such as polyester, rayon, acrylic fibres and polyamide. Materials such as hemp, jute, silk, flax and rags may be important or even predominate in some areas. The Working Group was concerned that so little published information was available on exposures in the textile industry in areas other than Europe, Japan and the USA, especially in view of the fact that exposures may be higher in areas where old technologies are still used.

The term 'textile industry' as used in this volume was considered to exclude manufacture of garments and of synthetic fibres. In addition, two specific textile processes that had been evaluated previously — manufacture of asbestos textiles (IARC, 1977) and mule spinning with exposure to mineral oils (IARC, 1984) — were excluded.

The main criterion for including biological data in this monograph was that the individuals or populations studied be textile workers, with the exclusions mentioned above. Detailed descriptions of biological data on specific chemical agents used or present in textile mills were considered to be outside the scope of this monograph. Chemical agents used currently or in the past in the textile industry are listed in Table 1 to facilitate the interpretation of possible carcinogenic risks among textile workers.

Since 1975, benign nodular hepatoproliferative lesions in rats have been classified as 'neoplastic nodules' by the National Cancer Institute and subsequently by the National Toxicology Program of the USA. Recently, the term 'hepatocellular adenoma' has been reintroduced (Maronpot *et al.*, 1986). Therefore, in this volume 'adenoma' has been indicated in square brackets whenever 'neoplastic nodules' of the liver were reported.

In evaluating studies of carcinogenicity in experimental animals, the occurrence of dose-related increases in tumour incidence was considered to be more relevant than the finding only of differences between treated and control animals. Tests for trend were therefore presented whenever possible.

## References

Anon. (1988) Better times ahead for US dye producers. *Chem. Eng. News*, July 25, 7-14

Boyland, E., Busby, E.R., Dukes, C.E., Grover, P.L. & Manson, D. (1964) Further experiments on implantation materials into the urinary bladder of mice. *Br. J. Cancer*, 18, 575-581

Brusick, D., Matheson, D., Jagannath, D.R., Goode, S., Lebowitz, H., Reed, M., Roy, G. & Benson, S. (1980) A comparison of the genotoxic properties of tris(2,3-dibromopropyl)phosphate and tris(1,3-dichloro-2-propyl)phosphate in a battery of short-term bioassays. *J. environ. Pathol. Toxicol.*, 3, 207-226

Elliott, W.C., Lynn, R.K., Houghton, D.C., Kennish, J.M. & Bennett, W.M. (1982) Nephrotoxicity of the flame retardant, tris(2,3-dibromopropyl) phosphate, and its metabolites. *Toxicol. appl. Pharmacol.*, 62, 179-182

Gold, M.D., Blum, A. & Ames, B.N. (1978) Another flame retardant, tris-(1,3-dichloro-2-propyl)phosphate, and its expected metabolites are mutagens. *Science*, 200, 785-787

IARC (1975) *IARC Monographs on the Evaluation of Carcinogenic Risk of Chemicals to Man*, Vol. 8, *Some Aromatic Azo Compounds*, Lyon

IARC (1977) *IARC Monographs on the Evaluation of Carcinogenic Risk of Chemicals to Man*, Vol. 14, *Asbestos*, Lyon

IARC (1978) *IARC Monographs on the Evaluation of the Carcinogenic Risk of Chemicals to Man*, Vol. 16, *Some Aromatic Amines and Related Nitro Compounds — Hair Dyes, Colouring Agents and Miscellaneous Industrial Chemicals*, Lyon

IARC (1979) *IARC Monographs on the Evaluation of the Carcinogenic Risk of Chemicals to Humans*, Vol. 20, *Some Halogenated Hydrocarbons*, Lyon, pp. 575-588

IARC (1984) *IARC Monographs on the Evaluation of the Carcinogenic Risk of Chemicals to Humans*, Vol. 33, *Polynuclear Aromatic Compounds, Part 2, Carbon Blacks, Mineral Oils and Some Nitroarenes*, Lyon, pp. 87-168

IARC (1986) *IARC Monographs on the Evaluation of the Carcinogenic Risk of Chemicals to Humans*, Vol. 41, *Some Halogenated Hydrocarbons and Pesticide Exposures*, Lyon, pp. 261-292

IARC (1987) *IARC Monographs on the Evaluation of Carcinogenic Risks to Humans*, Suppl. 7, *Overall Evaluations of Carcinogenicity: An Updating of* IARC Monographs *Volumes 1 to 42*, Lyon, pp. 321-322, 369-370

IARC (1989) *IARC Monographs on the Evaluation of Carcinogenic Risks to Humans*, Vol. 47, *Some Organic Solvents, Resin Monomers and Related Compounds, Pigments and Occupational Exposures in Paint Manufacture and Painting*, Lyon, pp. 291-305

Ishidate, M., Jr, Sofuni, T. & Yoshikawa, K. (1981) Chromosomal aberration tests *in vitro* as a primary screening tool for environmental mutagens and/or carcinogens. *Gann Monogr. Cancer Res.*, 27, 95-108

Kawachi, T., Komatsu, T., Kada, T., Ishidate, M., Sasaki, M., Sugiyama, T. & Tazima, Y. (1980a) Results of recent studies on the relevance of various short-term screening tests in Japan. *Appl. Methods Oncol.*, 3, 253-268

Kawachi, T., Yahagi, T., Kada, T., Tazima, T., Ishidate, M., Sasaki, M. & Sugiyama, T. (1980b) Cooperative programme on short-term assays for carcinogenicity in Japan. In: Montesano, R., Bartsch, H. & Tomatis, L., eds, *Molecular and Cellular Aspects of Carcinogen Screening Tests* (IARC Scientific Publications No. 27), Lyon, IARC, pp. 323-330

Kluwe, W.M., Huff, J.E., Matthews, H.B., Irwin, R. & Haseman, J.K. (1985) Comparative chronic toxicities and carcinogenic potentials of 2-ethylhexyl-containing compounds in rats and mice. *Carcinogenesis*, 6, 1577-1583

Lynn, R.K., Garvie-Gould, C., Wong, K. & Kennish, J.M. (1982) Metabolism, distribution and excretion of the flame retardant, tris(2,3-dibromopropyl)phosphate (tris-BP) in the rat: identification of mutagenic and nephrotoxic metabolites. *Toxicol. appl. Pharmacol.*, 63, 105-119

Maronpot, R.R., Montgomery, C.A., Jr, Boorman, G.A. & McConnell, E.E. (1986) National Toxicology Program nomenclature for hepatoproliferative lesions of rats. *Toxicol. Pathol.*, 14, 263-273

Mortelmans, K., Haworth, S., Lawlor, T., Speck, W., Tainer, B. & Zeiger, E. (1986) *Salmonella* mutagenicity tests: II. Results from the testing of 270 chemicals. *Environ. Mutagenesis*, 8 (Suppl. 7), 1-119

Nakamura, A., Tateno, N., Kojima, S., Kaniva, M.-A. & Kawamura, T. (1979) The mutagenicity of halogenated alkanols and their phosphoric acid esters for *Salmonella typhimurium*. *Mutat. Res.*, 66, 373-380

Nakamura, A., Tateno, N., Iwata, T., Kojima, S., Kaniwa, M.-A. & Kawamura, T. (1983) Mutagenicity of bis- and mono(2,3-dibromopropyl)phosphate, and their salts used as flame retardants, in the *Salmonella*/microsome system. *Mutat. Res.*, *117*, 1-8

National Toxicology Program (1984) *Carcinogenesis Studies of Sodium 2-ethylhexyl Sulfate (CAS No. 126-92-1) in F344/N Rats and B6C3F₁ Mice (Feed Study) (NTP Technical Report 256; NIH Publ. No. 83-2512)*, Research Triangle Park, NC

Priha, E., Vuorinen, R., Schimberg, R. & Ahonen, I. (1988) [*Textile Finishing Agents*] (Finn.) (*Series on Working Conditions No. 65*), Helsinki, Institute of Occupational Health

Smyth, H.F., Jr, Seaton, J. & Fischer, L. (1941) Some pharmacological properties of the 'Tergitol' penetrants. *J. ind. Hyg. Toxicol.*, *23*, 478-483

Smyth, H.F., Jr, Carpenter, C.P., Weil, C.S. & King, J.M. (1970) Experimental toxicity of sodium 2-ethylhexyl sulfate. *Toxicol. appl. Pharmacol.*, *17*, 53-59

Søderlund, E., Nelson, S.D. & Dybing, E. (1982) Mutagenicity and nephrotoxicity of two tris(2,3-dibromopropyl)phosphate analogues: bis(2,3-dibromopropyl)phosphate and 2,3-dibromopropylphosphate. *Acta pharmacol. toxicol.*, *51*, 76-80

Søderlund, E.J., Dybing, E., Holme, J.A., Hongslo, J.K., Rivedal, E., Sanner, T. & Nelson, S.D. (1985) Comparative genotoxicity and nephrotoxicity studies of the two halogenated flame retardants tris(1,3-dichloro-2-propyl)phosphate and tris(2,3-dibromopropyl)phosphate. *Acta pharmacol. toxicol.*, *56*, 20-29

Ulsamer, A.G., Osterberg, R.E. & McLaughlin, J., Jr (1980) Flame-retardant chemicals in textiles. *Clin. Toxicol.*, *17*, 101-131

Zeiger, E., Haworth, S., Mortelmans, K. & Speck, W. (1985) Mutagenicity testing of di(2-ethylhexyl)phthalate and related chemicals in *Salmonella*. *Environ. Mutagenesis*, *7*, 213-232

# THE MONOGRAPHS

# FLAME RETARDANTS

# CHLORENDIC ACID

## 1. Chemical and Physical Data

### 1.1 Synonyms

*Chem. Abstr. Services Reg. No.*: 115-28-6
*Chem. Abstr. Name*: Bicyclo[2.2.1]hept-5-ene-2,3-dicarboxylic acid, 1,4,5,6,7,7-hexachloro-
*IUPAC Systematic Name*: 1,4,5,6,7,7-Hexachloro-5-norbornene-2,3-dicarboxylic acid
*Synonyms*: HET acid; hexachloro-*endo*-methylenetetrahydrophthalic acid; 1,4,5,6,7,7-hexachlorobicyclo[2.2.1]-5-heptene-2,3-dicarboxylic acid

### 1.2 Structural and molecular formulae and molecular weight

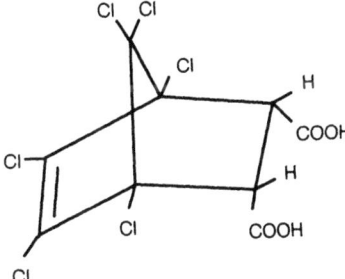

$C_9H_4Cl_6O_4$    Mol. wt: 388.85

### 1.3 Chemical and physical properties of the pure substance

(a) *Description*: White crystalline powder (Occidental Chemical Corp., 1987)

(b) *Melting-point*: 208-210°C, sealed tube; 230-235°C, open tube (Gupta *et al.*, 1978; Occidental Chemical Corp., 1987)

(c) *Spectroscopy data*: Infrared (prism [14020], grating [28088]), nuclear magnetic resonance (proton [12020]) and mass spectral data have been reported (Sadtler Research Laboratories, 1980; Chemical Information Systems, 1988).

(d) *Solubility*: Slightly soluble in water (0.3% by weight at 21°C) and in nonpolar organic solvents (e.g., benzene); readily soluble in methanol, ethanol and acetone (National Toxicology Program, 1987; Occidental Chemical Corp., 1987)

(e) *Stability*: Loses water in a heated open system to give the anhydride (Gupta *et al.*, 1978); emits chlorine when heated to decomposition (Occidental Chemical Corp., 1987)

(f) *Octanol/water partition coefficient (P)*: log P, 2.30 (Chemical Information Systems, 1988)

### 1.4 Technical products and impurities

*Trade names*: Hetron 92; Hetron 92C

Chlorendic acid is available at >97% purity (Morton Thiokol, 1985). Common impurities in technical-grade chlorendic acid are maleic anhydride (maximum, 0.25%), water (maximum, 0.25%) and hexachlorocyclopentadiene (maximum, 50 ppm; Occidental Chemical N.V., 1988). Commercial chlorendic anhydride typically contains 1-3% chlorendic acid (Velsicol Chemical Corp., 1982).

## 2. Production, Use, Occurrence and Analysis

### 2.1 Production and use

(a) *Production*

Chlorendic acid is prepared in a closed system by the Diels-Alder reaction of hexachlorocyclopentadiene and maleic anhydride in a solvent, followed by hydrolysis of the anhydride (Larsen, 1980).

The US Environmental Protection Agency (1986) reported that, in 1977, 1400-14 000 tonnes of chlorendic acid were produced in the USA. In 1980, less than 4% of the 140 thousand tonnes of maleic anhydride produced in the USA was used in the manufacture of chlorendic acid and anhydride (Anon., 1980; US International Trade Commission, 1981).

Chlorendic acid is currently manufactured in Belgium (Occidental Chemical N.V., 1988), and chlorendic anhydride is manufactured in the USA, in each case by a single manufacturer. Combined production in 1987 was over 2000 tonnes but has been declining since the early 1980s (US International Trade Commission, 1988).

(b) *Use*

Chlorendic acid is used primarily as a chemical intermediate in the manufacture of unsaturated polyester resins, with special applications in electrical systems, panelling, engineering plastics and paints (Makhlouf, 1982). A major use is in fibreglass-reinforced resins for process equipment in chemical industries. Chlorendic acid is also used to impart flame resistance to polyurethane foams when reacted with nonhalogenated glycols to form halogenated polyols and can be used in the manufacture of alkyd resins for special paints and inks (Gupta *et al.*, 1978; Larsen, 1980; Talbot, 1984; Occidental Chemical N.V., 1988).

In Europe, 80% of the chlorendic acid produced is used in composites for flame-retardant building and transport materials. The remainder is used in composites for the manufacture of anti-corrosion equipment, such as tanks, piping and scrubbers. In the USA, Latin America and the Far East, the usage pattern is reversed; 70-80% is used for anti-corrosion equipment and 20-30% for flame-retardant applications (Occidental Chemical N.V., 1988).

In the textile industry, the primary use for chlorendic acid is for flame-retardant treatment of wool fabrics. The natural flame resistance of wool is enhanced by finishing treatments with chlorendic acid in dimethylformamide (see Friedman *et al.*, 1973; Whitfield & Friedman, 1973; Seredina & Kryazhev, 1987; IARC, 1989).

(c) *Regulatory status and guidelines*

No data were available to the Working Group.

## 2.2 Occurrence

(a) *Natural occurrence*

Chlorendic acid is not known to occur as a natural product.

(b) *Occupational exposure*

No data were available to the Working Group.

(c) *Environmental exposure*

It has been suggested that chlorendic acid may be released by hydrolytic degradation of polyesters that contain it. Chlorendic acid has been reported in the leachate of a landfill (National Toxicology Program, 1987). It is also an oxidation product of heptachlor and its metabolites (Cochrane & Forbes, 1974) and of endosulfan (Martens, 1972).

## 2.3 Analysis

In a method for determining chlorendic anhydride in water (also applicable to the acid), the sample is adsorbed on activated charcoal, extracted with ethanol in a Soxhlet apparatus, concentrated by evaporation and analysed by gas chromatography with a flame ionization detector (Ermolaeva *et al.*, 1976).

In a method for the determination of chlorendic anhydride in air (also applicable to the acid), the anhydride is separated and hydrolysed to the acid, which is methylated with diazomethane; the methyl ester is estimated by gas chromatography (Pilenkova & Fat'yanova, 1980).

# 3. Biological Data Relevant to the Evaluation of Carcinogenic Risk to Humans

## 3.1 Carcinogenicity studies in animals

*Oral administration*

*Mouse*: Groups of 50 male and 50 female B6C3F$_1$ mice, eight weeks of age, were fed 0, 620 or 1250 ppm (mg/kg) chlorendic acid (purity, >98%) in the diet for 103 weeks. All survivors were killed at 112 weeks of age. The estimated mean daily intakes of chlorendic acid were 89 and 185 mg/kg bw for low-dose and high-dose males and 100 and 207 mg/kg bw for low-dose and high-dose females, respectively. Survival and feed consumption of treated mice of each sex were similar to those of controls, although mean body weights of high-dose males and females were lower than those of controls. The incidences of hepatocellular adenomas and carcinomas were significantly increased (incidental tumour test for trend) in males: adenomas occurred in 5/50 controls, 9/49 low-dose animals and 10/50 at the high dose ($p = 0.041$); carcinomas occurred in 9/50 controls, 17/49 low-dose animals and 20/50 high-dose animals ($p = 0.023$). Hepatocellular carcinomas metastasized to the lung in 2/50 male controls, 4/49 low-dose males and 7/50 high-dose males. The combined incidence of alveolar/bronchiolar adenomas and carcinomas in females was 1/50 controls, 5/50 low-dose animals and 6/50 high-dose animals ($p = 0.037$). The incidence of follicular-cell adenomas of the thyroid was significantly elevated in high-dose females: control, 0/50; low-dose, 0/47; high-dose, 3/50 ($p = 0.039$; National Toxicology Program, 1987).

*Rat*: Groups of 50 male and 50 female Fischer 344/N rats, eight weeks of age, were fed 0, 620 or 1250 ppm (mg/kg) chlorendic acid (purity, >98%) in the diet for 103 weeks. All survivors were killed at 112 weeks of age. The estimated mean daily intakes of chlorendic acid were 27 and 56 mg/kg bw for low-dose and high-dose males and 39 and 66 mg/kg bw for low-dose and high-dose females, respectively. Survival and feed consumption of treated rats were similar to those of controls, although mean body weights of high-dose males and females were lower than those of controls. The incidences of neoplastic nodules of the liver [adenomas; Maronpot *et al.*, 1986] were significantly increased (incidental tumour test for trend) in both males and females: in males they occurred in 2/50 controls, 21/50 low-dose and 23/50 high-dose animals ($p < 0.001$); and in females in 1/50 controls, 3/49 low-dose and 11/50 high-dose animals ($p = 0.001$); the incidence of hepatocellular carcinomas was significantly increased in females: in 0/50 controls, 3/49 low-dose and 5/50 high-dose animals ($p = 0.023$). In males, the incidence of acinar-cell adenomas of the pancreas was significantly increased: in 0/49 controls, 4/50 low-dose and 6/50 high-dose animals ($p = 0.014$), as was the incidence of alveolar/bronchiolar adenomas: in 0/50 controls, 3/50 low-dose and 5/50 high-dose animals ($p = 0.014$). The incidences of carcinomas of the preputial gland in males were: control, 1/50; low-dose, 8/50; high-dose, 4/50; the trend is not significant (National Toxicology Program, 1987).

## 3.2 Other relevant data

(a) *Experimental systems*

(i) *Absorption, distribution, excretion and metabolism*

$^{14}$C-Chlorendic acid in a solution of a polyoxyethylated vegetable oil, ethanol and water (3 mg/kg bw) was given to male Fischer 344 rats by intravenous injection or oral intubation. Following intravenous injection, more than 50% of the administered radioactivity was found in the liver within 15 min. Biliary excretion was the primary route of removal of radioactivity from the liver, which occurred with a half-life of 1.19 h. The blood contained 20% of the administered radioactivity at 1 h, and this declined with a half-life of 0.84 h. Muscle contained 14% of the administered radioactivity at 15 min, and this level fell rapidly, with a half-life of 0.57 h. Smaller amounts were detected in other organs. The highest specific activity per gram of tissue (wet weight) was noted in the adrenal gland early after administration. Administration of the same solution of $^{14}$C-chlorendic acid by oral intubation resulted in a somewhat higher liver concentration and a lower blood concentration at 24 h than those seen after the same time following intravenous administration. The majority of the radioactivity was found in the faeces (78% of the total dose) or large intestine. The $^{14}$C-chlorendic acid-derived radioactivity in the bile, urine and faeces was attached mainly to parent compound or conjugates resistant to β-glucuronidase and aryl sulfatase (Decad & Fields, 1982).

(ii) *Toxic effects*

Male and female Fischer 344/N rats and B6C3F$_1$ mice were fed diets containing chlorendic acid for 14 days, 13 weeks or two years. In the 14-day studies, animals received diets containing 3100-50 000 ppm (mg/kg); deaths occurred only in male and female rats and in male mice given the highest dose. No treatment-related gross lesion was observed at necropsy (National Toxicology Program, 1987).

In the 13-week studies, rats received concentrations of 620-10 000 ppm (mg/kg) in the diet and mice received 1250-20 000 ppm (mg/kg); all animals survived, but reduced weight gain was noted at the higher doses. In rats, the occurrence of hepatocytomegaly and bile-duct hyperplasia was dose-dependent. Liver lesions also occurred in mice and included centrolobular cytomegaly and coagulative necrosis. The liver lesions occurred mainly in rats given 5000 and 10 000 ppm and in mice given 10 000 and 20 000 (National Toxicology Program, 1987).

Non-neoplastic lesions observed in the two-year studies (see section 3.1) included increased incidences of liver cystic degeneration and bile-duct hyperplasia in male rats and liver granulomatous inflammation and pigmentation and bile-duct hyperplasia in female rats. Liver lesions also occurred in mice and included increased incidences of necrosis in treated males (National Toxicology Program, 1987).

(iii) *Effects on reproduction and prenatal toxicity*

No data were available to the Working Group.

(iv) *Genetic and related effects* (see Appendix 1)

Chlorendic acid was not mutagenic to several strains of *Salmonella typhimurium* in the presence or absence of an exogenous metabolic system from Aroclor 1254-induced rat liver and Syrian hamster liver (National Toxicology Program, 1987).

Chlorendic acid was mutagenic at the TK locus in cultured L5178Y mouse lymphoma cells in the absence of an exogenous metabolic system (National Toxicology Program, 1987).

(b) *Humans*

No data were available to the Working Group.

## 3.3 Case reports and epidemiological studies of carcinogenicity to humans

No data were available to the Working Group.

# 4. Summary of Data Reported and Evaluation

## 4.1 Exposure data

Chlorendic acid is used primarily as a chemical intermediate in the manufacture of unsaturated polyester resins that have applications in electrical systems, panelling, engineering plastics and paints. It is also used in the textile industry for flame-retardant treatment of wool. No data on occupational exposure levels were available.

## 4.2 Experimental carcinogencity data

Chlorendic acid was tested for carcinogenicity by oral administration in one strain of mice and one strain of rats. It produced hepatocellular adenomas and carcinomas in male mice and an increase in the incidence of alveolar/bronchiolar tumours and follicular-cell adenomas of the thyroid gland in female mice. In rats, it induced hepatocellular adenomas in animals of each sex and hepatocellular carcinomas in females; in male rats, it induced an increase in the incidence of alveolar/bronchiolar adenomas and of acinar-cell adenomas of the pancreas.

## 4.3 Human carcinogenicity data

No data were available to the Working Group.

## 4.4 Other relevant data

Hepatocytomegaly was observed in mice and rats fed chlorendic acid for 13 weeks.

In single studies, chlorendic acid induced mutations in mammalian cells in culture but was not mutagenic to bacteria in the presence or absence of an exogenous metabolic system.

## 4.5 Evaluation[1]

There is *sufficient evidence* for the carcinogenicity of chlorendic acid in experimental animals.

No data were available from studies in humans on the carcinogenicity of chlorendic acid.

### Overall evaluation

Chlorendic acid is *possibly carcinogenic to humans (Group 2B)*.

---

[1] For description of the italicized terms and criteria for making the evaluation, see Preamble pp. 25-29.

## Summary table of genetic and related effects of chlorendic acid

| Nonmammalian systems | | | | | | | | | | | | | | | Mammalian systems | | | | | | | | | | | | | | | | | | | | |
|---|---|---|---|---|---|---|---|---|---|---|---|---|---|---|---|---|---|---|---|---|---|---|---|---|---|---|---|---|---|---|---|---|---|---|---|
| Prokaryotes | | | Lower eukaryotes | | | | Plants | | | | Insects | | | | | In vitro | | | | | | | | | | | | | In vivo | | | | | | |
| | | | | | | | | | | | | | | | Animal cells | | | | | | | Human cells | | | | | | | Animals | | | | | Humans | |
| D | G | R | D | G | R | G | A | D | G | C | R | G | C | A | D | G | S | M | C | A | T | I | D | G | S | M | C | A | T | I | D | G | S | M | C | DL | A | D | S | M | C | A |
| −¹ | | | −¹ | | | | | | | | | | | | | | +¹ | | | | | | | | | | | | | | | | | | | | | | | | | |

A, aneuploidy; C, chromosomal aberrations; D, DNA damage; DL, dominant lethal mutation; G, gene mutation; I, inhibition of intercellular communication; M, micronuclei; R, mitotic recombination and gene conversion; S, sister chromatid exchange; T, cell transformation

*In completing the table, the following symbols indicate the consensus of the Working Group with regard to the results for each endpoint:*

−¹ considered to be negative, but only one valid study was available to the Working Group
+¹ considered to be positive, but only one valid study was available to the Working Group.

## 5. References

Anon. (1980) Chemical profile: maleic anhydride. *Chem. Mark. Rep.*, *218*, 9, 32

Chemical Information Systems (1988) *Information System for Hazardous Organics in Water (ISHOW), Infrared Search System (IRSS), Mass Spectral Search System (MSSS)*, Baltimore, MD

Cochrane, W.P. & Forbes, M.A. (1974) Oxidation products of heptachlor and its metabolites — a chemical study. *Chemosphere*, *3*, 41-46

Decad, G.M. & Fields, M.T. (1982) Disposition and excretion of chlorendic acid in Fischer 344 rats. *J. Toxicol. environ. Health*, *9*, 911-920

Ermolaeva, L.P., Luzyanin, B.P., Il'icheva, I.A. & Novikov, E.A. (1976) Chromatographic method for determination of epichlorohydrin, tetrachlorobenzene, and chlorendic anhydride in water. *Met. Opredeleniya Zagryaznyayushch. Veshchestv v Poverkhnostn. Vokakh*, 129-132 [*Chem. Abstr.*, *86*, 160921e]

Friedman, M., Whitfield, R.E. & Tillin, S. (1973) Enhancement of the natural flame-resistance of wool. *Text. Res. J.*, *43*, 212-217

Gupta, S.K., Krishnan, M. & Thampy, R.T. (1978) Preparation of chlorendic acid based polyester resins. *Ind. J. Text. Res.*, *3*, 124-128

IARC (1989) *IARC Monographs on the Evaluation of Carcinogenic Risks to Humans*, Vol. 47, *Some Solvents, Resin Monomers and Related Compounds, Pigments and Occupational Exposures in Paint Manufacture and Painting*, Lyon, pp. 171-197

Larsen, E.R. (1980) Flame retardants (halogenated). In: Mark, H.F., Othmer, D.F., Overberger, C.G., Seaborg, G.T. & Grayson, M., eds, *Kirk-Othmer Encyclopedia of Chemical Technology*, 3rd ed., Vol. 10, New York, John Wiley & Sons, pp. 388-389

Makhlouf, J. (1982) Polyesters, unsaturated. In: Mark, H.F., Othmer, D.F., Overberger, C.G., Seaborg, G.T. & Grayson, M., eds, *Kirk-Othmer Encyclopedia of Chemical Technology*, 3rd ed., Vol. 18, New York, John Wiley & Sons, pp. 575-594

Maronpot, R.R., Montgomery, C.A., Jr, Boorman, G.A. & McConnell, E.E. (1986) National Toxicology Program nomenclature for hepatoproliferative lesions of rats. *Toxicol. Pathol.*, *14*, 263-273

Martens, R. (1972) Degradation of endosulfan by soil microorganisms (Ger.). *Schriftenr. Ver. Wasser Boden Lufthyg. Berlin Dahlem*, *37*, 167-173

Morton Thiokol (1985) *Material Safety Data Sheet 22422: 1,4,5,6,7,7-Hexachlorobicyclo(2.2.1)-5-heptene-2,3-dicarboxylic Acid*, Danvers, MA, Alfa Products Division

National Toxicology Program (1987) *Toxicology and Carcinogenesis Studies of Chlorendic Acid (CAS No. 115-28-6) in F344/N Rats and B6C3F$_1$ Mice (Feed Studies)* (Technical Report No. 304; NIH Publ. No. 87-2560), Research Triangle Park, NC, US Department of Health and Human Services

Occidental Chemical Corp. (1987) *Material Safety Data Sheet M8584: HET Acid*, Niagara Falls, NY

Occidental Chemical N.V. (1988) *HET Acid*, Brussels

Pilenkova, I.I. & Fat'yanova, A.D. (1980) Determination of chlorendic anhydride in production premises air (Russ.). *Zh. anal. Khim.*, *35*, 2047-2049

Sadtler Research Laboratories (1980) *Standard Spectra Collection, 1980 Cumulative Index*, Philadelphia, PA

Seredina, M.A. & Kryazhev, Y.G. (1987) Flame-resistant treatment of wool materials with solutions of halogenated organic acids. *Tekhnol. Tekst. Prom-st'.*, *5*, 76-79

Talbot, R.C. (1984) Using fiberglass-reinforced plastics. *Chem. Eng.*, *91*, 76-82

US Environmental Protection Agency (1986) *Chemical Hazard Information Profile*, Washington DC, Office of Toxic Substances

US International Trade Commission (1981) *Synthetic Organic Chemicals, US Production and Sales, 1980 (USITC Publ. 1183)*, Washington DC, US Government Printing Office, p. 261

US International Trade Commission (1988) *Synthetic Organic Chemicals US Production and Sales, 1987 (USITC Publ. 2118)*, Washington DC, US Government Printing Office, p. 3-9

Velsicol Chemical Corp. (1982) *Product Information Bulletin, Specialty Chemicals, Velsicol Chlorendic Anhydride*, Rosemont, IL

Whitfield, R.E. & Friedman, M. (1973) Flame resistant wool. III. Chemical modification of wool with chlorendic and related halo-organic acid anhydrides. *Text. Chem. Color*, *5*, 76-78

# CHLORINATED PARAFFINS

## 1. Chemical and Physical Data

Chlorinated paraffins are manufactured by the chlorination of specified normal paraffin fractions (straight-chain hydrocarbons) obtained from petroleum refining. Ordinary commercial chlorinated paraffins are not single compounds but are mixtures, each containing several homologous *n*-alkanes corresponding to their manufacture from *n*-paraffin fractions with several different degrees of chlorination.

Chlorinated paraffins are characterized to a first approximation by the carbon-chain length range of their *n*-alkanes and by the chlorine content of the product. An average chain length for the hydrocarbon feedstock or an average molecular weight is often stated as well. For example, a chlorinated paraffin referred to as $C_{12}$, 60% chlorine, would be a product with an average chain length of 12 carbons with approximately 60% chlorine.

A general classification of chlorinated paraffins by carbon-chain length and degree of chlorination is presented in Table 1.

Table 1. Chlorinated paraffin categories[a]

| Carbon–chain length | Feedstock | Chlorination by weight (%) | | |
|---|---|---|---|---|
| | | 40–50 | 50–60 | 60–70 |
| $C_{10-13}$ | $C_{12}$ | A1 | A2 | A3 |
| $C_{14-19}$ | $C_{15}$ | B1 | B2 | B3 |
| $C_{20-30}$ | $C_{24}$ | C1 | C2 | C3 |

[a]From Chlorinated Paraffins Industry Association (1988)

### 1.1 Synonyms

*Chem. Abstr. Services Reg. Nos and Chem Abstr. Services Names*:

| | |
|---|---|
| 63449-39-8 | Paraffin waxes and hydrocarbon waxes, chloro |
| 85422-92-0 | Paraffin oils and hydrocarbon oils, chloro |
| 61788-76-9 | Alkanes, chloro |
| 68920-70-7 | Alkanes, $C_{6-18}$, chloro |
| 71011-12-6 | Alkanes, $C_{12-13}$, chloro |

| | |
|---|---|
| 84082-38-2 | Alkanes, $C_{10-21}$, chloro |
| 84776-06-7 | Alkanes, $C_{10-32}$, chloro |
| 84776-07-8 | Alkanes, $C_{16-27}$, chloro |
| 85049-26-9 | Alkanes, $C_{16-35}$, chloro |
| 85535-84-8 | Alkanes, $C_{10-13}$, chloro |
| 85535-85-9 | Alkanes, $C_{14-17}$, chloro |
| 85535-86-0 | Alkanes, $C_{18-28}$, chloro |
| 85536-22-7 | Alkanes, $C_{12-14}$, chloro |
| 85681-73-8 | Alkanes, $C_{10-14}$, chloro |
| 97659-46-6 | Alkanes, $C_{10-26}$, chloro |
| 97553-43-0 | Paraffins (petroleum), normal C > 10, chloro |
| 106232-85-3 | Alkanes, $C_{18-20}$, chloro |
| 106232-86-4 | Alkanes, $C_{22-40}$, chloro |
| 108171-26-2 | Alkanes, $C_{10-12}$, chloro |
| 108171-27-3 | Alkanes, $C_{22-26}$, chloro |

*Synonyms*: Alkanes, chlorinated; alkanes ($C_{10-12}$), chloro (60%); alkanes ($C_{10-13}$), chloro (50-70%); alkanes ($C_{14-17}$), chloro (40-52%); alkanes ($C_{18-28}$), chloro (20-50%); alkanes ($C_{22-26}$), chloro (43%); $C_{12}$, 60% chlorine; $C_{23}$, 43% chlorine; chlorinated alkanes; chlorinated hydrocarbon waxes; chlorinated paraffin waxes; chlorinated waxes; chloroalkanes; chlorocarbons; chloroparaffin waxes; paraffin, chlorinated; paraffins, chloro; paraffin waxes, chlorinated; paroils, chlorinated; polychlorinated alkanes; polychloro alkanes

## 1.2 Molecular formula

$$C_xH_{(2x-y+2)}Cl_y$$

## 1.3 Chemical and physical properties of chlorinated paraffins

Chlorinated paraffins that have been manufactured from pure *n*-paraffins are generally unreactive and stable during storage at normal temperatures.

Depending on their chain length and degree of chlorination, chlorinated paraffins are colourless or yellowish, mobile to highly viscous liquids or waxy to glassy solidified substances.

Chlorinated paraffins are practically insoluble in water, although they can form emulsions and/or suspensions (Schenker, 1979).

Selected chemical and physical properties of some chlorinated paraffin products are summarized in Table 2.

Table 2. Chemical and physical properties of representative chlorinated paraffins[a]

| Paraffin feedstock | Average chain length | Chlorine content (%) | Density (25°C, g/ml) | Refractive index | Viscosity (25°C, P) | Pour-point[b] (°C) | Heat stability (% HCl after 4 h at 175°C) |
|---|---|---|---|---|---|---|---|
| $C_{10}$–$C_{13}$ | $C_{12}$ | 60 | 1.36 | 1.516 | 35 | -10 | 0.10 |
| $C_{13}$–$C_{17}$ | $C_{15}$ | 52 | 1.25 | 1.510 | 16 | -10 | 0.10 |
| $C_{17}$–$C_{30}$ | $C_{24}$ | 39 | 1.12 | 1.501 | 7 | -20 | 0.20 |
|  |  | 42 | 1.17 | 1.505 | 30 | 0 | 0.20 |
|  |  | 48 | 1.23 | 1.516 | 125 | 10 | 0.25 |
|  |  | 70 | 1.65 | – | Solid | NA | 0.15 |

[a]From Schenker (1979)
[b]Lowest temperature at which a substance flows under specified conditions
–, not reported; NA, not applicable

### 1.4 Technical products and impurities

*Trade names*: The following generic trade names are usually accompanied by a suffix indicating a specific product: A 70; A 70 (wax); Adekacizer E; Arubren; Cereclor; Chlorcosane; Chlorez; Chlorofin; Chloroflo; Chlorparaffin; Chlorowax; Cloparin; Cloparol; Clorafin; CW; Derminolfett; Derminolöl; EDC-tar; Electrofine; Enpara; Hordaflam; Hordaflex; Hordalub; Hulz; KhP; Meflex; Monocizer; Paroil; Poliks; Tenekil; Toyoparax; Unichlor

Chlorinated paraffins are marketed in a variety of mixtures comprising a combination of different carbon-chain lengths with varying degrees of chlorination. Products may be classified according to the scheme in Table 1.

The chain lengths of commercial paraffin products are between ten and 38 carbon atoms and chlorine contents between 10 and 72%. The chlorinated paraffins most frequently used are those with chain lengths of $C_{10-17}$ and a chlorine content of 45–55% (40–70%; Schenker, 1979). Very few products contain less than 35% chlorine. At a chlorine content of approximately 72%, all of the carbon atoms are singly chlorinated and further chlorination is very difficult (Strack, 1986). For a given average chlorine content, the distribution of individual chlorinated homologues is distributed around this average value. For example, Zitko (1974) described the distribution of chlorinated paraffins in a commercial chlorinated paraffin product ($C_{20}$–$C_{30}$, 26% chlorine) as shown in Table 3.

Analysis of a $C_{26}$ paraffin chlorinated in the laboratory showed that with a chlorine content or more than about 40%, less than 1% of the chloroparaffins contained fewer than three chlorine atoms per molecule (Könnecke & Hahn, 1962).

Isoparaffins (usually less than 1%), aromatic compounds (usually less than 100 ppm) and low levels of metal contamination may be present in technical products (Schenker, 1979).

Table 3. Distribution of chlorinated homologues in a commercial chlorinated paraffin[a]

| No. of chlorine atoms per molecule | Vol. % |
|---|---|
| 0 | 1.1 |
| 1 | 3.7 |
| 2 | 11.0 |
| 3 | 14.2 |
| 4 | 24.1 |
| 5 | 25.2 |
| 6 | 12.2 |
| More than 6 | 8.2 |

[a]From Zitko (1974)

Chlorinated paraffins are relatively inert materials, but prolonged exposure to heat and light or the presence of aluminium, zinc or iron can result in dehydrochlorination, resulting in a darkening of the material. Stabilizers are therefore usually added for storage. The most common stabilizers used are epoxidized soya bean oils. Others used in the past include pentaerythritol, organometallic tin compounds, and certain lead and cadmium compounds (Schenker, 1979; see IARC, 1976, 1980).

## 2. Production, Use, Occurrence and Analysis

### 2.1 Production and use

*(a) Production*

Chlorinated paraffins have been produced commercially since the 1930s. These mixtures of chlorinated *n*-alkanes are produced by reacting normal paraffin fractions obtained from petroleum distillation with gaseous chlorine exothermically at 80–120°C in the liquid phase (Chlorinated Paraffins Industry Association, 1988). Ultraviolet light is often used to promote chlorination, particularly at higher chlorine levels. The linings of the reactor vessels must be inert (e.g., glass or steel; Strack, 1986) to avoid the formation of metal chlorides, which cause darkening of the product by decomposition. Production of resinous chlorinated paraffins (70% chlorine content) requires the use of a solvent such as carbon tetrachloride during chlorination. Additional procedures include solvent stripping and grinding of the products as necessary (Zitko, 1974; Schenker, 1979).

Approximately 45 000 tonnes of chlorinated paraffins were produced in the USA in 1987 (US International Trade Commission, 1988). In 1985, 95 000 tonnes were produced in western Europe (SRI International, 1986) and more than 300 000 tonnes worldwide (Strack, 1986).

Chlorinated paraffins are produced in Argentina, Australia, Brazil, Bulgaria, Canada, Czechoslovakia, China, the Federal Republic of Germany, France, the German Democratic Republic, India, Italy, Japan, Mexico, Poland, Romania, Spain, South Africa, Taiwan, the UK, the USA and the USSR.

*(b) Use*

Data are from the European Chemical Industry Ecology and Toxicology Centre (1989), unless otherwise specified.

Chlorinated paraffins are used as secondary plasticizers for polyvinyl chloride (PVC) in applications such as electrical cables when the inherent low inflammability of PVC would be impaired by primary plasticizers (e.g., dioctyl phthalate). Chlorinated paraffins are used on a large scale as extreme-pressure additives in metal-machining fluids, e.g., in the automobile industry, precision engineering industry and in machinery construction. As additives to paints, coatings and sealants, chlorinated paraffins improve resistance to water and chemicals. Systems of this kind are especially suitable for marine paints, as coatings for industrial flooring, vessels and swimming pools (e.g., rubber and chlorinated rubber coatings), and as road marking paints. The flame-retarding properties of highly chlorinated paraffins are important for their use in plastics, fabrics, paints and coatings. Chlorinated paraffins are also used with decabromodiphenyl oxide and antimony trioxide in polyester fabrics for tents (Priha *et al.*, 1988).

Approximately 50% of the chlorinated paraffins consumed in the USA is used as extreme-pressure lubricant additives in the metal working industry. The remainder is used in plastics, fire-retardant and water-repellent fabric treatments, and in paint, rubber, caulks and sealants. In contrast, 50% of the chlorinated paraffins consumed in western Europe is as secondary plasticizers in PVC and other plastics (Schenker, 1979).

The chlorinated paraffins most frequently used as plasticizers for plastics are those with a medium chain length ($C_{14-17}$), with chlorine contents between 45 and 52% (40 and 50%; Zitko, 1974). $C_{10-13}$ or $C_{>20}$ paraffins are also used, depending on the PVC or plastics type. $C_{10-13}$ chlorinated paraffins are suitable for water- and chemical-resistant, low-inflammability and abrasion-resistant paints, either as plasticizer or as a constituent of the binder. Special medium-chain length $C_{14-17}$ grades are used for sealants. Chlorinated paraffin grades with good solubility in mineral oils ($C_{10-17}$) and chlorine contents of 40–60% are preferred for use as extreme-pressure additives to metal machining fluids, pastes, emulsions and lubricants. For flame-retardant applications, chlorinated paraffins with approximately 70% chlorine are used; the chain length depends on the substrate: $C_{10-13}$ for rubber and soft plastics and $C_{18-30}$ for rigid plastics such as polyesters and polystyrene (Zitko, 1974).

*(c) Regulatory status and guidelines*

No regulatory standard or guideline has been established for chlorinated paraffins.

## 2.2 Occurrence

*(a) Natural occurrence*

Chlorinated paraffins are not known to occur as natural products.

*(b) Occupational exposure*

Approximately 1 500 000 workers were potentially exposed to chlorinated paraffins in the USA in 1972–74 (National Institute for Occupational Safety and Health, 1977).

No data on levels of exposure to chlorinated paraffins were available to the Working Group.

*(c) Water and sediment*

Chlorinated paraffins have been identified in marine and fresh water and in sediments in the UK. Concentrations ranged from < 0.5 to 4 µg/l (w/w) in water and from < 0.05 to 10 mg/l in sediments. Near industrialized areas, maximal levels of 6 mg/l (water) and 15 mg/l (sediment) have been detected (Campbell & McConnell, 1980).

*(d) Biological samples*

Short-chain chlorinated paraffins were found at levels of 6–12 mg/kg in mussels from waterways contaminated with chlorinated paraffins close to the point of discharge. In contrast, the values in seals, marine shellfish and fresh- and salt-water fish from unpolluted areas were less than 0.2 mg/kg $C_{20-30}$ and 0.4 mg/kg $C_{10-20}$. Seabird eggs contained up to 2 mg/kg $C_{10-20}$ and up to 0.1 mg/kg $C_{20-30}$ (detection limit, 0.05 mg/kg). $C_{20-30}$ chlorinated paraffins were detected in only a few samples of human food, whereas 70% of the samples contained up to 0.5 mg/kg $C_{10-20}$, with up to 0.3 mg/kg in milk products, 0.15 mg/kg in vegetable oils and 0.025 mg/kg in fruit and vegetables. Liver samples from sheep that had been pastured near a chlorinated paraffin factory contained up to 0.2 mg/kg. Chlorinated paraffins were also found in human tissues *post mortem*: $C_{10-20}$ compounds were often found in liver, adipose tissues and kidneys, whereas long-chain chlorinated paraffins were found in only a few samples. The maximal value was 1.5 mg/kg in a liver sample; most values were below 0.09 mg/kg (Campbell & McConnell, 1980).

## 2.3 Analysis

Selected methods for the analysis of chlorinated paraffins in various matrices are presented in Table 4.

Table 4. Analytical methods for the determination of chlorinated paraffins in various matrices

| Sample matrix | Sample preparation | Assay procedure[a] | Limit of detection | Reference |
|---|---|---|---|---|
| Adipose tissue | Homogenize in dichloromethane; percolate through anhydrous $Na_2SO_4$; remove solvent; dissolve residue in pentane; wash, dry and concentrate; purify by alumina chromatography | GC/MS | 5 ng | Schmid & Müller (1985) |
| Sediment | Extract with acetone:hexane (1:1, v:v); wash, dry and concentrate; purify by alumina chromatography | GC/MS | 5 ng | Schmid & Müller (1985) |
| Sewage sludge | Homogenize with acetone; extract with pentane; wash, dry and concentrate; purify by alumina chromatography | GC/MS | 5 ng | Schmid & Müller (1985) |
| Environmental and biota samples | Clean up by irradiating extracts with high-intensity UV light (90 min, <20°C) in aliphatic hydrocarbons | GC/CD | NR | Friedman & Lombardo (1975) |
| | Introduce extract directly into mass spectrometer | NICIMS | NR | Gjos & Gustavsen (1982) |
| Air | Adsorb on charcoal; desorb with carbon disulfide | GC/FID | 0.01 mg/sample | Eller (1985) |

[a]Abbreviations: GC/MS, gas chromatography/mass spectrometry; GC/CD, gas chromatography/coulometric detection; NICIMS, negative-ion chemical ionization mass spectrometry; NR, not reported; GC/FID, gas chromatography/flame ionization detection

# 3. Biological Data Relevant to the Evaluation of Carcinogenic Risk to Humans

## 3.1 Carcinogenicity studies in animals

*Oral administration*

(i) *Chlorinated paraffin; average carbon-chain length, $C_{12}$; average degree of chlorination, 60%*

*Mouse*: Groups of 50 male and 50 female B6C3F$_1$ mice, eight to nine weeks of age, were treated by gavage with 0, 125 or 250 mg/kg bw of a commercial-grade chlorinated paraffin product dissolved in corn oil on five days a week for 103 weeks. All survivors were killed at 112–114 weeks of age. Body weights of treated females were about 10% lower than those of controls during the second year. Survival of treated males was not significantly different from that of controls, but fewer high-dose females were still alive after week 100 as compared to controls. The incidences of tumours at various sites that are significantly greater than those in controls are shown in Table 5. The incidences of hepatocellular adenomas and of hepatocellular adenomas and carcinomas combined were significantly increased in treated mice. The incidence of alveolar/bronchiolar carcinomas was significantly increased in males, and the combined incidence of follicular-cell adenomas and carcinomas of the thyroid in females was significantly elevated. The incidences of adenomas of the Harderian gland in females were 1/50 controls, 6/50 in low-dose animals and 2/50 in high-dose animals; the trend with dose is not significant (National Toxicology Program, 1986a; Bucher et al., 1987).

Table 5. Incidences of tumours in mice administered $C_{12}$, 60% chlorine chlorinated paraffin

| Dose (mg/kg bw) | Hepatocellular adenomas | Hepatocellular adenomas and carcinomas | Alveolar/bronchiolar carcinomas | Follicular-cell tumours of the thyroid |
|---|---|---|---|---|
| Males | | | | |
| Control | 11/50 | 20/50 | 0/50 | |
| 125 | 20/50 | 34/50 | 3/50 | |
| 250 | 29/50 | 38/50 | 6/50 | |
| | $p < 0.001^a$ | $p < 0.001^a$ | $p < 0.011^a$ | |
| Females | | | | |
| Control | 0/50 | 3/50 | | 8/50 |
| 125 | 18/50 | 22/50 | | 12/49 |
| 250 | 22/50 | 28/50 | | 13/49 |
| | $p < 0.001^a$ | $p < 0.001^a$ | | $p < 0.024^a$ |

[a]Incidental tumour test for trend

*Rat*: Groups of 50 male and 50 female Fischer 344/N rats, six to seven weeks of age, were treated by gavage with 0, 312 or 625 mg/kg bw of a commercial-grade chlorinated paraffin product dissolved in corn oil on five days a week for 104 weeks. All survivors were killed at 111–113 weeks of age. Body weights of high-dose males were 10–23% lower than those of controls after week 37, and survival of treated males was shorter than that of controls after about week 90; survival of low-dose females was shorter than that of controls after week 92. The incidences of tumours that are significantly greater than those in controls are shown in Table 6. The incidences of hepatic neoplastic nodules [adenomas; Maronpot et al., 1986] and of hepatic neoplastic nodules and hepatocellular carcinomas combined was significantly increased in treated animals. Hepatocellular carcinomas occurred in 0/50 control males and in 3/50 at the low dose and 2/48 at the high dose. The combined incidences of renal tubular-cell adenomas and adenocarcinomas in males were 0/50 controls and 9/50 low-dose and 3/49 high-dose animals; two of the tumours in the low-dose group were carcinomas. The

Table 6. Incidences of tumours in rats administered $C_{12}$, 60% chlorine chlorinated paraffin

| Dose (mg/kg bw) | Hepatocellular carcinomas | Hepatocellular adenomas and carcinomas | Follicular-cell adenomas and carcinomas of the thyroid | Mononuclear cell leukaemia |
|---|---|---|---|---|
| Males |  |  |  |  |
| Control | 0/50 | 0/50 |  | 7/50 |
| 312 | 10/50 | 13/50 |  | 12/50 |
| 625 | 16/48 | 16/48 |  | 14/50 |
|  | $p < 0.001^a$ | $p < 0.001^a$ |  | $p = 0.001^b$ |
| Females |  |  |  |  |
| Control | 0/50 | 0/50 | 0/50 |  |
| 312 | 4/50 | 5/50 | 6/50 |  |
| 625 | 7/50 | 7/50 | 6/50 |  |
|  | $p = 0.005^a$ | $p = 0.008^a$ | $p = 0.02^a$ |  |

[a] Incidental tumour test for trend
[b] Life table test

combined incidence of follicular-cell adenomas and carcinomas of the thyroid was significantly increased in treated females; three in the high-dose group were carcinomas. The incidence of mononuclear-cell leukaemia was significantly increased in treated males; in females, mononuclear-cell leukaemia was observed in 11/50 controls and 22/50 low-dose and 16/50 high-dose animals. The combined incidences of acinar-cell adenomas and adenocarcinomas of the pancreas in males were 11/50 controls and 22/50 low-dose and 17/49 high-dose animals; two of the pancreatic tumours in the high-dose group were carcinomas (National Toxicology Program, 1986a; Bucher et al., 1987).

(ii) *Chlorinated paraffin; average carbon length, $C_{23}$; average degree of chlorination, 43%*

*Mouse*: Groups of 50 male and 50 female B6C3F$_1$ mice, eight to nine weeks of age, were treated by gavage with 0, 2500 or 5000 mg/kg bw of a commercial-grade chlorinated paraffin product dissolved in corn oil on five days a week for 103 weeks. All survivors were killed at 113–114 weeks of age. Low-dose males and females had lower weight gains than controls or high-dose animals. Survival in treated and control groups was similar for animals of each sex, but median survival was shorter in females (90–95 weeks) than in males (more than 105 weeks). The authors commented that the lower survival in females may have decreased the potential of the study to detect a carcinogenic effect. The incidence of malignant lymphomas was significantly increased in males: they occurred in 6/50 controls and in 12/50 low-dose and 16/50 high-dose animals ($p = 0.009$, life-table test for trend; $p = 0.011$, incidental tumour test for trend). The combined incidences of hepatocellular adenomas and carcinomas in females were 4/50 controls, 3/49 low-dose and 10/50 high-dose animals (trend not significant; National Toxicology Program, 1986b; Bucher et al., 1987).

*Rat*: Groups of 50 male and 50 female Fischer 344/N rats, six to seven weeks of age, were treated by gavage with 0, 1875 or 3750 mg/kg bw (males) and 0, 100, 300 or 900 (females) mg/kg bw of a commercial-grade chlorinated paraffin product dissolved in corn oil on five days a week for 103 weeks. All survivors were killed at 111-112 weeks of age. No significant difference in body weight gain or survival was observed between treated and control animals. The incidence of phaeochromocytomas of the adrenal medulla was significantly increased in females: control, 1/50; low-dose, 4/50; mid-dose, 6/50; high-dose, 7/50 ($p = 0.046$, incidental tumour test for trend; National Toxicology Program, 1986b; Bucher *et al.*, 1987).

## 3.2 Other relevant data

(a) *Experimental systems*

The Working Group noted the lack of systematic investigation of the influence of carbon-chain length and degree of chlorination in the reported studies on toxicokinetics and toxic effects.

(i) *Absorption, distribution, excretion and metabolism*

The Working Group noted that in these studies labelled material was isolated from tissues or excreta but was not characterized, and the kinetics of parent compounds and metabolites were not studied; thus, the metabolic pathways involved in the degradation of chlorinated paraffins remain largely unknown.

Percutaneous absorption of two $^{14}$C-labelled paraffins ($C_{18}$, 50-53% chlorine; $C_{28}$, 47% chlorine) was evaluated in Sprague-Dawley rats; absorption of the $C_{18}$ paraffin over four days was 0.7% of the applied radioactivity in males and less than 0.7% in females and that of the $C_{28}$ paraffin was less than 0.1% (Yang *et al.*, 1987).

Studies in which the disposition of radiolabel was determined following intravenous or oral administration to C57Bl mice of three $^{14}$C-labelled chlorododecanes of different chlorine content (17.5%, 55.9% and 68.5%) demonstrated marked uptake of label on all three paraffins in liver, fat, salivary glands, bone marrow and thymus. The concentration of radioactivity in the tissues and the amount of exhaled $^{14}$C-$CO_2$ were inversely related to the degree of chlorination of the paraffins (Darnerud *et al.*, 1982).

In C57Bl mice, a $^{14}$C-$C_{16}$, 34% chlorine paraffin in a fat emulsion was readily absorbed after oral administration and the label was distributed to tissues that exhibit high metabolic activity, e.g., intestinal mucosa, bone marrow and exocrine glands. Exhaled $CO_2$ contained 33% of the $^{14}$C-label within 12 h of administration, compared with 44% of the label when the material was given by intravenous administration (Darnerud & Brandt, 1982).

By following the disappearance of radioactivity after feeding a $^{36}$Cl-labelled $C_{14-17}$, 52% chlorine paraffin to Wistar rats for ten weeks, the half-life for its elimination was estimated to be less than one week from the liver and approximately eight weeks from fat (Birtley *et al.*, 1980).

Injection of a $^{14}$C-$C_{16}$, 65% chlorine paraffin into the portal vein of Sprague-Dawley rats *via* cannulated bile ducts resulted in excretion of conjugates of the paraffin with *N*-acetylcysteine and glutathione into the bile. The parent compound constituted less than 3% of the total label excreted (Åhlman *et al.*, 1986).

In studies in C57Bl mice with a $^{14}$C-labelled $C_{12}$, 68.5% chlorine paraffin, exhaled $^{14}$C-$CO_2$ was quantified following administration of inducers and inhibitors of cytochrome P450. Pretreatment with the inhibitors piperonyl butoxide and metyrapone inhibited $CO_2$ production by 84 and 60%, respectively. Induction with phenobarbital stimulated the peak exhalation rate to 152% of that in controls. Studies with differently chlorinated dodecanes (17.4, 55.9 and 68.5% chlorine) suggested a more prominent role for cytochrome P450 in the metabolism of more heavily chlorinated paraffins (Darnerud, 1984). These studies suggest that cytochrome P450 catalyses a de-chlorination reaction which is followed by β-oxidation and incorporation of the carbon chain into cellular metabolism.

(ii) *Toxic effects*

The toxicity of chlorinated paraffins in fish and birds has been studied extensively (Howard *et al.*, 1975; Lombardo *et al.*, 1975; Svanberg *et al.*, 1978; Madeley & Birtley, 1980). The acute toxicity of chlorinated paraffins is low; in rats the oral $LD_{50}$ value for a $C_{12}$, 59% chlorine paraffin was reported to be greater than 21.5 ml/kg bw, and no death resulted from oral dosing of rats with 10 ml/kg bw of a $C_{24}$, 40% chlorine paraffin or with 50 g/kg bw of a $C_{24}$, 70% chlorine paraffin (Howard *et al.*, 1975).

It has been reported that in 14-day and 90-day feed and gavage studies in Fischer 344 rats with a $C_{10-13}$, 58% chlorine paraffin, livers were enlarged and showed hepatocellular hypertrophy at doses of 100 mg/kg bw per day and above; in 90-day studies, chronic nephropathy and thyroid hyperplasia [unspecified] were also observed with doses of 100 mg/kg bw per day and above (Serrone *et al.*, 1987).

In 16-day studies with a $C_{12}$, 60% chlorine paraffin, deaths and reduced body weight gains occurred in male and female rats at doses of 7500 mg/kg bw per day, and all mice receiving doses of 3750 mg/kg bw per day or above died. Livers were enlarged in all groups of treated rats (low dose, 469 mg/kg bw per day) and mice (low dose, 938 mg/kg bw per day). In 90-day gavage studies, no death was considered to be related to treatment (highest doses, 5000 mg/kg bw per day for rats and 2000 mg/kg bw per day for mice). Liver weights were increased in treated rats and mice, and hypertrophy of hepatocytes was evident microscopically; focal hepatic necrosis was observed in mice. Nephrosis was more severe in high-dose rats than in controls. In two-year studies in rats (see also section 3.1), non-neoplastic lesions, including minimal necrosis, hypertrophy and angiectasis of the liver, were associated with treatment. Severe chronic renal disease with secondary parathyroid hyperplasia and subsequent fibrous osteodystrophy and inflammation and hyperkeratosis of the forestomach were seen in male rats. Nephropathy was also increased in incidence in female rats. In similar studies in mice, the incidence of nephrosis was slightly increased in females (National Toxicology Program, 1986a; Bucher *et al.*, 1987).

Liver enlargement was reported in 14- and 90-day dietary studies (at up to 15 000 and 625 ppm, respectively), and chronic nephropathy and thyroid hyperplasia [unspecified] were observed in 90-day dietary studies in Fischer 344 rats administered a $C_{14-17}$, 52% chlorine paraffin (Serrone *et al.*, 1987).

In 90-day studies in which Wistar rats were fed diets containing up to 5000 ppm of a $C_{14-17}$, 52% chlorine paraffin, no effect on survival, clinical signs, haematological measurements or efficiency of food utilization was noted; however, liver and kidney weights were elevated, and microscopic examination of the liver showed proliferation of smooth endoplasmic reticulum. Similar results were observed in male beagle dogs fed diets providing up to 100 mg/kg bw per day of the same paraffin for up to 90 days, but no effect was seen in females (Birtley et al., 1980).

In 14- and 90-day gavage studies in Fischer 344 rats with a longer-chain paraffin ($C_{20-30}$, 43% chlorine), no compound-related effect was reported in the 14-day study, but females in the 90-day study showed an increase in liver weight and lesions described as multifocal granulomatous hepatitis at doses of 100 mg/kg bw per day and above. Males showed increased nephrosis and females increased kidney mineralization at 3750 mg/kg bw per day (Serrone et al., 1987)

A $C_{23}$, 43% chlorine paraffin was evaluated in 16-day, 90-day and two-year studies by oral gavage in corn oil in Fischer 344 rats and B6C3F$_1$ mice of each sex. No significant toxicity was observed in the 16-day or 90-day studies at doses of up to 3750 mg/kg bw per day in rats and 7500 mg/kg bw per day in mice, with the exception of granulomatous inflammation of the livers in female rats in the 90-day study. In the two-year studies (see also section 3.1), non-neoplastic lesions in rats of each sex included lymphocytic infiltration and granulomatous inflammation of the liver and mesenteric and pancreatic lymph nodes, with associated lymphoid hyperplasia and splenic congestion. Increased kidney-tubule pigmentation and nephropathy occurred in female rats. No significant non-neoplastic lesion was seen in mice treated with up to 5000 mg/kg bw per day (National Toxicology Program, 1986b; Bucher et al., 1987).

Feeding of Fischer 344 rats with a $C_{22-26}$, 70% chlorine paraffin was reported to induce no toxicity in 14-day studies but slight increases in serum enzyme levels, liver weight, hepatocellular hypertrophy and cytoplasmic fat vacuolization at 3750 mg/kg bw per day in the 90-day studies (Serrone et al., 1987).

The effects of chlorinated paraffins of varying chain lengths ($C_{10-13}$, 49% chlorine, 59% chlorine, 71% chlorine; $C_{14-17}$, 50% chlorine; $C_{18-26}$, 49% chlorine) on proliferation of hepatocyte smooth endoplasmic reticulum and induction of various forms of cytochrome P450 have been examined in rats by intraperitoneal injection. Cytochrome P450 induction and proliferation of smooth endoplasmic reticulum were stimulated to a greater extent by shorter-chain than by longer-chain paraffins (Nilsen & Toftgård, 1981; Nilsen et al., 1981). An increase in the occurrence of lipid droplets followed by proliferation of peroxisomes and mitochondria was observed in the livers of the rats given the $C_{10-13}$, 49% chlorine and $C_{18-26}$, 49% chlorine paraffins (Nilsen et al., 1980). Administration of a highly chlorinated mixture of paraffins ($C_{10-23}$, 70% chlorine) to C57Bl/6 mice resulted in an increase in the level of hepatic cytosolic epoxide hydrolase (Meijer & DePierre, 1987).

As reported in an abstract, administration by gavage for 14 days of 2 g/kg bw per day to male rats and of 1 g/kg bw per day to female rats and male and female mice of $C_{12}$, 60% chlorine, $C_{10-12}$, 56% chlorine or $C_{14-17}$, 40% chlorine caused increases in liver weight and proliferation of hepatocellular smooth endoplasmic reticulum and peroxisomes. A $C_{23}$, 40% chlorine compound did not induce similar effects on peroxisome proliferation (Elcombe *et al.*, 1990).

*(iii) Effects on reproduction and prenatal toxicity*

In a series of studies on chlorinated paraffins ($C_{10-13}$, 58% chlorine; $C_{14-17}$, 52% chlorine; $C_{20-30}$, 43% chlorine; and $C_{22-26}$, 70% chlorine), pregnant Charles River rats and pregnant rabbits were treated by gavage on gestation days 6–19 and 6–27, respectively. No teratogenic effect was reported (Serrone *et al.*, 1987). [The Working Group noted that the data given did not allow an evaluation of the study for reproductive effects.]

*(iv) Genetic and related effects* (see Appendix 1)

Chlorinated paraffins $C_{10-13}$, 50% chlorine (Birtley *et al.*, 1980); $C_{12}$, 60% chlorine (National Toxicology Program, 1986a); $C_{14-17}$, 52% chlorine (Birtley *et al.*, 1980); $C_{20-30}$, 42% chlorine (Birtley *et al.*, 1980); $C_{23}$, 43% chlorine (National Toxicology Program, 1986b); and $C_{10-23}$, 70% chlorine (Meijer *et al.*, 1981) were not mutagenic to several strains of *Salmonella typhimurium* in the presence or absence of an exogenous metabolic system from Aroclor 1254-induced rat liver (Birtley *et al.*, 1980; Meijer *et al.*, 1981; National Toxicology Program, 1986a,b) or Syrian hamster liver (National Toxicology Program, 1986a,b).

Chlorinated paraffins ($C_{14-17}$, 52% chlorine; $C_{20-30}$, 43% chlorine; $C_{22-26}$, 70% chlorine; $C_{10-13}$, 58% chlorine) were reported not to cause chromosomal aberrations in rat bone marrow when given by gavage at toxic doses of up to 5 g/kg bw per day for five days. A $C_{10-13}$, 58% chlorine chlorinated paraffin at up to 2 g/kg bw per day did not cause dominant lethal mutations in rats (Serrone *et al.*, 1987). [The Working Group noted that the data reported did not allow an evaluation of the study with regard to genetic and related effects.]

*(b) Humans*

No data relevant to an evaluation of carcinogenicity were available to the Working Group.

## 3.3 Case reports and epidemiological studies of carcinogenicity to humans

No data were available to the Working Group.

# 4. Summary of Data Reported and Evaluation

## 4.1 Exposure data

Chlorinated paraffins are mixtures of polychlorinated *n*-alkanes produced by the reaction of chlorine with specific normal paraffin fractions from petroleum distillation. Carbon-chain lengths of commercial products are generally between $C_{10}$ and $C_{30}$, and the chlorine content is typically between 40 and 70%. Chlorinated paraffins are used as plasticizers for polyvinyl chloride, as extreme-pressure additives in metal-machining fluids, as additives to paints, coatings and sealants to improve their resistance to chemicals and to water, and as flame retardants for plastics, fabrics, paints and coatings. No data on occupational exposure levels were available. Chlorinated paraffins have been detected in water and sediments, in tissues of marine animals, in human foods and in human tissues *post mortem*.

### 4.2 Experimental carcinogenicity data

A commercial chlorinated paraffin product of average carbon-chain length $C_{12}$ and average degree of chlorination 60% was tested for carcinogenicity by oral administration in one strain of mice and in one strain of rats. In mice, it increased the incidence of hepatocellular tumours in animals of each sex and of alveolar/bronchiolar carcinomas in males and of follicular-cell tumours of the thyroid gland in females. In rats, it increased the incidences of hepatocellular tumours in animals of each sex, of follicular-cell tumours of the thyroid in females and of mononuclear-cell leukaemia in males.

A commercial chlorinated paraffin product of average carbon-chain length $C_{23}$ and average degree of chlorination 43% was tested for carcinogenicity by oral administration in one strain of mice and in one strain of rats. It increased the incidence of malignant lymphomas in male mice. In rats, it induced phaeochromocytomas of the adrenal medulla in females.

### 4.3 Human carcinogenicity data

No data were available to the Working Group.

### 4.4 Other relevant data

Administration of some chlorinated paraffins to rodents resulted in nephrotoxicity and proliferation of smooth endoplasmic reticulum and peroxisomes in hepatocytes.

None of six chlorinated paraffins tested was mutagenic to bacteria either in the presence or absence of an exogenous metabolic system

### 4.5 Evaluation[1]

There is *sufficient evidence* for the carcinogenicity of a commercial chlorinated paraffin product of average carbon-chain length $C_{12}$ and average degree of chlorination 60% in experimental animals.

---

[1]For description of the italicized terms and criteria for making the evaluation, see Preamble, pp. 25-29.

## Summary table of genetic and related effects of chlorinated paraffins

| Nonmammalian systems | | | | | | | | | | | Mammalian systems | | | | | | | | | | | | | | | | | | |
|---|---|---|---|---|---|---|---|---|---|---|---|---|---|---|---|---|---|---|---|---|---|---|---|---|---|---|---|---|---|
| Proka-ryotes | | Lower eukaryotes | | | | Plants | | | | Insects | In vitro | | | | | | | | | | | | | In vivo | | | | | |
| | | | | | | | | | | | Animal cells | | | | | | Human cells | | | | | | | Animals | | | | | Humans |
| D | G | D | R | G | A | D | G | C | R | G | C | A | D | G | S | M | C | A | T | I | D | G | S | M | C | A | T | I | D | G | S | M | C | DL | A | D | S | M | C | A |
| | | - | | | | | | | | | | | | | | | | | | | | | | | | | | | | | | | | | | | | | | |

A, aneuploidy; C, chromosomal aberrations; D, DNA damage; DL, dominant lethal mutation; G, gene mutation; I, inhibition of intercellular communication; M, micronuclei; R, mitotic recombination and gene conversion; S, sister chromatid exchange; T, cell transformation

*In completing the table, the following symbol indicates the consensus of the Working Group with regard to the results for each endpoint:*
- considered to be negative

There is *limited evidence* for the carcinogenicity of a commercial chlorinated paraffin product of average carbon-chain length $C_{23}$ and average degree of chlorination 43% in experimental animals.

No data were available from studies in humans on the carcinogenicity of chlorinated paraffins.

**Overall evaluation**

Chlorinated paraffins of average carbon-chain length $C_{12}$ and average degree of chlorination approximately 60% are *possibly carcinogenic to humans (Group 2B)*.

# 5. References

Åhlman, M., Bergman, Å., Darnerud, P.O., Egestad, B. & Sjövall, J. (1986) Chlorinated paraffins: formation of sulphur-containing metabolites of polychlorohexadecane in rats. *Xenobiotica*, *16*, 225-232

Birtley, R.D.N., Conning, D.M., Daniel, J.W., Ferguson, D.M., Longstaff, E. & Swan, A.A.B. (1980) The toxicological effects of chlorinated paraffins in mammals. *Toxicol. appl. Pharmacol.*, *54*, 514-525

Bucher, J.R., Alison, R.H., Montgomery, C.A., Huff, J., Haseman, J.K., Farnell, D., Thompson, R. & Prejean, J.D. (1987) Comparative toxicity and carcinogenicity of two chlorinated paraffins in F344/N rats and B6C3F$_1$ mice. *Fundam. appl. Toxicol.*, *9*, 454-468

Campbell, I. & McConnell, G. (1980) Chlorinated paraffins and the environment. 1. Environmental occurrence. *Environ. Sci. Technol.*, *14*, 1209-1214

Chlorinated Paraffins Industry Association (1988) *Chlorinated Paraffins: Status Report*, Washington DC

Darnerud, P.O. (1984) Chlorinated paraffins: effects of some microsomal enzyme inducers and inhibitors on the degradation of 1-$^{14}$C-chlorododecanes to $^{14}CO_2$ in mice. *Acta pharmacol. toxicol.*, *55*, 110-115

Darnerud, P.O. & Brandt, I. (1982) Studies on the distribution and metabolism of a $^{14}$C-labelled chlorinated alkane in mice. *Environ. Pollution (Ser. A)*, *27*, 45-56

Darnerud, P.O., Biessmann, A. & Brandt, I. (1982) Metabolic fate of chlorinated paraffins: degree of chlorination of [1-$^{14}$C]chlorododecanes in relation to degradation and excretion in mice. *Arch. Toxicol.*, *50*, 217-226

Elcombe, C.R., Watson, S.C., Soames, A.R. & Foster, J.R. (1990) Hepatic effects of chlorinated paraffins. *Arch. Toxicol.* (in press)

Eller, P.M. (1985) *NIOSH Manual of Analytical Methods*, 3rd ed. (*DHHS (NIOSH) Publ. No. 84-1000*), Washington DC, US Government Printing Office, pp. 5013-1–5013-5

European Chemical Industry Ecology and Toxicology Centre (1989) *Chlorinated Paraffins*, Brussels

Friedman, D. & Lombardo, P. (1975) Photochemical technique for the elimination of chlorinated aromatic interferences in the gas-liquid chromatographic analysis for chlorinated paraffins. *J. Assoc. off. anal. Chem.*, *58*, 703-706

Gjos, N. & Gustavsen, K.O. (1982) Determination of chlorinated paraffins by negative ion chemical ionization mass spectrometry. *Anal. Chem.*, *54*, 1316-1318

Howard, P.H., Santodonato, J. & Saxena, J. (1975) *Investigation of Selected Potential Environmental Contaminants: Chlorinated Paraffins (EPA-560/2-75-007; PB248 634)*, Washington DC, US Environmental Protection Agency

IARC (1976) *IARC Monographs on the Evaluation of Carcinogenic Risk of Chemicals to Man*, Vol. 11, *Cadmium, Nickel, Some Epoxides, Miscellaneous Industrial Chemicals and General Considerations on Volatile Anaesthetics*, Lyon, pp. 39–74

IARC (1980) *IARC Monographs on the Evaluation of the Carcinogenic Risk of Chemicals to Humans*, Vol. 23, *Some Metals and Metallic Compounds*, Lyon, pp. 325–415

Könnecke, H.-G. & Hahn, P. (1962) Chromatographic separation of chloroalkanes obtained by chlorination of hexakontane (Ger.). *J. prakt. Chem.*, 16, 37–41

Lombardo, P., Dennison, J.L. & Johnson, W.W. (1975) Bioaccumulation of chlorinated paraffin residues in fish fed Chlorowax 500C. *J. Assoc. off. anal. Chem.*, 58, 707–710

Madeley, J.R. & Birtley, R.D.N. (1980) Chlorinated paraffins and the environment. 2. Aquatic and avian toxicology. *Environ. Sci. Technol.*, 14, 1215–1221

Maronpot, R.R., Montgomery, C.A., Jr, Boorman, G.A. & McConnell, E.E. (1986) National Toxicology Program nomenclature for hepatoproliferative lesions of rats. *Toxicol. Pathol.*, 14, 263–273

Meijer, J. & DePierre, J.W. (1987) Hepatic levels of cytosolic, microsomal and 'mitochondrial' epoxide hydrolases and other drug-metabolizing enzymes after treatment of mice with various xenobiotics and endogenous compounds. *Chem.-biol. Interactions*, 62, 249–269

Meijer, J., Rundgren, M., Åström, A., DePierre, J.W., Sundvall, A. & Rannug, U. (1981) Effects of chlorinated paraffins on some drug-metabolizing enzymes in rat liver and in the Ames test. *Adv. exp. Med. Biol.*, 136, 821–828

National Institute for Occupational Safety and Health (1977) *National Occupational Hazard Survey (NOHS)*, Cincinnati, OH

National Toxicology Program (1986a) *Toxicology and Carcinogenesis Studies of Chlorinated Paraffins ($C_{12}$, 60% Chlorine) (CAS No. 63449-39-8) in F344/N Rats and B6C3F$_1$ Mice (Gavage Studies) (Tech. Rep. Ser. No. 308)*, Research Triangle Park, NC

National Toxicology Program (1986b) *Toxicology and Carcinogenesis Studies of Chlorinated Paraffins ($C_{23}$, 43% Chlorine) (CAS No. 63449-39-8) in F344/N Rats and B6C3F$_1$ Mice (Gavage Studies) (Tech. Rep. Ser. No. 305)*, Research Triangle Park, NC

Nilsen, O.G. & Toftgård, R. (1981) Effects of polychlorinated terphenyls and paraffins on rat liver microsomal cytochrome P-450 and in vitro metabolic activities. *Arch. Toxicol.*, 47, 1–11

Nilsen, O.G., Toftgård, R. & Glaumann, H. (1980) Changes in rat liver morphology and metabolic activities after exposure to chlorinated paraffins. *Dev. Toxicol. environ. Sci.*, 8, 525–528

Nilsen, O.G., Toftgård, R. & Glaumann, H. (1981) Effects of chlorinated paraffins on rat liver microsomal activities and morphology: importance of the length and the degree of chlorination of the carbon chain. *Arch. Toxicol.*, 49, 1–13

Priha, E., Vuorinen, R., Schimberg, R. & Ahonen, I. (1988) *Tekstiilien Viimeistysaineet* (Textile Finishing Agents) (*Series on Working Conditions No. 65*) (Finn.), Helsinki, Institute of Occupational Health

Schenker, B.A. (1979) Chlorocarbons, -hydrocarbons (paraffins). In: Mark, H.F., Othmer, D.F., Overberger, C.G., Seaborg, G.T. & Grayson, M., eds, *Kirk-Othmer Encyclopedia of Chemical Technology*, 3rd ed., Vol. 5, New York, John Wiley & Sons, pp. 786–791

Schmid, P.P. & Müller, M.D. (1985) Trace level detection of chlorinated paraffins in biological and environmental samples, using gas chromatography/mass spectrometry with negative-ion chemical ionization. *J. Assoc. off. anal. Chem.*, 68, 427–430

Serrone, D.M., Birtley, R.D.N., Weigand, W. & Millischer, R. (1987) Toxicology of chlorinated paraffins. *Food chem. Toxicol.*, 25, 553-562

SRI International (1986) *Chemical Economics Handbook*, Menlo Park, CA

Strack, H. (1986) Chlorinated paraffins. In: *Ullmann's Encyclopedia of Industrial Chemistry*, Vol. A6, 5th ed., Weinheim, VCH Verlagsgesellschaft, pp. 323-330

Svanberg, O., Bengtsson, B.-E. & Lindén, E. (1978) Chlorinated paraffins — a case of accumulation and toxicity to fish. *Ambio*, 7, 64-65

US International Trade Commission (1988) *Synthetic Organic Chemicals, US Production and Sales, 1987 (USITC Publ. 2118)*, Washington DC, US Government Printing Office, pp. 15-7, 15-29

Yang, J.J., Roy, T.A., Neil, W., Krueger, A.J. & Mackerer, C.R. (1987) Percutaneous and oral absorption of chlorinated paraffins in the rat. *Toxicol. ind. Health*, 3, 405-412

Zitko, V. (1974) *Chlorinated Paraffins: Properties, Uses and Pollution Potential (Environ. Canada, Fish. Mar. Serv. tech. Rep. No. 491)*, St Andrews, New Brunswick, Fisheries and Marine Services, pp. 1-38

# DECABROMODIPHENYL OXIDE

## 1. Chemical and Physical Data

### 1.1 Synonyms

*Chem. Abstr. Services Reg. No.*: 1163-19-5
*Chem. Abstr. Name*: Benzene, 1,1'-oxybis[2,3,4,5,6-pentabromo]-
*IUPAC Systematic Name*: Bis(pentabromophenyl) ether
*Synonyms*: DBDPO; decabrom; decabromobiphenyl ether; decabromobiphenyl oxide; decabromodiphenyl ether; decabromophenyl ether; ether, bis(pentabromophenyl); pentabromophenyl ether

### 1.2 Structural and molecular formulae and molecular weight

$C_{12}Br_{10}O$    Mol. wt: 959.17

### 1.3 Chemical and physical properties of the pure substance

(a) *Description*: White powder (AmeriBrom, 1987; White Chemical Co., 1988)
(b) *Boiling-point*: Decomposes at 425°C (US Environmental Protection Agency, 1988)
(c) *Melting-point*: 290-305°C (AmeriBrom, 1987; White Chemical Co., 1988)
(d) *Spectroscopy data*: Infrared (prism [635D]; prism-FT [1057D]) and ultraviolet spectral data have been reported (Pouchert, 1981, 1985; National Toxicology Program, 1986).
(e) *Solubility*: Very slightly soluble (20-30 ppb [µg/l]) in water at 25°C; slightly soluble in acetone, benzene, dichloromethane, *ortho*-xylene, methanol, methyl ethyl ke-

tone, pentane and toluene (AmeriBrom, 1987; US Environmental Protection Agency, 1988; White Chemical Co., 1988; AmeriBrom, undated)

(f) *Volatility*: Vapour pressure, < 1 mm Hg at 250°C (Tabor & Bergman, 1975; AmeriBrom, 1987)

(g) *Stability*: Stable under normal temperatures and pressures (White Chemical Co., 1988); thermal or light-catalysed decomposition of decabromodiphenyl oxide may release carbon monoxide, carbonyl bromide and hydrogen bromide, lower congeners of brominated diphenyl oxide (1-8 bromines/molecule) and polybrominated dibenzodioxins and dibenzofurans (1-6 bromines/molecule) (AmeriBrom, 1987; Watanabe & Tatsukawa, 1987; Aldrich Chemical Co., 1988; US Environmental Protection Agency, 1988; White Chemical Co., 1988)

(h) *Specific gravity*: 3.0 at 20°C (AmeriBrom, 1987)

(i) *Octanol/water partition coefficient (P)*: log P, 5.24 (US Environmental Protection Agency, 1988)

## 1.4 Technical products and impurities

*Trade names*: AFR 1021; Berkflam B 10E; BR 55N; Bromkal 81; Bromkal 82-ODE; Bromkal 83-10DE; Caliban F/R-P 39P; Caliban F/R-P 44; DE 83; DE 83R; DP 10F; EB 10FP; EBR 700; Flame Cut BR 100; FR 300; FR 300BA; FR P-39; FR 1210; FRP 53; FR-PE; FR-PE(H); Planelon DB 100; Saytex 102; Saytex 102E; Tardex 100

Decabromodiphenyl oxide is available at purities usually greater than 97% (Tabor & Bergman, 1975; AmeriBrom, 1987; Aldrich Chemical Co., 1988; Ethyl Corp., 1988a,b; White Chemical Co., 1988). The commercial products typically contain a minimum of 81-83% bromine (83% theoretical; Tabor & Bergman, 1975; AmeriBrom, undated). Differences in manufacturing processes may affect the nature and amounts of impurities in the product (Larsen, 1980). Isomers of nonabromodiphenyl oxide and octabromodiphenyl oxide have been reported as impurities in decabromodiphenyl oxide (Timmons & Brown, 1988). Up to four impurities were reported in four lots of a commercial decabromodiphenyl oxide with purities ranging from 94% to 99%. Two isomers of nonabromodiphenyl oxide were identified as the major impurities (National Toxicology Program, 1986). A technical product of 88.1% purity containing 11% nonabromodiphenyl oxide, 0.5% octabromodiphenyl oxide and 0.1% hexabromobenzene is available (Klusmeier *et al.*, 1988). A company in Japan has produced decabromodiphenyl oxide with about 3% nonabromodiphenyl oxide as an impurity (Watanabe & Tatsukawa, 1987).

# 2. Production, Use, Occurrence and Analysis

## 2.1 Production and use

(a) *Production*

Decabromodiphenyl oxide is produced by bromination of diphenyl oxide in the presence of a Friedel-Crafts catalyst (Larsen, 1980). Decabromodiphenyl oxide has been reported to be manufactured in a batch process involving closed vessels during the reaction and drying cycle (US Environmental Protection Agency, 1988).

Commercial production of decabromodiphenyl oxide in the USA began in 1976. The production quantity ranks second among brominated flame retardants, after tetrabromobisphenol A; the combined world-wide capacity is approximately 18 000 tonnes. Five manufacturers have been reported in Japan (Anon., 1984), three in the USA (US Environmental Protection Agency, 1988), two in Belgium and one each in Israel, Switzerland and the UK.

*(b) Use*

Decabromodiphenyl oxide is an unreactive, additive flame retardant widely used for its thermal stability and its low cost in thermoplastic resins, thermoset resins, textiles and adhesives. The major applications are in high-impact polystyrene, glass-reinforced thermoplastic polyester moulding resins, low-density polyethylene extrusion coatings, polypropylene (homo- and copolymers), acrylonitrile-butadiene-styrene rubber, nylon and polyvinyl chloride (Tabor & Bergman, 1975; AmeriBrom, undated).

Approximately 12 thousand tonnes of decabromodiphenyl oxide are used annually world-wide, about two-thirds in high-impact polystyrene applications such as television and radio cabinets. Textile applications, such as in polyester fibres and in coatings for automobile fabrics, tarpaulins and tents, account for a further 900 tonnes.

A mixture of decabromodiphenyl oxide and antimony trioxide has been used to treat nylon and polyester/cotton fabrics destined for industrial safety apparel and tents (Mischutin, 1977; LeBlanc, 1979). Decabromodiphenyl oxide is also used in insulation for wire and electrical cable (Ethyl Corp., 1988b).

*(c) Regulatory status and guidelines*

The recommended occupational exposure limit for decabromodiphenyl oxide in the USA in 1980 was 5 mg/m$^3$ as an 8-h time-weighted average. The maximum allowable concentration in workplace air in the USSR in 1987 was 3 mg/m$^3$ (Cook, 1987).

## 2.2 Occurrence

*(a) Natural occurrence*

Decabromodiphenyl oxide is not known to occur as a natural product.

*(b) Occupational exposure*

Analysis of wipe samples collected during an industrial hygiene survey in 1977 and 1978 in a decabromodiphenyl oxide manufacturing plant in Sayreville, NJ, USA, indicated that workers in the reactor area were exposed to 3.6 mg/cm$^2$ and those in the distillation area to 5.9 mg/m$^2$. Analysis of personal samples collected on workers in the mill area indicated that the airborne levels of decabromodiphenyl oxide were 0.08-0.21 mg/m$^3$ as an 8-h time-weighted average. Following a spill in the mill area, personal airborne levels were 1.3-1.9 mg/m$^3$ (Bialik, 1982).

*(c) Other*

Decabromodiphenyl oxide was found at 33-375 μg/kg (dry-weight basis) in river sediment from the Neya River and Second Neya River in Osaka, Japan. Marine sediment from Osaka Bay, however, did not contain detectable levels. Decabromodiphenyl oxide was identified at 20 μg/kg (dry-weight basis) in one of three estuary sediment samples from Osaka but was not detected in samples from Tokyo, Matsuyama or Hiroshima (Watanabe *et al.*, 1986, 1987a,b).

Decabromodiphenyl oxide was reported to occur at 1.4 μg/kg (wet-weight basis) in one of three mussels collected from Osaka Bay. It was not found in mullet, goby, sea bass or horse mackerel from this area or in mussel, mullet, goby, sardine, mackerel or hairtail from other locations. It was not found in human adipose tissue obtained from a hospital in Osaka (Watanabe *et al.*, 1987a,b).

Zweidinger *et al.* (1978) reported levels of none detected to 1 g/kg decabromodiphenyl oxide in sediment samples near a flame-retardant manufacturing facility in the USA. Decabromodiphenyl oxide was also found (limit of detection, 10 μg/kg) in sediment from the vicinity of bromine facilities in El Dorado and Magnolia, AR, and in sludge samples from a discharge-treatment zone of a polybrominated biphenyl facility in Bayonne, NJ (DeCarlo, 1979).

Decabromodiphenyl oxide was detected at concentrations up to 5 μg/kg in samples of human hair obtained from barber shops in the same towns in Arkansas. The author estimated that at least 5% of these populations had detectable levels of decabromodiphenyl oxide in their hair (DeCarlo, 1979).

## 2.3 Analysis

Selected methods for the analysis of decabromodiphenyl oxide are presented in Table 1.

# 3. Biological Data Relevant to the Evaluation of Carcinogenic Risk to Humans

## 3.1 Carcinogenicity studies in animals

*Oral administration*

*Mouse*: Groups of 50 male and 50 female B6C3F$_1$ mice, nine weeks of age, were fed 0, 2.5 or 5.0% decabromodiphenyl oxide (purity, 94-97%; two lots) in the diet for 103 weeks, and all survivors were killed at 112-113 weeks of age. Body weights and survival of treated animals were comparable to those of controls. The combined incidence of hepatocellular adenomas and carcinomas in males was 8/50 in controls, 22/50 in low-dose and 18/50 in high-dose animals (trend not significant). The combined incidence of thyroid gland follicular-cell adenomas and carcinomas was: 0/50 in control males, 4/50 in low-dose males and 3/50 in high-dose males, and 1/50 in control females, 3/50 in low-dose females and 3/50 in high-dose females (neither trend significant; National Toxicology Program, 1986).

**Table 1. Methods for the analysis of decabromodiphenyl oxide**

| Sample matrix | Sample preparation | Assay procedure[a] | Limit of detection | Reference |
|---|---|---|---|---|
| Air | Collect on glass fibre filter; extract with acetone | GC/MS<br>GC/ECD<br>TLC/SD | 20-100 ng/m$^{3}$[b]<br>Not given<br>Not given | Zweidinger et al. (1979) |
| | Collect on glass fibre filter/Florisil solvent system; desorb with hexane | GC/ECD | 0.3 µg/sample | Eller (1985) |
| Sewage | Extract with chloroform, evaporate; dissolve residue in ethanol | GC/MS | 0.06 mg/dm$^{3}$ | Kaart & Kokk (1987) |
| Sediment | Extract with diethyl ether; decant; extract with acetone and toluene | GC/MS and TLC/SD | 100 µg/kg | Zweidinger et al. (1978) |
| | Extract with acetone; chromatograph on Florisil | NAA and GC/ECD | < 5 µg/kg | Watanabe et al. (1986, 1987a,b) |
| Human adipose tissue | Grind with excess anhydrous sodium sulfate; extract with hexane; chromatograph on Florisil | NAA and GC/ECD | < 100 µg/kg | Watanabe et al. (1987a) |
| Marine organisms | Homogenize; extract with acetone/hexane mixture; chromatograph on Florisil | GC/ECD and GC/MS | < 0.5 µg/kg | Watanabe et al. (1987b) |
| Fish | Grind tissue; extract; clean on Florisil column | GC/ECD | 10 µg/kg | Miller & Puma (1979) |
| Feed | Extract with tetrahydrofuran; filter; elute isocratically with methanol or water/acetonitrile | HPLC | Not given | National Toxicology Program (1986) |

[a]Abbreviations: GC/MS, gas chromatography/mass spectrometry; GC/ECD, gas chromatography/electron capture detection; TLC/SD, thin-layer chromatography/spectrophotometric determination; NAA, neutron activation analysis; HPLC, high-performance liquid chromatography
[b]Variable, due to daily fluctuations

*Rat*: Groups of 25 male and 25 female Sprague-Dawley rats, six to seven weeks of age, were fed 0, 0.01, 0.1 or 1.0 mg/kg bw per day decabromodiphenyl oxide (purity, 77.4%; nonabromodiphenyl oxide, 21.8%; octabromodiphenyl oxide, 0.8%) in the diet for 100-105 weeks. Ingestion of decabromodiphenyl oxide did not influence survival rates, and mean body weights of treated groups were similar to those of controls. No discernible toxicological effect was produced by decabromodiphenyl oxide, and no significant difference in the number of rats developing tumours (total number of tumours or specific type of tumour) was observed between treated and control groups when evaluated by Fisher's exact probability test (Kociba et al., 1975). [The Working Group noted the very low dose levels used.]

Groups of 50 male and 50 female Fischer 344/N rats, seven to eight weeks of age, were fed 0, 2.5 or 5.0% decabromodiphenyl oxide (purity, 94-97%; two lots) in the diet for 103 weeks, and all survivors were killed at 111-112 weeks of age. Body weights of treated rats were not significantly different from those of controls, but after week 75 survival in the treated groups was lower than that in controls. Significant increases in the incidences of neoplastic nodules of the liver [adenomas (Maronpot *et al.*, 1986)] were seen in animals of each sex: they occurred in 1/50 control males and 7/50 at the low dose and 15/49 at the high dose ($p < 0.001$, incidental tumour test for trend); and in females they occurred in 1/50 controls, 3/49 at the low dose and 9/50 at the high dose ($p = 0.002$, incidental tumour test for trend). No difference in the incidence of hepatocellular carcinomas was seen among the groups. The incidence of acinar-cell adenomas of the pancreas was significantly increased in males: control, 0/49; low-dose, 0/50; high-dose, 4/49 ($p = 0.017$, incidental tumour test for trend). A high incidence of mononuclear-cell leukaemia was observed in treated and control rats of each sex: in males, the overall rates were 30/50 controls and 33/50 low-dose and 35/50 high-dose animals; the adjusted rates were 67.9%, 81.9% and 82.8%, respectively ($p = 0.028$, life-table test for trend; National Toxicology Program, 1986).

## 3.2 Other relevant data

### (a) Experimental systems

#### (i) *Absorption, distribution, excretion and metabolism*

$^{14}$C-Labelled decabromodiphenyl oxide suspended in corn oil was given by gavage to male and female Sprague-Dawley rats at a dose of 1 mg/kg bw. Less than 1% of the label appeared in the urine over 16 days; over 99% of the label appeared in the faeces within two days. Trace amounts of label were detected in the adrenal gland and spleen after sacrifice on day 16 (Norris *et al.*, 1975). When concentrations of 0.025-5% $^{14}$C-labelled decabromodiphenyl oxide were given in the diet to male Fischer 344 rats, more than 99% of the radioactivity was recovered in the faeces and gut contents after 72 h. The liver contained approximately 0.5% of the consumed dose 24 h after feeding; for the high dose, this level declined to 0.016% after 72 h. Labelled material extracted from the liver was found to be mainly unchanged decabromodiphenyl oxide. Trace amounts of label were found in the kidney, spleen, lung, brain, muscle, fat and skin. By 72 h after an intravenous dose of $^{14}$C-labelled decabromodiphenyl oxide, the faeces and gut contents contained 74% of the dose, suggesting significant biliary excretion. Of the extracted faecal label, 63% was metabolites of decabromodiphenyl oxide and 37% was the parent compound. Labelled materials were found in the muscle, skin, liver, fat, kidney and lungs (El Dareer *et al.*, 1987).

Bromine concentrations were determined periodically in selected tissues in two-year dietary studies in male and female Sprague-Dawley rats. A slight increase in the bromine content of liver was observed with 1% in the diet, and increases were seen in adipose tissue with concentrations of 0.1 and 1% (Kociba *et al.*, 1975).

#### (ii) *Toxic effects*

Decabromodiphenyl oxide has low acute toxicity (Norris *et al.*, 1973; Kociba *et al.*, 1975; Norris *et al.*, 1975).

Daily administration of 0.1 mmol (96 mg)/kg bw decabromodiphenyl oxide in corn oil by gavage to male Sprague-Dawley rats for 14 days resulted in significantly increased liver weights but did not significantly induce NADPH cytochrome c reductase or cytochrome P450 activities (Carlson, 1980).

In 30-day studies in which male Sprague-Dawley rats were maintained on diets containing 0.01-1% decabromodiphenyl oxide (approximately 8-800 mg/kg bw per day), microscopic examination of the livers was reported to have revealed centrilobular cytoplasmic enlargement and vacuolization (with the 1% dose). Other treatment-related lesions were reported to include hyaline degenerative cytoplasmic changes in the kidney (with the 1% dose) and thyroid hyperplasia (with the 0.1 and 1% doses; Norris *et al.*, 1975).

Fourteen-day studies in which concentrations of up to 10% decabromodiphenyl oxide were administered in the diet to Fischer 344 rats and B6C3F$_1$ mice resulted in no death, no compound-related clinical sign and no gross pathological effect. Similarly, no toxic effect was seen in 90-day studies in which doses of up to 5% were administered in the diet. Liver weights were not recorded in these studies, but, in supplementary studies, liver weights of Fischer 344 rats were increased by up to about 40% following consumption of diets containing 0, 2.5 or 5% decabromodiphenyl oxide for 11 days (National Toxicology Program, 1986).

Non-neoplastic changes observed in two-year studies in which dietary concentrations of 2.5 and 5.0% decabromodiphenyl oxide were fed to Fischer 344 rats and B6C3F$_1$ mice (see also section 3.1) included slightly increased incidences of thrombosis, degeneration of the liver, fibrosis of the spleen and acanthosis of the forestomach in male rats. In mice, an increased incidence of centrilobular hypertrophy of the liver and a slight increase in the frequency of granulomas of the liver were observed in treated males. Follicular-cell hyperplasia of the thyroid gland was more prevalent in male and female mice treated with either dose. The incidence of gastric ulcers was increased in female mice fed the high dose (National Toxicology Program, 1986).

(iii) *Effects on reproduction and prenatal toxicity*

Sprague-Dawley rats were administered 10-1000 mg/kg bw decabromodiphenyl oxide per day by gavage on gestation days 6-15. Some embryotoxicity but no malformation was reported (Norris *et al.*, 1973, 1975). [The Working Group noted that details were not given.]

(iv) *Genetic and related effects* (see Appendix 1)

Decabromodiphenyl oxide was not mutagenic to several strains of *Salmonella typhimurium*, in the presence or absence of an exogenous metabolic system from Aroclor 1254-induced rat liver and Syrian hamster liver. It was not mutagenic at the TK locus in L5178Y mouse lymphoma cells and did not cause sister chromatid exchange or chromosomal aberrations in the Chinese hamster CHO cell line (National Toxicology Program, 1986).

No increase in the incidence of chromosomal aberrations was reported in parental or neonate bone-marrow cells of rats given 3-100 mg/kg bw decabromodiphenyl oxide per day in the diet for 90 days (Norris *et al.*, 1975). [The Working Group noted that details were not reported.]

*(b) Humans*

No data were available to the Working Group.

## 3.3 Case reports and epidemiological studies of carcinogenicity to humans

No data were available to the Working Group.

# 4. Summary of Data Reported and Evaluation

## 4.1 Exposure data

Decabromodiphenyl oxide has been produced since the late 1970s as a flame retardant for use in plastics, especially high-impact polystyrene, and to treat textiles, such as automotive fabrics and tents. Occupational exposure to decabromodiphenyl oxide may occur during its production and use. It has also been detected in environmental samples collected near some production facilities.

## 4.2 Experimental carcinogenicity data

Decabromodiphenyl oxide was tested for carcinogenicity by oral administration in one strain of mice and in two strains of rats. In one study in rats, it induced hepatocellular adenomas in animals of each sex and acinar-cell adenomas of the pancreas and mononuclear-cell leukaemia in males.

## 4.3 Human carcinogenicity data

No data were available to the Working Group.

## 4.4 Other relevant data

In single studies, decabromodiphenyl oxide did not induce sister chromatid exchange or chromosomal aberrations in Chinese hamster cells in culture or mutations in mouse cells in culture. In one study, decabromodiphenyl oxide was not mutagenic to bacteria in the presence or absence of an exogenous metabolic system.

## Summary table of genetic and related effects of decabromodiphenyl oxide

| Nonmammalian systems | | | | | | | | | | | | | | Mammalian systems | | | | | | | | | | | | | | | | | | | | |
|---|---|---|---|---|---|---|---|---|---|---|---|---|---|---|---|---|---|---|---|---|---|---|---|---|---|---|---|---|---|---|---|---|---|---|
| Proka-ryotes | | Lower eukaryotes | | | | Plants | | | | Insects | | | | In vitro | | | | | | | | | | | | | | | In vivo | | | | | |
| | | | | | | | | | | | | | | Animal cells | | | | | | | | Human cells | | | | | | | Animals | | | | Humans | | |
| D | G | D | R | G | A | A | D | G | C | R | G | C | A | A | D | G | S | M | C | A | T | I | D | G | S | M | C | A | T | I | D | G | S | M | C | DL | A | D | S | M | C | A |
| –¹ | | –¹ | | | | | | | | | | | | | | –¹ –¹ | | | | | –¹ | | | | | | | | | | | | | | | | | | | | | |

A, aneuploidy; C, chromosomal aberrations; D, DNA damage; DL, dominant lethal mutation; G, gene mutation; I, inhibition of intercellular communication; M, micronuclei; R, mitotic recombination and gene conversion; S, sister chromatid exchange; T, cell transformation

*In completing the table, the following symbol indicates the consensus of the Working Group with regard to the results for each endpoint:*
¹ considered to be negative, but only one valid study was available to the Working Group

### 4.5 Evaluation[1]

There is *limited evidence* for the carcinogenicity of decabromodiphenyl oxide in experimental animals.

No data were available from studies in humans on the carcinogenicity of decabromodiphenyl oxide.

**Overall evaluation**

Decabromodiphenyl oxide is *not classifiable as to its carcinogenicity to humans* (Group 3).

# 5. References

Aldrich Chemical Co. (1988) *Material Safety Data Sheet: Pentabromophenyl Ether*, Milwaukee, WI

AmeriBrom (1987) *Material Safety Data Sheet: FR-1210*, New York, NY

AmeriBrom (undated) *Technical Product Data Sheet: Decabromodiphenyl Oxide*, New York, NY

Anon. (1984) *Specialty Chemicals Handbook*, Tokyo, The Chemical Daily Co., pp. 39-40

Bialik, O. (1982) *Endocrine Function of Workers Exposed to PBB and PBBO (Terminal Progress Report)*, Cincinnati, OH, National Institute for Occupational Safety and Health

Carlson, G.P. (1980) Induction of xenobiotic metabolism in rats by short-term administration of brominated diphenyl ethers. *Toxicol. Lett.*, 5, 19-25

Cook, W.A. (1987) *Occupational Exposure Limits—Worldwide*, Washington DC, American Industrial Hygiene Association

DeCarlo, V.J. (1979) Studies on brominated chemicals in the environment. *Ann. N.Y. Acad. Sci.*, 320, 678-681

El Dareer, S.M., Kalin, J.R., Tillery, K.F. & Hill, D.L. (1987) Disposition of decabromodiphenyl ether in rats dosed intravenously or by feeding. *J. Toxicol. environ. Health*, 22, 405-415

Eller, P.M. (1985) *NIOSH Manual of Analytical Methods*, 3rd ed. *(DHHS (NIOSH) Publ. No. 84-1000)*, Washington DC, US Government Printing Office, pp. 5013-1-5013-5

Ethyl Corp. (1988a) *Product Information: Saytex 102*, Baton Rouge, LA, Bromine Chemicals Division

Ethyl Corp. (1988b) *Product Information: Saytex 102E*, Baton Rouge, LA, Bromine Chemicals Division

Kaart, K.S. & Kokk, K.Y. (1987) Spectrophotometric determination of decabromodiphenyl oxide in industrial sewage. *Ind. Labor*, 53, 289-290

Klusmeier, W., Vögler, P., Ohrbach, K.-H., Weber, H. & Kettrup, A. (1988) Thermal decomposition of decabromodiphenyl ether. *J. anal. appl. Pyrol.*, 13, 277-285

Kociba, R.J., Frauson, L.O., Humiston, C.G., Norris, J.M., Wade, C.E., Lisowe, R.W., Quast, J.F., Jersey, G.C. & Jewett, G.L. (1975) Results of a two-year dietary feeding study with decabromodiphenyl oxide (DBDPO) in rats. *J. Combust. Toxicol.*, 2, 267-285

Larsen, E.R. (1980) Flame retardants (halogenated). In: Mark, H.F., Othmer, D.F., Overberger, C.G., Seaborg, G.T. & Grayson, M., eds, *Kirk-Othmer Encyclopedia of Chemical Technology*, 3rd ed., Vol. 10, New York, John Wiley & Sons, pp. 385-386

---

[1]For description of the italicized terms and criteria for making the evaluation, see Preamble, pp. 25-29.

LeBlanc, R.B. (1979) What's available for FR textiles. *Text. Ind., 143,* 78-83

Maronpot, R.R., Montgomery, C.A., Jr, Boorman, G.A. & McConnell, E.E. (1986) National Toxicology Program nomenclature for hepatoproliferative lesions of rats. *Toxicol. Pathol., 14,* 263-273

Miller, L.J. & Puma, B.J. (1979) Analytical characteristics of late-eluting halogenated flame retardants. *J. Assoc. off. anal. Chem., 62,* 1319-1326

Mischutin, V. (1977) Safe flame retardant. *Am. Dyest. Rep., 66,* 51-56

National Toxicology Program (1986) *Toxicology and Carcinogenesis Studies of Decabromodiphenyl Oxide (CAS No. 1163-19-5) in F344/N Rats and B6C3F$_1$ Mice (Feeding Studies)* (Tech. Rep. Ser. No. 309), Research Triangle Park, NC

Norris, J.M., Ehrmantraut, J.W., Gibbons, C.L., Kociba, R.J., Schwetz, B.A., Rose, J.Q., Humiston, C.G., Jewett, G.L., Crummett, W.B., Gehring, P.J., Tirsell, J.B. & Brosier, J.S. (1973) Toxicological and environmental factors involved in the selection of decabromodiphenyl oxide as a fire retardant chemical. *Appl. Polym. Symp., 22,* 195-219

Norris, J.M., Kociba, R.J., Schwetz, B.A., Rose, J.Q., Humiston, C.G., Jewett, G.L., Gehring, P.J. & Mailhes, J.B. (1975) Toxicology of octabromobiphenyl and decabromodiphenyl oxide. *Environ. Health Perspect., 11,* 152-161

Pouchert, C.J., ed. (1981) *The Aldrich Library of Infrared Spectra,* 3rd ed., Milwaukee, WI, Aldrich Chemical Co., p. 635

Pouchert, C.J., ed. (1985) *The Aldrich Library of FT-IR Spectra,* Milwaukee, WI, Aldrich Chemical Co., p. 1057

Tabor, T.E. & Bergman, S. (1975) Decabromodiphenyl oxide—a new fire retardant additive for plastics. In: Bhatnagan, V.M., ed., *Fire Retardants: Proceedings of 1974 International Symposium on Flammability and Fire Retardants, May 1-2, 1974, Cornwall, Ontario, Canada,* Westport, CT, Technomic Publishing, pp. 162-179

Timmons, L.L. & Brown, R.D. (1988) Analysis of the brominated fire retardant decabromodiphenyl oxide for low and trace levels impurities. *Chemosphere, 17,* 217-233

US Environmental Protection Agency (1988) *Information Review: Brominated Diphenyl Ethers (Report No. IR-516),* Washington DC, TSCA Interagency Testing Committee

Watanabe, I. & Tatsukawa, R. (1987) Formation of brominated dibenzofurans from the photolysis of flame retardant decabromobiphenyl ether in hexane solution by UV and sun light. *Bull. environ. Contam. Toxicol., 39,* 953-959

Watanabe, I., Kashimoto, T. & Tatsukawa, R. (1986) Confirmation of the presence of the flame retardant decabromobiphenyl ether in river sediment from Osaka, Japan. *Bull. environ. Contam. Toxicol., 36,* 839-842

Watanabe, I., Kashimoto, T., Kawano, M. & Tatsukawa, R. (1987a) A study of organic bound halogens in human adipose, marine organisms and sediment by neutron activation and gas chromatographic analysis. *Chemosphere, 16,* 849-857

Watanabe, I., Kashimoto, T. & Tatsukawa, R. (1987b) Polybrominated biphenyl ethers in marine fish, shellfish and river and marine sediments in Japan. *Chemosphere, 16,* 2389-2396

White Chemical Co. (1988) *Material Safety Data Sheet: Decabromodiphenyl Oxide,* Newark, NJ

Zweidinger, R.A., Cooper, S.D. & Pellizzari, E.D. (1978) Identification and quantitation of brominated fire retardants. In: Van Hall, C.E., ed., *Measurement of Organic Pollutants in Water and Wastewater, Symposium of the American Society for Testing and Materials, 19-20 June 1978, Denver, CO (ASTM Technical Publication No. 686),* Philadelphia, PA, American Society for Testing and Materials, pp. 234-250

Zweidinger, R.A., Cooper, S.D., Erickson, M.D., Michael, L.C. & Pellizzari, E.D. (1979) Sampling and analysis for semivolatile brominated organics in ambient air. In: Schuetzle, D., ed., *Monitoring Toxic Substances (ACS Symposium Series 94)*, Washington DC, American Chemical Society, pp. 217-231

# DIMETHYL HYDROGEN PHOSPHITE

## 1. Chemical and Physical Data

### 1.1 Synonyms

*Chem. Abstr. Services Reg. No.*: 868-85-9
*Chem. Abstr. Name*: Dimethyl phosphonate
*IUPAC Systematic Name*: Dimethyl phosphonate
*Synonyms*: Bis(hydroxymethyl)phosphine oxide; dimethoxyphosphine oxide; dimethyl phosphite; dimethyl acid phosphite; O,O-dimethyl phosphonate; dimethyl phosphorous acid; DMHP; hydrogen dimethyl phosphite; methyl phosphonate; phosphorous acid dimethyl ester

### 1.2 Structural and molecular formulae and molecular weight

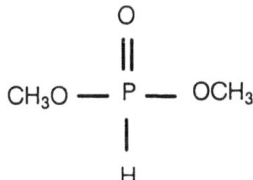

C₂H₇O₃P                      Mol. wt: 110.05

### 1.3 Chemical and physical properties of the pure substance

(a) *Description*: Colourless liquid with mild odour (Hawley, 1981)
(b) *Boiling-point*: 170-171°C (Weast & Astle, 1985)
(c) *Density*: 1.2004 at 20°C (Weast & Astle, 1985)
(d) *Spectroscopic data*: Infrared (prism, Sadtler [3003, 61328], Aldrich [549D]; prism-FT [912D]; grating [42253P], nuclear magnetic resonance (proton, Sadtler [6652], Aldrich [864C]; C-13 [529]) and ultraviolet spectral data have been reported (Sadtler Research Laboratories, 1980; Pouchert, 1981, 1983; National Toxicology Program, 1985; Pouchert, 1985).
(e) *Solubility*: Soluble in water; miscible with most common organic solvents (Hawley, 1981)

(f) *Volatility*: Vapour pressure, < 1.0 mm Hg at 20°C (Albright & Wilson Americas, 1987)

(g) *Flash-point*: 96°C (Hawley, 1981)

(h) *Reactivity*: Hydrolyses in water with a half-life of approximately ten days at 25°C and 19 days at 20°C; basic conditions accelerate hydrolysis (TOXNET, 1988)

(i) *Conversion factor*: mg/m³ = 4.5 × ppm[1]

## 1.4 Technical products and impurities

*Trade name*: TL 585

Commercial dimethyl hydrogen phosphite is marketed as a high-purity liquid (99%) for industrial use. Trace levels of dimethyl methyl phosphonate, trimethyl phosphate and methanol have been reported in the technical product (Albright & Wilson Americas, 1987).

# 2. Production, Use, Occurrence and Analysis

## 2.1 Production and use

### (a) Production

Dimethyl hydrogen phosphite is manufactured by the reaction of phosphorous trichloride with methanol or with sodium methoxide (US Environmental Protection Agency, 1985).

Between 95 and 950 thousand tonnes of dimethyl hydrogen phosphite were produced or imported in the USA in 1977, when two companies reported production and one reported importation of the compound (US Environmental Protection Agency, 1985). More recently, two manufacturers have been identified in the UK and one each in Canada, France, the Federal Republic of Germany, Switzerland (SRI International, 1986) and the USA (US International Trade Commission, 1988).

### (b) Use

Dimethyl hydrogen phosphite is used as a flame retardant on Nylon 6 fibres (see IARC, 1979) and, in combination with guanidine and formaldehyde (see IARC, 1982), to impart flame and crease resistance to cotton textiles. The compound is also used to increase fire resistance to cellulosic textiles, acrolein-grafted polyamide fibres and γ-irradiated polyethylene. It is used as a lubricant additive, as a chemical intermediate in the production of organophosphorous pesticides and as an adhesive. Dimethyl hydrogen phosphite has also been used as a stabilizer in oil and plaster and, in combination with pyrocatechol, as a corrosion

---

[1] Calculated from mg/m³ = (molecular weight/24.45) x ppm, assuming standard temperature (25°C) and pressure (760 mm Hg)

inhibitor on steel (Hawley, 1981; National Toxicology Program, 1985; US Environmental Protection Agency, 1985).

(c) *Regulatory status and guidelines*

No regulatory standard or guideline has been established for dimethyl hydrogen phosphite.

## 2.2 Occurrence

(a) *Natural occurrence*

Dimethyl hydrogen phosphite is not known to occur as a natural product.

(b) *Occupational exposure*

No data were available to the Working Group.

(c) *Other*

Dimethyl hydrogen phosphite is a degradation product of the pesticides trichlorphon and malathion and may be released into the environment following their application. It is a contaminant (approximately 2%) in the chemical intermediate trimethyl phosphite, which hydrolyses readily to dimethyl hydrogen phosphite in the presence of moist air or water (US Environmental Protection Agency, 1985).

## 2.3 Analysis

No data were available to the Working Group on methods for the analysis of dimethyl hydrogen phosphite in the workplace or the environment. Capillary gas chromatography and high-performance liquid chromatography have been used to analyse this compound under conditions simulating a physiological environment (Nomeir *et al.*, 1988).

# 3. Biological Data Relevant to the Evaluation of Carcinogenic Risk to Humans

## 3.1 Carcinogenicity studies in animals

*Oral administration*

*Mouse*: Groups of 50 male and 50 female $B6C3F_1$ mice, six to eight weeks of age, were administered 0, 100 or 200 mg/kg bw dimethyl hydrogen phosphite (purity, >97-98%) dissolved in corn oil by gavage on five days a weeks for 103 weeks. All survivors were killed at 110-112 weeks of age. Survival of high-dose males was significantly shorter and mean body weights of high-dose males lower than those of vehicle controls. Hepatocellular adenomas were observed in 0/50 female controls and in 6/49 at the low dose and 3/50 at the high dose (trend not significant). No other tumour was observed that could be attributed to treatment (National Toxicology Program, 1985; Dunnick *et al.*, 1986).

*Rat*: Groups of 50 male and 50 female Fischer 344/N rats, seven weeks of age, were administered 0, 100 or 200 (males) and 0, 50 or 100 (females) mg/kg bw dimethyl hydrogen phosphite (purity, >97-98%) dissolved in corn oil by gavage on five days a week for 103 weeks. All survivors were killed at 111 weeks of age. Survival of high-dose males was significantly shorter and mean body weights of high-dose males lower than those of vehicle controls. The incidences of squamous-cell carcinomas of the lung in males were 0/50 controls, 0/50 low-dose and 5/50 high-dose animals ($p = 0.034$, incidental tumour test for trend). The incidences of alveolar/bronchiolar carcinomas were significantly increased in males: controls, 0/50; low-dose animals, 1/50; high-dose animals, 20/50 ($p < 0.001$, incidental tumour test for trend). Alveolar/bronchiolar carcinomas were also observed in 0/50 female controls, and 1/49 at the low dose and 3/50 at the high dose ($p = 0.047$, incidental tumour test for trend. The combined incidences of squamous-cell papillomas and carcinomas of the forestomach were significantly increased in males: controls, 0/50; low-dose, 1/50; high-dose, 6/50 ($p = 0.006$, incidental tumour test for trend; National Toxicology Program, 1985; Dunnick *et al.*, 1986).

## 3.2 Other relevant data

(a) *Experimental systems*

(i) *Absorption, distribution, excretion and metabolism*

No data were available to the Working Group.

(ii) *Toxic effects*

The acute oral $LD_{50}$s for dimethyl hydrogen phosphite were 3283 and 3040 mg/kg bw for male and female Fischer 344/N rats, respectively, and 2815 mg/kg bw for male $B6C3F_1$ mice. In 15-day gavage studies, deaths of male and female rats occurred at 500 mg/kg bw and above, and deaths of male and female mice occurred at 2000 mg/kg bw and above. Gastritis, epithelial ulceration and squamous atrophy of the stomach appeared to be related to treatment in mice (National Toxicology Program, 1985).

In 90-day studies in which Fischer 344/N rats were administered 25-400 mg/kg bw dimethyl hydrogen phosphite by gavage (five days per week), deaths occurred at 400 and 200 mg/kg bw. Urinary bladder calculi were seen in two of ten high-dose males. In $B6C3F_1$ mice administered 95-1500 mg/kg bw dimethyl hydrogen phosphite by gavage, deaths occurred at concentrations of 375 mg/kg bw and above. Mice showed increased hepatocellular vacuolization, cardiac mineralization, testicular atrophy and lung congestion, which may have been related to treatment (National Toxicology Program, 1985).

Non-neoplastic lesions observed in two-year studies in rats (see also section 3.1) included alveolar epithelial hyperplasia, adenomatous hyperplasia of the lung and chronic interstitial chemical pneumonia in animals of each sex, as well as hyperkeratosis of the forestomach in high-dose males and hyperplasia of the forestomach in treated males and high-dose females. In mice, focal calcification of the testis was associated with administration of dimethyl hydrogen phosphite (National Toxicology Program, 1985).

A dose of 200 mg/kg bw dimethyl hydrogen phosphite was administered in corn oil to male Fischer 344/N rats by gavage for up to six weeks to evaluate early microscopic and biochemical changes related to the lung and forestomach lesions noted in the two-year study (section 3.1). No lung change was seen, but epithelial hyperplasia, hyperkeratosis, subepithelial inflammation and submucosal oedema were observed microscopically in the forestomach. Levels of serum angiotensin converting enzyme (an indicator of lung injury) were elevated in treated rats from week 4 onwards but returned to control levels when treatment was stopped. Levels of soluble nonprotein sulfhydryls in the forestomach were elevated; a similar effect was produced by a single oral or intravenous administration of 1000 mg/kg bw. Microsomal cytochrome P450 activity in liver and kidney was unchanged, as were the activities of *para*-nitroanisole demethylase, soluble superoxide dismutase and glutathione *S*-transferase in liver, kidney, lung, forestomach and glandular stomach (Nomeir & Uraih, 1988).

(iii) *Effects on reproduction and prenatal toxicity*

No data were available to the Working Group.

(iv) *Genetic and related effects* (see Appendix 1)

Dimethyl hydrogen phosphite was not mutagenic to several strains of *Salmonella typhimurium* in the presence or absence of an exogenous metabolic system from Aroclor 1254-induced rat liver or Syrian hamster liver. It did not induce sex-linked recessive mutation in *Drosophila melanogaster* after feeding or injection (National Toxicology Program, 1985). It was reported not to induce unscheduled DNA synthesis in a primary culture of rat hepatocytes [details not given] (Tennant *et al.*, 1987a). It induced mutation at the TK locus in L5178Y mouse lymphoma cells in culture; an exogenous metabolic system from Aroclor 1254-induced rat liver was not required for activity but increased the response (McGregor *et al.*, 1988). It caused sister chromatid exchange and chromosomal aberrations in the Chinese hamster CHO cell line, both in the presence and absence of an exogenous metabolic system from Aroclor 1254-induced rat liver (Tennant *et al.*, 1987b).

(b) *Humans*

No data were available to the Working Group.

## 3.3 Case reports and epidemiological studies of carcinogenicity to humans

No data were available to the Working Group.

## 4. Summary of Data Reported and Evaluation

### 4.1 Exposure data

Dimethyl hydrogen phosphite is used as a flame retardant on Nylon 6 fibres, as a chemical intermediate in the production of pesticides and in lubricant additives and adhesives. No data on occupational exposure levels were available. A potential source of exposure to this chemical is from its occurrence as a degradation product of the chemical intermediate trimethyl phosphite and of pesticides such as trichlorphon and malathion.

### 4.2 Experimental carcinogenicity data

Dimethyl hydrogen phosphite was tested for carcinogenicity by oral administration in one strain of mice and in one strain of rats. In rats, it caused an increase in the incidence of alveolar/bronchiolar carcinomas in animals of each sex and of squamous-cell carcinomas of the lung and of papillomas and carcinomas of the forestomach in males.

### 4.3 Human carcinogenicity data

No data were available to the Working Group.

### 4.4 Other relevant data

In single studies, dimethyl hydrogen phosphite induced sister chromatid exchange and chromosomal aberrations in Chinese hamster cells in culture and mutations in mouse cells in culture but did not induce sex-linked recessive lethal mutation in *Drosophila*. It was not mutagenic to bacteria in the presence or absence of an exogenous metabolic system.

### 4.5 Evaluation[1]

There is *limited evidence* for the carcinogenicity of dimethyl hydrogen phosphite in experimental animals.

No data were available from studies in humans on the carcinogenicity of dimethyl hydrogen phosphite.

#### Overall evaluation

Dimethyl hydrogen phosphite is *not classifiable as to its carcinogenicity to humans (Group 3)*.

---

[1]For description of the italicized terms and criteria for making the evaluation, see Preamble, pp. 25-29.

## Summary table of genetic and related effects of dimethyl hydrogen phosphite

| Nonmammalian systems | | | | | | | | | | | | | | | Mammalian systems | | | | | | | | | | | | | | | | | | | | | |
|---|---|---|---|---|---|---|---|---|---|---|---|---|---|---|---|---|---|---|---|---|---|---|---|---|---|---|---|---|---|---|---|---|---|---|---|
| Proka-ryotes | | Lower eukaryotes | | | | Plants | | | | Insects | | | | | In vitro | | | | | | | | | | | | | | | In vivo | | | | | |
| | | | | | | | | | | | | | | | Animal cells | | | | | | | | | Human cells | | | | | | Animals | | | | | Humans | |
| D | G | D | R | G | A | D | G | C | A | C | R | G | C | A | D | G | S | M | C | A | T | I | D | G | S | M | C | A | T | I | D | G | S | M | C | DL | A | D | S | M | C | A |
|   | $-^1$ |   |   |   |   |   |   |   |   |   | $-^1$ |   |   |   |   | $+^1$ | $+^1$ |   |   |   | $+^1$ |   |   |   |   |   |   |   |   |   |   |   |   |   |   |   |   |   |   |   |   |   |

A, aneuploidy; C, chromosomal aberrations; D, DNA damage; DL, dominant lethal mutation; G, gene mutation; I, inhibition of intercellular communication; M, micronuclei; R, mitotic recombination and gene conversion; S, sister chromatid exchange; T, cell transformation

*In completing the tables, the following symbols indicate the consensus of the Working Group with regard to the results for each endpoint:*

$-^1$  considered to be negative, but only one valid study was available to the Working Group
$+^1$  considered to be positive, but only one valid study was available to the Working Group.

## 5. References

Albright & Wilson Americas (1987) *Material Safety Data Sheet: Albrite (Dimethyl Hydrogen Phosphite)*, Richmond, VA

Dunnick, J.K., Boorman, G.A., Haseman, J.K., Langloss, J., Cardy, R.H. & Manus, A.G. (1986) Lung neoplasms in rodents after chronic administration of dimethyl hydrogen phosphite. *Cancer Res.*, 46, 264-270

Hawley, G.G. (1981) *Hawley's Condensed Chemical Dictionary*, 10th ed., New York, Van Nostrand Reinhold, p. 371

IARC (1979) *IARC Monographs on the Evaluation of the Carcinogenic Risk of Chemicals to Humans*, Vol. 19, *Some Monomers, Plastics and Synthetic Elastomers, and Acrolein*, Lyon, pp. 120-130

IARC (1982) *IARC Monographs on the Evaluation of the Carcinogenic Risk of Chemicals to Humans*, Vol. 29, *Some Industrial Chemicals and Dyestuffs*, Lyon, pp. 345-389

McGregor, D.B., Brown, A., Cattanach, P., Edwards, I., McBride, D. & Caspary, W.J. (1988) Responses of the L5178Y tk+/tk− mouse lymphoma cell forward mutation assay. II: 18 coded chemicals. *Environ. mol. Mutagenesis*, 11, 91-118

National Toxicology Program (1985) *Toxicology and Carcinogenesis Studies of Dimethyl Hydrogen Phosphite (CAS No. 868-85-9) in F344/N Rats and B6C3F$_1$ Mice (Gavage Studies)* (Technical Report No. 287; HIN Publ. No. 86-2543), Research Triangle Park, NC, US Department of Health and Human Services

Nomeir, A.A. & Uraih, L.C. (1988) Pathological and biochemical effects of dimethyl hydrogen phosphite in Fischer 344 rats. *Fundam. appl. Toxicol.*, 10, 114-124

Nomeir, A.A., Burka, L.T. & Matthews, H.B. (1988) Analysis of dimethyl hydrogen phosphite and its stability under simulated physiological conditions. *J. anal. Toxicol.*, 12, 334-338

Pouchert, C.J., ed. (1981) *The Aldrich Library of Infrared Spectra*, 3rd ed., Milwaukee, WI, Aldrich Chemical Co., p. 549

Pouchert, C.J., ed. (1983) *The Aldrich Library of NMR Spectra*, 2nd ed., Milwaukee, WI, Aldrich Chemical Co., p. 864

Pouchert, C.J., ed. (1985) *The Aldrich Library of FT-IR Spectra*, Milwaukee, WI, Aldrich Chemical Co., p. 912

Sadtler Research Laboratories (1980) *Standard Spectra Collection, 1980 Cumulative Index*, Philadelphia, PA

SRI International (1986) *Chemical Economics Handbook*, Menlo Park, CA

Tennant, R.W., Spalding, J.W., Stasiewicz, S., Caspary, W.D., Mason, J.M. & Resnick, M.A. (1987a) Comparative evaluation of genetic toxicity patterns of carcinogens and noncarcinogens: strategies for predictive use of short-term assays. *Environ. Health Perspect.*, 75, 87-95

Tennant, R.W., Margolin, B.H., Shelby, M.D., Zeiger, E., Haseman, J.K., Spalding, J., Caspary, W., Resnick, M., Stasiewicz, S., Anderson, B. & Minor, R. (1987b) Prediction of chemical carcinogenicity in rodents from in vitro genetic toxicity assays. *Science*, 236, 933-941

TOXNET (1988) *Hazardous Substances Data Bank (HSDB)*, Bethesda, MD, National Library of Medicine

US Environmental Protection Agency (1985) *Chemical Hazard Information Profile: Dimethyl Hydrogen Phosphite*, Washington DC, TSCA Interagency Testing Committee

US International Trade Commission (1988) *Synthetic Organic Chemicals US Production and Sales, 1987 (USITC Publ. 2118)*, Washington DC, US Government Printing Office, p. 15-26

Weast, R.C. & Astle, M.J., eds (1985) *CRC Handbook of Data on Organic Compounds*, Vol. 2, Boca Raton, FL, CRC Press, p. 110

# TETRAKIS(HYDROXYMETHYL) PHOSPHONIUM SALTS

## 1. Chemical and Physical Data

### 1.1 Synonyms

**Tetrakis(hydroxymethyl) phosphonium sulfate**
*Chem. Abstr. Services Reg. No.*: 55566-30-8
*Chem. Abstr. Name*: Phosphonium, tetrakis(hydroxymethyl)-, sulfate (2:1) (salt)
*IUPAC Systematic Name*: Bis[tetrakis(hydroxymethyl) phosphonium] sulfate (salt)
*Synonyms*: Octakis(hydroxymethyl) phosphonium sulfate; THPS

**Tetrakis(hydroxymethyl) phosphonium chloride**
*Chem. Abstr. Services Reg. No.*: 124-64-1
*Chem. Abstr. Name*: Phosphonium, tetrakis(hydroxymethyl)-, chloride
*IUPAC Systematic Name*: Tetrakis(hydroxymethyl) phosphonium chloride
*Synonyms*: Tetrahydroxymethylphosphonium chloride; THPC

**Tetrakis(hydroxymethyl) phosphonium acetate/phosphate**
*Chem. Abstr. Services Reg. No.*: 55818-96-7
*Chem. Abstr. Name*: Phosphonium, tetrakis(hydroxymethyl)-, acetate (salt), mixture with tetrakis(hydroxymethyl) phosphonium phosphate (3:1) (salt)
*IUPAC Systematic Name*: Tetrakis(hydroxymethyl) phosphonium acetate (salt), mixture with tris[tetrakis(hydroxymethyl) phosphonium] phosphate (salt)

See Table 1 for CAS numbers and names of other tetrakis(hydroxymethyl) phosphonium salts.

Table 1. Chemical Abstracts Services Registry numbers of tetrakis(hydroxymethyl) phosphonium salts

| Salt | CAS No. |
|---|---|
| Acetate | 7580-37-2 |
| Acetate-phosphate (1:1) | 62588-94-7 |
| Bromide | 5940-69-2 |
| 6-Carboxycellulose salt | 73082-49-2 |
| Cellulose carboxymethyl ether salt | 73083-23-5 |
| Formate | 25151-36-4 |
| Hydroxybutanedioate | 39734-92-4 |
| 2-Hydroxypropionate | 39686-78-7 |
| Iodide | 69248-12-0 |
| 1-Naphthalenesulfonate | 79481-21-3 |
| 2-Naphthalenesulfonate | 79481-22-4 |
| Oxalate (1:1) | 53211-22-6 |
| Oxalate (2:1) | 52221-67-7 |
| Phosphate | 22031-17-0 |
| Tetraphenylborate-tetraacetate | 15652-65-0 |
| *para*-Toluenesulfonate | 75019-90-8 |

## 1.2 Structural and molecular formulae and molecular weights

**Tetrakis(hydroxymethyl) phosphonium sulfate**

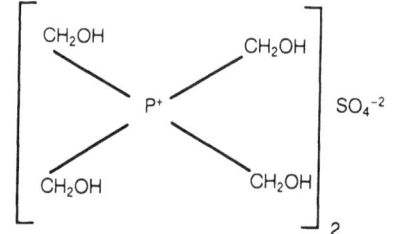

$C_8H_{24}O_{12}P_2S$              Mol. wt: 406.28

**Tetrakis(hydroxymethyl) phosphonium chloride**

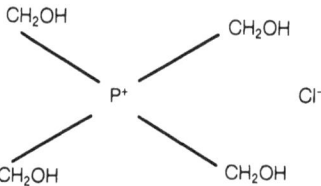

$C_4H_{12}ClO_4P$              Mol. wt: 190.56

### Tetrakis(hydroxymethyl) phosphonium acetate/phosphate

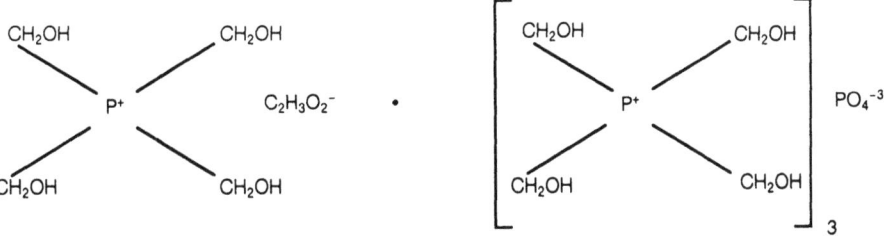

C$_4$H$_{12}$O$_4$P · C$_2$H$_3$O$_2$/(C$_4$H$_{12}$O$_4$P)$_3$ · PO$_4$  Mol. wt: 214.16/560.30

### 1.3 Chemical and physical properties of the pure substance

**Tetrakis(hydroxymethyl) phosphonium sulfate**
(a) *Description*: Crystalline solid (Weil, 1980)
(b) *Solubility*: Soluble in water (Weil, 1980)

**Tetrakis(hydroxymethyl) phosphonium chloride**
(a) *Description*: Crystalline solid (Weil, 1980)
(b) *Melting-point*: 154°C (Grasseli & Ritchey, 1975)
(c) *Spectroscopy data*: Infrared (prism [13510]; grating [47569P]), ultraviolet and nuclear magnetic resonance (proton [11664]) spectral data have been reported (Sadtler Research Laboratories, 1980; National Toxicology Program, 1987).
(d) *Solubility*: Soluble in water (Weil, 1980)

**Tetrakis(hydroxymethyl) phosphonium acetate/phosphate**
No data were available to the Working Group.

### 1.4 Technical products and impurities

**Tetrakis(hydroxymethyl) phosphonium sulfate**
*Trade names*: Pyroset TKO; Retardol S

**Tetrakis(hydroxymethyl) phosphonium chloride**
*Trade names*: Proban CC; Pyroset TKC; Retardol C

**Tetrakis(hydroxymethyl) phosphonium acetate/phosphate**
*Trade names*: Pyroset Flame Retardant TKP; Pyroset TKP

Tetrakis(hydroxymethyl) phosphonium chloride (THPC) and tetrakis(hydroxymethyl) phosphonium sulfate (THPS) are marketed in concentrated aqueous solutions at approximately 80 and 75 wt%, respectively (Albright & Wilson Americas, Inc., 1988a,b). Commercial THPC has been reported to contain free formaldehyde (see IARC, 1982; 3.8% at the pH at which THPS is available, pH 0.4; Ulsamer *et al.*, 1980). Tetrakis(hydroxymethyl) phosphonium acetate/phosphate (THPA/P) was available in the USA as a clear, nearly colourless solution with a pH of approximately 5, containing 10% active phosphorus (Hooper et al., 1976a).

## 2. Production, Use, Occurrence and Analysis

### 2.1 Production and use

(a) *Production*

Tetrakis(hydroxymethyl) phosphonium salts have been produced for commercial use since the 1950s. The first, THPC, was introduced in 1953. The salts are produced by the reaction of formaldehyde with phosphine in the appropriate aqueous acid (Weil, 1980; Hawley, 1981).

Two US companies supply THPS and THPC. Combined annual use of each compound in the USA is 900-4500 tonnes (National Toxicology Program, 1987).

(b) *Use*

Tetrakis(hydroxymethyl) phosphonium salts are used to produce crease-resistant flame-retardant finishes on cotton textiles and cellulosic fabrics (Hooper, 1973; Hooper et al., 1976a,b). THPC, THPS and THPA/P can be cured on the fabric with amine compounds (e.g., ammonia, urea, melamine-formaldehyde resins) to form durable, cross-linked flame-retardant resin finishes (Weil, 1980). Recently, THPS has largely replaced THPC in commercial use (Duffy, 1983); THPA/P has never been a major commercial product. Many co-reactants have been used to form flame-retardant finishes with these compounds. One of the most popular processes has been the tetrakis(hydroxymethyl) phosphonium hydroxide-ammonia finish, in which THPS is converted to a free organic base and then cured on the fabric by reaction with ammonia gas (Weil, 1980).

In 1974, over 14 million metres of cotton flannel for children's nightwear were estimated to have been treated with tetrakis(hydroxymethyl) phosphonium salts in the USA (Hooper et al., 1976a).

(c) *Regulatory status and guidelines*

No regulatory standard or guideline has been established for tetrakis(hydroxymethyl) phosphonium salts.

### 2.2 Occurrence

(a) *Natural occurrence*

These compounds are not known to occur as natural products.

(b) *Occupational exposure*

Approximately 100 workers were potentially exposed to THPC in the USA in 1972-74 (National Institute for Occupational Safety and Health, 1977).

No data on levels of exposure were available to the Working Group.

## 2.3 Analysis

A number of analytical methods have been used to identify and characterize THPC-based flame-retardant polymers on fabric. These include potassium iodate-thiosulfate titration (Frank, 1977), thermogravimetric and differential thermal analysis, differential scanning calorimetry, scanning and transmission electron microscopy, electron spin resonance and energy dispersive X-ray analysis (Frank *et al.*, 1982).

No data were available to the Working Group on methods for the analysis of tetrakis(hydroxymethyl) phosphonium salts in the workplace or in the environment.

# 3. Biological Data Relevant to the Evaluation of Carcinogenic Risk to Humans

## 3.1 Carcinogenicity studies in animals

### Tetrakis(hydroxymethyl) phosphonium sulfate

*Oral administration*

*Mouse*: Groups of 50 male and 50 female $B6C3F_1$ mice, seven weeks of age, received 0, 5 or 10 mg/kg bw THPS dissolved in distilled water (72:28 vol%) by gavage on five days a week for 104 weeks; all survivors were killed at 112 weeks of age. No difference in survival or mean body weight was observed between control and treated mice. The incidence of malignant lymphomas in males showed a negative trend: control, 2/50; low-dose, 9/50; high-dose, 0/50 (National Toxicology Program, 1987).

*Rat*: Groups of 49 or 50 male and female Fischer 344/N rats, six weeks of age, received 0, 5 or 10 mg/kg bw THPS in distilled water (72:28 vol%) by gavage on five days a week for 104 weeks. All survivors were killed at 112 weeks of age. Survival of treated males was reduced as compared to controls; mean body weights of treated animals were comparable to those of controls. The incidence of mononuclear-cell leukaemia in males showed a negative trend: control, 30/50; low-dose, 36/50; high-dose, 20/50 (National Toxicology Program, 1987).

### Tetrakis(hydroxymethyl) phosphonium chloride

*(a) Oral administration*

*Mouse*: Groups of 50 male and 50 female $B6C3F_1$ mice, eight weeks of age, received 0, 7.5 or 15 (males) and 0, 15 or 30 (females) mg/kg bw THPC dissolved in deionized water (75:25 vol%) by gavage on five days a week for 103 weeks; all survivors were killed at 112-113 weeks of age. No difference in survival or in mean body weight was observed between control and treated mice. There was no significant increase in the incidence of any tumour in any organ in treated mice of either sex (National Toxicology Program, 1987).

*Rat*: Groups of 50 male and 50 female Fischer 344/N rats, seven weeks of age, received 0, 3.5 or 7.5 mg/kg bw THPC in deionized water (75:25 vol%) by gavage on five days a week for 103 weeks; all survivors were killed at 111 weeks of age. Survival of high-dose females after week 70 was lower than that of controls; mean body weights of treated animals were comparable to those of controls. The incidence of mononuclear-cell leukaemia in males showed a negative trend: control, 19/50; low-dose, 25/50; high-dose, 16/50 (National Toxicology Program, 1987).

(b)  *Skin application*

*Mouse*: Groups of 20 female ICR/Ha Swiss mice, six to eight weeks of age, received skin applications of 2 mg/mouse THPC in dimethyl sulfoxide (DMSO) to examine the initiating (I), promoting (II) and complete carcinogenic (III) potential in skin carcinogenesis. Two groups of 20 mice (I) received a single application of THPC in DMSO followed by applications of 2.5 μg/animal phorbol myristyl acetate (TPA) in acetone or acetone alone three times a week for 57 weeks. No skin tumour occurred in either group. Three groups of 20 mice (II) received a single application of 20 μg 7,12-dimethylbenz[a]anthracene in acetone followed by applications of either 2 mg/animal THPC in DMSO, 2.5 μg/animal TPA in acetone (positive control) or DMSO alone three times a week for 57 weeks. The numbers of mice with squamous-cell papillomas and carcinomas of the skin were 3/20 (three with a carcinoma [$p > 0.05$]), 19/20 (nine with a carcinoma) and 0/20, respectively. A further group of mice (III) received applications of 2 mg/animal THPC in DMSO alone three times a week for 57 weeks; one squamous-cell carcinoma of the skin developed, whereas no skin tumour was observed in an untreated group (Loewengart & Van Duuren, 1977).

A group of 60 female ICR/Ha Swiss mice, six to eight weeks of age, received skin applications of 2 mg/mouse THPC in acetone three times a week for 71 weeks. Control groups of 249 and 29 mice (effective numbers necropsied) received no treatment and treatment with 0.1 ml acetone, respectively. The numbers of mice with papillary tumours of the lung were 90/249 (36%), 7/29 (24%) and 17/59 (29%) in the two control and the THPC-treated groups, respectively; the numbers with papillomas of the forestomach were 6/249 (2%) and 1/59 (2%) in the untreated control and the treated groups, respectively (Van Duuren *et al.*, 1978).

### Tetrakis(hydroxymethyl) phosphonium acetate/phosphate

*Skin application*

*Mouse*: In a two-stage carcinogenicity study, groups of 20 female ICR/Ha Swiss mice, six to eight weeks of age, received a single application of 20 μg 7,12-dimethylbenz[a]anthracene in acetone followed by applications of 7 mg/animal Pyroset TKP (THPA/P), 2.5 μg/animal TPA (positive control) or acetone three times a week for 57 weeks. The numbers of mice with squamous-cell papillomas and carcinomas of the skin in the THPA/P-, TPA- and acetone-treated groups were 7/20 (two with a carcinoma [$p = 0.004$]), 19/20 (nine with a carcinoma) and 0/20, respectively. When THPA/P was given alone, no skin tumour was observed (Loewengart & Van Duuren, 1977).

## 3.2 Other relevant data

(a) *Experimental systems*

(i) *Absorption, distribution, excretion and metabolism*

No data were available to the Working Group.

(ii) *Toxic effects*

**Tetrakis(hydroxymethyl) phosphonium sulfate**

Administration by gavage of 2-50 mg/kg bw per day THPS in saline to male ICR Swiss mice for 14 days resulted in deaths in the group given 50 mg/kg bw after the fifth day. Application of 125-1000 mg/kg bw per day THPS to chemically depilated back skin of male ICR Swiss mice daily for up to 14 days resulted in reduced body weight, paralysis and superficial necrosis of the treated area at doses of 700 mg/kg and above (Connor *et al.*, 1980).

In gavage studies, Fischer 344/N rats and B6C3F$_1$ mice received single doses of 200-1600 mg/kg bw THPS; all rats at the highest dose and all mice receiving 400 mg/kg bw or more died. All rats and 8/10 mice that received doses of 100 mg/kg bw per day for 14 days died. Of animals dosed for 90 days on five days per week, male rats died after doses of 60 mg/kg bw per day and mice of each sex after 40 mg/kg bw per day or higher. In the last studies, hepatocyte vacuolar degeneration, which appeared to be related to treatment, was seen at doses of 10 mg/kg per day and above in rats and at 20 mg/kg per day and above in mice (National Toxicology Program, 1987).

In two-year studies (see also section 3.1), non-neoplastic lesions attributed to administration of THPS in rats included cystic degeneration of the liver in males and hepatocyte cytoplasmic vacuolization in animals of each sex. No significant non-neoplastic lesion attributable to the treatment was seen in mice (National Toxicology Program, 1987).

**Tetrakis(hydroxymethyl) phosphonium chloride**

The oral LD$_{50}$ for THPC was reported to be 282 mg/kg bw in male rats (Ulsamer *et al.*, 1980). The compound was irritating to rats and rabbits following dermal application, and daily dermal exposures to a 30% solution were fatal to rats nine days after the first dose (Aoyama, 1975).

In gavage studies, all Fischer 344/N rats and B6C3F$_1$ mice that received single doses of 150 mg/kg bw and 300 mg/kg bw THPC, respectively, died. In 14-day studies, deaths were observed in rats that received 75 mg/kg bw and in mice that received 300 mg/kg bw. Deaths also occurred in 90-day studies in rats that received 15 mg/kg bw and in mice that received 135 mg/kg bw per day on five days a week. In the last studies, clinical signs of neurotoxicity and hepatocellular necrosis and vacuolization were seen in rats and mice (National Toxicology Program, 1987).

In two-year studies (see also section 3.1), non-neoplastic lesions in mice and rats treated with THPC included hepatocyte cytoplasmic vacuolization in animals of each sex, cystic degeneration of the liver in male rats, haematopoiesis of the spleen in female rats and follicular-cell hyperplasia of the thyroid in female mice (National Toxicology Program, 1987).

THPC reacts *in vitro* with the 2-amino group of guanosine to form a stable product (Loewengart & Van Duuren, 1976).

(iii) *Effects on reproduction and prenatal toxicity*

No data were available to the Working Group.

(iv) *Genetic and related effects* (see Appendix 1)

**Tetrakis(hydroxymethyl) phosphonium sulfate**

THPS was not mutagenic to several strains of *Salmonella typhimurium* in the presence or absence of an exogenous metabolic system from Aroclor 1254-induced rat liver (Connor *et al.*, 1980; MacGregor *et al.*, 1980). Negative results in *S. typhimurium* strains TA1535, TA1537, TA1538, TA98 and TA100 were also obtained in mutagenicity assays performed on 200-μl samples of urine from male ICR Swiss mice treated with THPS by gavage (2 mg/kg bw or 50 mg/kg bw for 14 days, 50 mg/kg bw for five days) or by dermal application (125-1000 mg/kg bw, 13-16 days) or by feeding several doses of a cotton fabric treated with THPS and mixed in the diet over 14 days. These assays were conducted in the absence of exogenous metabolic activation and in the presence or absence of β-glucuronidase (Connor *et al.*, 1980).

THPS caused mutation at the TK locus in L5178Y mouse lymphoma cells in culture at 5 μg/ml in the absence of an exogenous metabolic system (National Toxicology Program, 1987).

This compound did not induce micronuclei in bone marrow of male ICR Swiss mice treated dermally. A two-fold increase in the incidence of chromatid breaks was seen, however, in bone marrow of mice treated orally with 10 mg/kg bw THPS, and a six-fold increase in polyploidy was seen in mice treated dermally with 1 g/kg (Connor *et al.*, 1980).

**Tetrakis(hydroxymethyl) phosphonium chloride**

THPC was not mutagenic to several strains of *S. typhimurium* in the presence or absence of an exogenous metabolic system from Aroclor 1254-induced rat liver (MacGregor *et al.*, 1980; National Toxicology Program, 1987) or Syrian hamster liver (National Toxicology Program, 1987).

The compound caused mutation at the TK locus in L5178Y mouse lymphoma cells at 5 μg/ml in the absence of an exogenous metabolic system (National Toxicology Program, 1987).

THPC induced sister chromatid exchange in the Chinese hamster CHO cell line in the presence and absence of an exogenous metabolic activation system from Aroclor 1254-induced rat liver at doses of 20 and 15 μg/ml (National Toxicology Program, 1987) and 40 and 50 μg/ml (Loveday *et al.*, 1989), respectively. It induced chromosomal aberrations in the CHO cell line, in the presence and absence of an exogenous metabolic system from Aroclor 1254-induced rat liver at 50 and 30 μg/ml, respectively (National Toxicology Program, 1987). In the absence of an exogenous metabolic system, it induced chromosomal aberrations in CHO cells at 30-50 μg/ml (Loveday *et al.*, 1989), in Chinese hamster lung cells at 30 μg/ml (Ishidate, 1983) and in the Chinese hamster DON cell line at 19 μg/ml (Sasaki *et al.*, 1980).

DMSO extracts of fabrics that had been treated with either THPS or THPC induced ouabain resistance in the Chinese hamster V79 cell line, in the presence and absence of an exogenous metabolic system from Aroclor 1254-induced rat liver, and cell transformation in mouse BALB/c 3T3 cells (Ehrlich *et al.*, 1980).

*(b) Humans*

No data were available to the Working Group.

### 3.3 Case reports and epidemiological studies of carcinogenicity to humans

No data were available to the Working Group.

## 4. Summary of Data Reported and Evaluation

### 4.1 Exposure data

Tetrakis(hydroxymethyl) phosphonium salts are used to produce crease-resistant and flame-retardant finishes on textile fabrics, including children's nightwear. No data on occupational exposure levels were available.

### 4.2 Experimental carcinogenicity data

Tetrakis(hydroxymethyl) phosphonium sulfate was tested for carcinogenicity by oral administration in one strain of mice and in one strain of rats. No dose-related increase in the incidence of any tumour was observed, but in males receiving the low dose there was an increased incidence of malignant lymphomas in mice and of mononuclear-cell leukaemia in rats.

Tetrakis(hydroxymethyl) phosphonium chloride was tested for carcinogenicity by oral administration in one strain of mice and in one strain of rats. No dose-related increase in the incidence of any tumour was observed; however, in male rats receiving the low dose there was an increased incidence of mononuclear-cell leukaemia. Tetrakis(hydroxymethyl) phosphonium chloride did not show significant promoting activity in a two-stage skin carcinogenicity test in mice.

A mixed acetate/phosphate salt of tetrakis(hydroxymethyl) phosphonium base showed weak promoting activity in a two-stage skin carcinogenicity study.

### 4.3 Human carcinogenicity data

No data were available to the Working Group.

### 4.4 Other relevant data

In single studies, tetrakis(hydroxymethyl) phosphonium sulfate did not induce micronuclei but caused a marginal increase in the frequency of chromosomal aberrations in mouse bone marrow *in vivo* and induced mutation in mouse cells *in vitro*. It was not mutagenic to bacteria either in the presence or absence of an exogenous metabolic system.

## Summary table of genetic and related effects of tetrakis(hydroxymethyl) phosphonium chloride

| Nonmammalian systems | | | | | | | | | | | | | Mammalian systems | | | | | | | | | | | | | | | | | |
|---|---|---|---|---|---|---|---|---|---|---|---|---|---|---|---|---|---|---|---|---|---|---|---|---|---|---|---|---|---|---|
| Proka-ryotes | | Lower eukaryotes | | | | Plants | | | | Insects | | | | In vitro | | | | | | | | | | | | In vivo | | | | |
| | | | | | | | | | | | | | | Animal cells | | | | | | | Human cells | | | | | Animals | | | | Humans |
| D | G | D | R | G | A | D | G | C | A | C | R | G | C | A | D | G | S | M | C | A | T | I | D | G | S | M | C | A | T | I | D | G | S | M | C | DL | A | D | S | M | C | A |
| – | | | | | | | | | | | | | | | | +¹ | + | | | | | | | | | | | | | | | | | | | | | | | | | |

A, aneuploidy; C, chromosomal aberrations; D, DNA damage; DL, dominant lethal mutation; G, gene mutation; I, inhibition of intercellular communication; M, micronuclei; R, mitotic recombination and gene conversion; S, sister chromatid exchange; T, cell transformation

*In completing the tables, the following symbols indicate the consensus of the Working Group with regard to the results for each endpoint:*

–    considered to be negative
+¹   considered to be positive, but only one valid study was available to the Working Group
+    considered to be positive for the specific endpoint and level of biological complexity

## Summary table of genetic and related effects of tetrakis(hydroxymethyl) phosphonium sulfate

| Nonmammalian systems | | | | | | | | | | | | | | | Mammalian systems | | | | | | | | | | | | | | | | | |
|---|---|---|---|---|---|---|---|---|---|---|---|---|---|---|---|---|---|---|---|---|---|---|---|---|---|---|---|---|---|---|---|---|
| Prokaryotes | | Lower eukaryotes | | | | Plants | | | | Insects | | | | | In vitro | | | | | | | | | | | | | In vivo | | | | |
| | | | | | | | | | | | | | | | Animal cells | | | | | | | Human cells | | | | | | Animals | | | | Humans |
| D | G | D | R | G | A | D | G | C | R | G | C | A | D | G | S | M | C | A | T | I | D | G | S | M | C | A | T | I | D | G | S | M | C | DL | A | D | S | M | C | A |
| − | | | | | | | | | | | | | | | +¹ | | | | | | | | | | | | | | | | −¹ | +¹ | | | | | | | | |

A, aneuploidy; C, chromosomal aberrations; D, DNA damage; DL, dominant lethal mutation; G, gene mutation; I, inhibition of intercellular communication; M, micronuclei; R, mitotic recombination and gene conversion; S, sister chromatid exchange; T, cell transformation

*In completing the tables, the following symbols indicate the consensus of the Working Group with regard to the results for each endpoint:*

− considered to be negative
+¹ considered to be positive, but only one valid study was available to the Working Group.
−¹ considered to be negative, but only one valid study was available to the Working Group

Tetrakis(hydroxymethyl) phosphonium chloride induced sister chromatid exchange and chromosomal aberrations in Chinese hamster cells *in vitro* and, in a single study, mutation in mouse cells *in vitro*. It was not mutagenic to bacteria either in the presence or absence of an exogenous metabolic system.

### 4.5 Evaluation[1]

There is *inadequate evidence* for the carcinogenicity of tetrakis(hydroxymethyl) phosphonium salts in experimental animals.

No data were available from studies in humans on the carcinogenicity of tetrakis(hydroxymethyl) phosphonium salts.

**Overall evaluation**

Tetrakis(hydroxymethyl) phosphonium salts *are not classifiable as to their carcinogenicity to humans (Group 3)*.

## 5. References

Albright & Wilson Americas, Inc. (1988a) *Material Safety Data Sheet: Retardol C*, Richmond, VA

Albright & Wilson Americas, Inc. (1988b) *Material Safety Data Sheet: Retardol S*, Richmond, VA

Aoyama, M. (1975) Effect of anti-flame treating agents on the skin. *Nagoya med. J.*, 20, 11-19

Connor, T.H., Meyne, J. & Legator, M.S. (1980) The mutagenic evaluation of tetrakis(hydroxymethyl)phosphonium sulfate using a combined testing approach. *J. environ. Pathol. Toxicol.*, 4, 145-158

Duffy, J.J. (1983) Source control: modification of a flame retardant chemical. *Plant/Oper. Progr.*, 2, 241-243

Ehrlich, K., Hulett, A. & Turnham, T. (1980) Mammalian cell culture mutagenicity and carcinogenicity testing of dimethyl sulfoxide extract of flame retardant-treated cotton fabrics. *J. Toxicol. environ. Health*, 6, 259-271

Frank, A.W. (1977) The iodometric determination of P(III) in flame retardants for cotton. 4. Reaction of THPC with iodate. *J. Text. Res.*, 47, 60-61

Frank A.W., Daigle, D.J. & Vail, S.L. (1982) Chemistry of hydroxymethyl phosphorus compounds. III. Phosphines, phosphine oxides, and phosphonium hydroxides. *J. Text. Res.*, 52, 738-750

Grasselli, J.G. & Ritchey, W.M., eds (1975) *CRC Atlas of Spectral Data and Physical Constants for Organic Compounds*, Vol. 4, Cleveland, OH, CRC Press, p. 120

Hawley, G.G. (1981) *Condensed Chemical Dictionary*, 10th ed., New York, Van Nostrand Reinhold, p. 1008

---

[1]For description of the italicized terms and criteria for making the evaluation, see Preamble, pp. 25-29.

Hooper, G. (1973) Phosphine-based fire retardants for cellulosic textiles. In: LeBlanc, R.B., ed., *Proceedings of the First Symposium on Textile Flammability*, East Greenwich, RI, LeBlanc Research Corp., pp. 50-66 [*Chem. Abstr., 84*, 32438z]

Hooper, G., Nakajima, W.N. & Herbes, W.F. (1976a) The use of various phosphonium salts for flame retardancy by the ammonia cure technique. In: Bhatnagar, V.M., ed., *Fire Retardants, Proceedings of 1975 International Symposium on Flammability and Fire Retardants, May 22-23, 1975, Montreal, Canada*, Westport, CT, Technomic Publishing Co., pp. 98-114

Hooper, G., Nakajima, W.N. & Herbes, W.F. (1976b) The use of various phosphonium salts for flame retardancy by the ammonia cure technique. *J. coated Fabr., 6*, 105-120 [*Chem. Abstr., 86*, 91593k]

IARC (1982) *IARC Monographs on the Evaluation of the Carcinogenic Risk of Chemicals to Humans*, Vol. 29, *Some Industrial Chemicals and Dyestuffs*, Lyon, pp. 345-389

Ishidate, M., ed. (1983) *Chromosomal Aberration Test In Vitro*, Tokyo, Realize, Inc., p. 539

Loewengart, C. & Van Duuren, B.L. (1976) The reaction of guanosine with tetrakis(hydroxymethyl)phosphonium chloride. *Tetrahedron Lett., 39*, 3473-3476

Loewengart, G. & Van Duuren, B.L. (1977) Evaluation of chemical flame retardants for carcinogenic potential. *J. Toxicol. environ. Health, 2*, 539-546

Loveday, K.S., Lugo, M.H., Resnick, M.A., Anderson, B.E. & Zeiger, E. (1989) Chromosome aberration and sister chromatid exchange tests in Chinese hamster ovary cells *in vitro*. II. Results with 20 chemicals. *Environ. mol. Mutagenesis, 13*, 60-94

MacGregor, J.T., Diamond, M.J., Mazzeno, L.W., Jr & Friedman, M. (1980) Mutagenicity tests of fabric-finishing agents in *Salmonella typhimurium*: fiber-reactive wool dyes and cotton flame retardants. *Environ. Mutagenesis, 2*, 405-418

National Institute for Occupational Safety and Health (1977) *National Occupational Hazard Survey (NOHS)*, Cincinnati, OH

National Toxicology Program (1987) *Toxicology and Carcinogenesis Studies of Tetrakis(hydroxymethyl) Phosphonium Sulfate (THPS) [CAS No. 55566-30-8] and Tetrakis(hydroxymethyl) Phosphonium Chloride (THPC) [CAS No. 124-64-1] in F344/N Rats and B6C3F$_1$ Mice (Gavage Studies)* (Technical Report No. 296; NIH Publ. No. 87-2552), Research Triangle Park, NC

Sadtler Research Laboratories (1980) *Standard Spectra Collection, 1980 Cumulative Index*, Philadelphia, PA

Sasaki, M., Sugimura, K., Yoshida, M.A. & Abe, S. (1980) Cytogenetic effects of 60 chemicals on cultured human and Chinese hamster cells. *Senshokutai, 20*, 574-584

Ulsamer, A.G., Osterberg, R.E. & McLaughlin, J., Jr (1980) Flame-retardant chemicals in textiles. *Clin. Toxicol., 17*, 101-131

Van Duuren, B.L., Loewengart, G., Seidman, I., Smith, A.C. & Melchionne, S. (1978) Mouse skin carcinogenicity tests of the flame retardants tris(2,3-dibromopropyl)phosphate, tetrakis(hydroxymethyl)phosphonium chloride, and polyvinyl bromide. *Cancer Res., 38*, 3236-3240

Weil, E.D. (1980) Flame retardants (phosphorous compounds). In: Mark, H.F., Othmer, D.F., Overberger, C.G., Seaborg, G.T. & Grayson, M., eds, *Kirk-Othmer Encyclopedia of Chemical Technology*, 3rd ed., Vol. 10, New York, John Wiley & Sons, pp. 411-412

# TRIS(2-CHLOROETHYL) PHOSPHATE

## 1. Chemical and Physical Data

### 1.1 Synonyms

*Chem. Abstr. Services Reg. No.*: 115-96-8
*Chem. Abstr. Name*: Tris(2-chloroethyl) phosphate
*IUPAC Systematic Name*: Tris(2-chloroethyl) phosphate
*Synonyms*: Phosphoric acid, tris(2-chloroethyl) ester; TCEP; tri(chloroethyl) phosphate; tri(β-chloroethyl) phosphate; tri(2-chloroethyl) phosphate; tris(2-chloroethyl) orthophosphate; tris(chloroethyl) phosphate; tris(β-chloroethyl) phosphate

### 1.2 Structural and molecular formulae and molecular weight

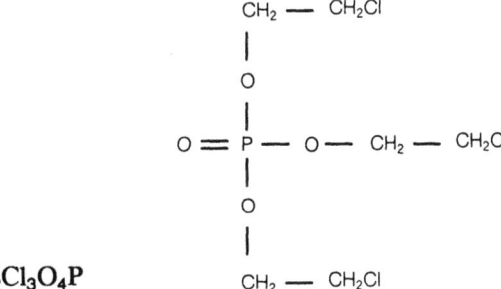

$C_6H_{12}Cl_3O_4P$   Mol. wt: 285.49

### 1.3 Chemical and physical properties of the pure substance

(a) *Description*: Clear, colourless liquid with a slight odour (Lefaux, 1968; Hawley, 1981)
(b) *Boiling-point*: 330°C (Aldrich Chemical Co., 1988)
(c) *Melting-point*: -55°C (Clayton & Clayton, 1981)
(d) *Density*: 1.425 at 20°C (Clayton & Clayton 1981; Hawley, 1981)
(e) *Spectroscopy data*: Mass (Chemical Information Systems, 1988), infrared (prism, Sadtler [6850], Aldrich [556E]; prism-FT [926C]; grating [33388]) and nuclear

magnetic resonance (proton, Sadtler [10547], Aldrich [876D]; C-13 [1036]) spectral data have been reported (Sadtler Research Laboratories, 1980; Pouchert, 1981, 1983, 1985).

(f) *Solubility*: Very slightly soluble in water (0.7 wt %) and aliphatic hydrocarbons; soluble in alcohols, esters, ketones and aromatic hydrocarbons (Lefaux, 1968; Clayton & Clayton, 1981)

(g) *Volatility*: Vapour pressure, < 10 mm Hg at 25°C (Akzo Chemicals, 1982)

(h) *Flash-point*: 216°C (Hawley, 1981)

(i) *Stability*: Thermally stable at temperatures below 150°C (Akzo Chemicals, 1982)

(j) *Reactivity*: When heated to decomposition, carbon monoxide, hydrogen chloride, phosphorus oxides, phosphine and/or phosgene may be released (Morton Thiokol/Alfa Products Division, 1981; Aldrich Chemical Co., 1988).

(k) *Refractive index*: 1.4721 (20°C) (Hawley, 1981)

(l) *Viscosity*: 45 cp (20°C) (Lefaux, 1968)

(m) *Octanol/water partition coefficient (P)*: log P, 1.7 (US Environmental Protection Agency, 1988)

(n) *Conversion factor*: mg/m$^3$ = 11.6 × ppm[1]

## 1.4 Technical products and impurities

*Trade names*: Celanese celluflex CEF; Celluflex CEF; 3CF; CLP; Disflamoll TCA; Fyrol CEF; Fyrol CF; Genomoll P; Niax 3CF; Niax Flame Retardant 3CF

Tris(2-chloroethyl) phosphate is available with a purity of 97% (Morton Thiokol/Alfa Products Division, 1981; Aldrich Chemical Co., 1988). One commercial product contains 10.8 wt% phosphorus, 36.7 wt% chlorine and a maximum of 0.10 wt% water (Akzo Chemicals, 1980).

# 2. Production, Use, Occurrence and Analysis

## 2.1 Production and use

(a) *Production*

Tris(2-chloroethyl) phosphate is produced by the reaction of phosphorus oxychloride with ethylene oxide (see IARC, 1985) or ethylene chlorohydrin (Weil, 1980; Anon., 1985).

---

[1]Calculated from: mg/m$^3$ = (molecular weight/24.45) x ppm, assuming standard temperature (25°C) and pressure (760 mm Hg)

It is available from five manufacturers in the USA, five in Japan and two in France. Total production by the major manufacturers in Japan was approximately 1100 tonnes in 1984 and 1200 tonnes in 1985 (Anon., 1985, 1986). No other data on production were available to the Working Group.

*(b) Use*

Tris(2-chloroethyl) phosphate combines the flame-retarding properties of chlorine and phosphorus compounds. It is used in the manufacture of polyester resins, polyacrylates, polyurethanes and cellulose derivatives, especially materials based on ethyl cellulose, nitrocellulose and cellulose acetate (Lefaux, 1968; Hawley, 1981). This compound is used as a flame-retardant additive for flexible and rigid polyurethane and polyisocyanate foams, carpet backing, paints and lacquers, epoxy, phenolic and amino resins, and wood-resin composites such as particle boards. When blended with binders such as vinyl or acrylic emulsions, it may also be used to coat the backs of upholstery (Weil, 1980). The major use appears to be in foams, such as the flexible foams used in automobiles and furniture and rigid foams for building insulation (US Environmental Protection Agency, 1988). In Japan, about 90-95% is reportedly utilized in urethane and polyvinyl chloride resin additives (Anon., 1986). Direct application to or use in formulations to be applied to fabrics intended for apparel use is not recommended (Akzo Chemicals, 1980).

*(c) Regulatory status and guidelines*

No regulatory standard or guideline has been established for tris(2-chloroethyl) phosphate.

## 2.2 Occurrence

*(a) Natural occurrence*

Tris(2-chloroethyl) phosphate is not known to occur as a natural product.

*(b) Occupational exposure*

No data were available to the Working Group.

*(c) Air*

Tris(2-chloroethyl) phosphate was detected at concentrations of 2-5 ng/m$^3$ in ambient air at Kitakyushu, Japan (Haraguchi *et al.*, 1985).

*(d) Water and sediments*

Tris(2-chloroethyl) phosphate has been detected in river water, seawater and sediment, presumably as an environmental pollutant from industrial and domestic wastewater. Nationwide surveys conducted in Japan in 1977 and 1978 by the Environmental Agency did not indicate the presence of tris(2-chloroethyl) phosphate in water or sediment from river estuaries or the sea; it was detected only at a level of 90 ng/l in a sample of sea-water. In a survey around Kitakyushu in 1980, however, tris(2-chloroethyl) phosphate was identified at levels of

17-347 ng/l in river water, 10-60 ng/l in sea-water and 13-28 ng/g in sediment (Ishikawa *et al.*, 1985a). Tris(2-chloroethyl) phosphate was also detected in river water and sewage sludge from the Okayama area (Kenmochi *et al.*, 1981).

Factory and domestic wastewater effluents in Kitakyushu, Japan, contained detectable levels of tris(2-chloroethyl) phosphate (detection limit, 30 ng/l). Concentrations of 83-87 ng/l were measured in effluents from two food factories, 43-740 ng/l at eight chemical factories, 170-14 000 ng/l at two steel factories, 45-11 000 ng/l at six other industrial sites, 40-560 ng/l at eight residences, 500-1200 ng/l at five sewage treatment plants and 51 ng/l in one metal processing plant. Although high levels were found in two factory effluents, the concentrations were not much higher than those in river water (17-350 ng/l; limit of detection, 10 ng/l), indicating that the pollution was due to a combination of municipal and industrial wastewater sources (Ishikawa *et al.*, 1985b).

Tris(2-chloroethyl) phosphate was detected in water from the River Rhine in the Netherlands at 1 μg/l in 1979 (Zoeteman *et al.*, 1980) and at 0.16-0.35 μg/l in 1986 (Brauch & Kühn, 1988). It was found at levels up to 5.5 μg/l in raw water samples from Trent, Torksey and Elsham, UK, in 1979-80 (Burchill *et al.*, 1983). The compound was also found in the River Waal at Brakel, The Netherlands, in 1974 (Meijers & van der Leer, 1976).

Tris(2-chloroethyl) phosphate was identified at a mean level of 0.57 μg/l in groundwater from two wells adjacent to a municipal wastewater infiltration system at Fort Devens, MA, USA, near Boston (Bedient *et al.*, 1983).

Tris(2-chloroethyl) phosphate has been identified in drinking-water throughout the world. It was found in one of 14 samples of drinking-water collected in 1976 in the UK (Fielding *et al.*, 1981); at 2.0-60.5 ng/l (mean, 17.4 ng/l) in drinking-water collected over a one-year period in Japan (Adachi *et al.*, 1984); at 0.3-9.2 ng/l in six eastern Ontario, Canada, treatment plants in 1978 (LeBel *et al.*, 1981); at 0.2-52 ng/l in 22 of 29 Canadian municipalities in 1979 (Williams & LeBel, 1981); at 0.3-13.8 ng/l in 11 of 12 Great Lakes municipalities in 1980 (Williams *et al.*, 1982); and at 3-9.6 ng/l in 1982 and 1983 in four of five Great Lakes areas (LeBel *et al.*, 1987).

*(e) Animal tissues*

Tris(2-chloroethyl) phosphate was identified at levels of < 0.005-0.019 μg/g in fish and shellfish captured in the Okayama, Japan, area (Kenmochi *et al.*, 1981).

## 2.3 Analysis

Selected methods for the analysis of tris(2-chloroethyl) phosphate are presented in Table 1.

**Table 1. Methods for the analysis of tris(2-chloroethyl) phosphate**

| Sample matrix | Sample preparation | Assay procedure[a] | Limit of detection | References |
|---|---|---|---|---|
| Air | Sample on glass-fibre filter or XAD-7 resin; prefractionate on silica gel column | GC/NPD | 0.04–0.1 ng | Haraguchi et al. (1985) |
| Water | Extract with dichloromethane; dry (anhydrous sodium sulfate); concentrate | GC/MS | 10 ng/l | Ishikawa et al. (1985a); Ishikawa & Baba (1988) |
| | Extract with dichloromethane | GC/FPD | 2 ng/l | Burchill et al. (1983) |
| Drinking-water | Adsorb on XAD resin cartridge; extract with dichloromethane; dry (anhydrous sodium sulfate); concentrate | GC/NPD | 0.3 ng/l | LeBel et al. (1981) |
| | Adsorb on XAD resin cartridge; elute with acetone/hexane; dry (anhydrous sodium sulfate); concentrate; extract (dichloromethane) | GC/MS and GC/NPD | 0.1 ng/l | LeBel et al. (1987) |
| Sediment | Extract with acetone; filter; add filtrate to purified water; extract with dichloromethane; dry (anhydrous sodium sulfate); concentrate | GC/MS | 5 ng/g | Ishikawa et al. (1985a) |
| Sea-water, fish, sea sediment | Extract with acetonitrile and dichloromethane; adsorb; extract on activated charcoal column; extract with sulfuric acid; wash with sodium hydroxide; purify by Florisil chromatography | GC/MS GC/FPD | 1–5 ng/g (fish) | Kenmotsu et al. (1980) |

[a]Abbreviations: GC/NPD, gas chromatography/nitrogen phosphorus detection; GC/MS, gas chromatography/mass spectrometry; GC/FPD, gas chromatography/flame photometric detection

## 3. Biological Data Relevant to the Evaluation of Carcinogenic Risk to Humans

### 3.1 Carcinogenicity studies in animals[1]

*Skin application*

*Mouse*: Groups of 35 female Swiss mice, nine weeks of age, received skin applications of tris(2-chloroethyl) phosphate (Genomoll P) [purity unspecified] in acetone to examine its initiating potential. One group of mice received a single application of 71 mg/mouse Genomoll P followed by applications of 1 μg/mouse tetradecanoyl phorbol acetate (TPA) twice a week for 78 weeks. A control group was treated with TPA alone. The incidence of squamous-cell papillomas of the skin was 17/33 (52%) Genomoll P plus TPA-treated animals and 12/28 (43%) TPA-treated mice; squamous-cell carcinomas of the skin developed in 2/33 Genomoll P plus TPA-treated animals but in none of the TPA-treated controls. The incidences of lung adenomas were 7/33 and 5/28 in Genomoll P plus TPA-treated and in TPA-treated groups, respectively (Sala *et al.*, 1982). [The Working Group noted that the promoting activity and complete carcinogenicity of Genomoll P could not be evaluated because of the lack of controls.]

### 3.2 Other relevant data

(a) *Experimental systems*

(i) *Absorption, distribution, excretion and metabolism*

No data were available to the Working Group.

(ii) *Toxic effects*

Acute oral $LD_{50}$s for tris(2-chloroethyl) phosphate have been reported to be 1230 for rats [sex unspecified] and 501 mg/kg bw for male rats; $LD_{50}$s for female rats were reported to be 794, 501 and 430 mg/kg bw with three different lots of the chemical (Ulsamer *et al.*, 1980).

Neurotoxic effects of tris(2-chloroethyl) phosphate have been reported in rats (Smith, 1936) and hens (Sprague *et al.*, 1981).

Tris(2-chloroethyl) phosphate did not react with DNA *in vitro* (Lown *et al.*, 1980).

(iii) *Effects on reproduction and prenatal toxicity*

Wistar rats were given 50, 100 or 200 mg/kg bw tris(2-chloroethyl) phosphate suspended in olive oil by gavage on days 7-15 of gestation. No change in maternal body weight gain, food

---

[1]The Working Group was aware of studies in progress by oral administration in mice and rats and by skin application in mice (IARC, 1988).

consumption or general appearance was found in the low- and mid-dose groups, but in the high-dose group, maternal food consumption was markedly suppressed; piloerection and general weakness occurred, and 7/30 dams died. On day 20 of gestation, no increase in fetal deaths or in malformations attributable to treatment was observed in any group, but there was some increase in the incidence of cervical and lumbar ribs in the high-dose group. [The Working group noted that this result may have been related to maternal toxicity.] Postnatal examination revealed normal development in the offspring of all groups; no disorder attributable to treatment was observed on morphological examination, and no effect on functional behaviour was seen (Kawashima *et al.*, 1983).

(iv) *Genetic and related effects* (see Appendix 1)

Tris(2-chloroethyl) phosphate was not mutagenic to several strains of *Salmonella typhimurium* in the presence or absence of an exogenous metabolic system from livers of untreated rats or from rats or Syrian hamsters treated with Aroclor 1254 (Prival *et al.*, 1977; Haworth *et al.*, 1983). In contrast, tris(2-chloroethyl) phosphate produced a dose-related increase in mutations (with a maximal 7.6-fold increase in the number of revertants over that in controls at 10 µmol/plate) in *S. typhimurium* TA1535 in the presence but not in the absence of an exogenous metabolic system from the livers of rats treated with Kanechlor 500. The same doses produced a dose-related increase in mutations in *S. typhimurium* TA100, with a maximal 1.8-fold increase in the number of revertants at 10 µmol/plate (Nakamura *et al.*, 1979).

Tris(2-chloroethyl) phosphate caused a dose-related (343-1000 µg/ml) increase in the incidence of sister chromatid exchange in the Chinese hamster V79 cell line. Doses up to 2 mg/ml did not induce mutation at the *hprt* locus in the same cell line. The compound induced dose-related (400-800 µg/ml) transformation in Syrian hamster embryo cells but only weakly transformed C3H 10T½ cells at 1.5 mg/ml. Equivocal results were obtained at 62.5-250 mg/kg bw in an assay for induction of micronuclei in Chinese hamsters *in vivo* (Sala *et al.*, 1982). It caused dominant lethal mutations in rats exposed by inhalation to 0.5 or 1.5 mg/m$^3$ for four months (Shepel'skaia & Dyshginevich, 1981).

(*b*) *Humans*

No data were available to the Working Group.

### 3.3 Case reports and epidemiological studies of carcinogenicity to humans

No data were available to the Working Group.

# 4. Summary of Data Reported and Evaluation

### 4.1 Exposure data

Tris(2-chloroethyl) phosphate is used as a flame retardant in plastics, especially in flexible foams used in automobiles and furniture, and in rigid foams used for building insulation.

No data on occupational exposure levels were available. Tris(2-chloroethyl) phosphate has been detected in drinking-water, river water, sea water and sediments in various parts of the world.

### 4.2 Experimental carcinogenicity data

Tris(2-chloroethyl) phosphate was tested for initiating and promoting activity and for complete carcinogenicity in one strain of mice by skin application. No initiating activity was found; promoting activity and complete carcinogenicity could not be evaluated.

### 4.3 Human carcinogenicity data

No data were available to the Working Group.

### 4.4 Other relevant data

In single studies, tris(2-chloroethyl) phosphate gave equivocal results in a micronucleus test in Chinese hamsters *in vivo* and caused dominant lethal mutation in rats. It caused cell transformation and, in single studies, sister chromatid exchange but not mutation in rodent cells *in vitro*. It was not mutagenic to bacteria in the absence of an exogenous metabolic system but gave equivocal results in the presence of an exogenous metabolic system.

### 4.5 Evaluation[1]

There is *inadequate evidence* for the carcinogenicity of tris(2-chloroethyl) phosphate in experimental animals.

No data were available from studies in humans on the carcinogenicity of tris(2-chloroethyl) phosphate.

#### Overall evaluation

Tris(2-chloroethyl) phosphate is *not classifiable as to its carcinogenicity to humans (Group 3)*.

## 5. References

Adachi, K., Mitsuhashi, M. & Ohkuni, N. (1984) Pesticides and trialkyl phosphates in tap water (Jpn.). *Hyogo-ken Eisei Kenkyusho Kenkyu Hokoku*, 19, 1-6

---

[1]For description of the italicized terms and criteria for making the evaluation, see Preamble, pp. 25–29.

## Summary table of genetic and related effects of tris(2-chloroethyl) phosphate

| Nonmammalian systems | | | | | | | | | | | | | | | Mammalian systems | | | | | | | | | | | | | | | | | | |
|---|---|---|---|---|---|---|---|---|---|---|---|---|---|---|---|---|---|---|---|---|---|---|---|---|---|---|---|---|---|---|---|---|---|
| Proka-ryotes | | Lower eukaryotes | | | | Plants | | | | Insects | | | | | In vitro | | | | | | | | | | | | | In vivo | | | | | |
| | | | | | | | | | | | | | | | Animal cells | | | | | | | Human cells | | | | | | Animals | | | | | Humans |
| D | G | D | R | G | A | D | G | C | R | G | C | A | D | G | S | M | C | A | T | I | D | G | S | M | C | A | T | I | D | G | S | M | C | DL | A | D | S | M | C | A |
| | ? | | | | | | | | | | | | | $-^1$ | $+^1$ | | | + | | | | | | | | | | | | | | ? | | $+^1$ | | | | | | |

A, aneuploidy; C, chromosomal aberrations; D, DNA damage; DL, dominant lethal mutation; G, gene mutation; I, inhibition of intercellular communication; M, micronuclei; R, mitotic recombination and gene conversion; S, sister chromatid exchange; T, cell transformation

*In completing the tables, the following symbols indicate the consensus of the Working Group with regard to the results for each endpoint:*

? considered to be equivocal or inconclusive (e.g., there were contradictory results from different laboratories; there were confounding exposures; the results were equivocal)
$-^1$ considered to be negative, but only one valid study was available to the Working Group
$+^1$ considered to be positive, but only one valid study was available to the Working Group
+ considered to be positive for the specific endpoint and level of biological complexity

Akzo Chemicals (1980) *Product Data Sheet: Fyrol CEF*, Chicago, IL

Akzo Chemicals (1982) *Product Safety Information: Fyrol CEF (Flame Retardant)*, Chicago, IL

Aldrich Chemical Co. (1988) *Material Safety Data Sheet Tris-(2-chloroethyl)phosphate*, Milwaukee, WI

Anon. (1985) Trichloroethyl phosphate (Abstract). *Fain Kem., 14*, 46-47

Anon. (1986) Tris(2-chloroethyl)phosphate (Abstract). *Fain Kem., 15*, 23-25

Bedient, P.B., Springer, N.K., Baca, E., Bouvette, T.C., Hutchins, S.R. & Tomson, M.B. (1983) Ground-water transport from wastewater infiltration. *J. environ. Eng. (NY), 109*, 485-501

Brauch, H.J. & Kühn, W. (1988) Organic micropollutants in the river Rhine and in drinking water treatment (Ger.). *Gas-Wasserfach: Wasser/Abwasser, 129*, 189-196

Burchill, P., Herod, A.A., Marsh, K.M. & Pritchard, E. (1983) Gas chromatography in water analysis -- II. Selective detection methods. *Water Res., 17*, 1905-1916

Chemical Information Systems (1988) *Mass Spectral Search System (MSSS), Infrared Spectral Search System (ISSS)*, Baltimore, MD

Clayton, G.D. & Clayton, F.E., eds (1981) *Patty's Industrial Hygiene and Toxicology*, 3rd rev. ed., Vol. 2A, *Toxicology*, New York, John Wiley & Sons, pp. 2362-2363

Fielding, M., Gibson, T.M., James, H.A., McLoughlin, K. & Steel, C.P. (1981) *Organic Micropollutants in Drinking Water (Technical Report TR159)*, Medmenham, UK, Water Research Centre

Haraguchi, K., Yamashita, T. & Shigemori, N. (1985) Sampling and analysis of phosphoric acid triesters in ambient air. *Air Pollut. ind. Hyg., 20*, 407-415 [*Chem. Abstr., 105*, 84345p]

Hawley, G.G. (1981) *Condensed Chemical Dictionary*, 10th ed., New York, Van Nostrand Reinhold, p. 1059

Haworth, S., Lawlor, T., Mortelmans, K., Speck, W. & Zeiger, E. (1983) *Salmonella* mutagenicity test results for 250 chemicals. *Environ. Mutagenesis, 5 (Suppl. 1)*, 3-142

IARC (1985) *IARC Monographs on the Evaluation of the Carcinogenic Risk of Chemicals to Humans*, Vol. 36, *Allyl Compounds, Aldehydes, Epoxides and Peroxides*, Lyon, pp. 189-226

IARC (1988) *Information Bulletin on the Survey of Chemicals Being Tested for Carcinogenicity*, No. 13, Lyon, pp. 122, 268-269

Ishikawa, S. & Baba, K. (1988) Reaction of organic phosphate esters with chlorine in aqueous solution. *Bull. environ. Contam. Toxicol., 41*, 143-150

Ishikawa, S., Taketomi, M. & Shinohara, R. (1985a) Determination of trialkyl and triaryl phosphates in environmental samples. *Water Res., 19*, 119-125

Ishikawa, S., Shigezumi, K., Yasuda, K. & Shigemori, N. (1985b) Determination of organic phosphate esters in factory effluent and domestic effluent (Jpn.). *Suishitsu Odaku Kenkyu, 8*, 529-535

Kawashima, K., Tanaka, S., Nakaura, S., Nagao, S., Endo, T., Onoda, K., Takanaka, A. & Omori, Y. (1983) Effect of oral administration of tris(2-chloroethyl)phosphate to pregnant rats on prenatal and postnatal developments. *Bull. natl Inst. Hyg. Sci., 101*, 55-61

Kenmochi, K., Matsunaga, K. & Ishida, R. (1981) The effects of environmental pollutants on biological systems. 6. Organic phosphates in environments (Jpn.). 2. *Okayama-ken Kankyo Hoken Senta Nenpo, 5*, 167-175

Kenmotsu, K., Matsunaga, K. & Ishida, T. (1980) Multiresidue determination of phosphoric acid triesters in fish, sea sediment and sea water. *Shokuhin Eiseigaku Zasshi, 2*, 18-31

LeBel, G.L., Williams, D.T. & Benoit, F.M. (1981) Gas chromatographic determination of trialkyl/aryl phosphates in drinking water, following isolation using macroreticular resin. *J. Assoc. off. anal. Chem., 64*, 991-998

LeBel, G.L., Williams, D.T. & Benoit, F.M. (1987) Use of large-volume resin cartridges for the determination of organic contaminants in drinking water derived from the Great Lakes. *Adv. Chem. Ser.*, 214, 309-325

Lefaux, R. (1968) *Practical Toxicology of Plastics*, London, Iliffe Books Ltd, pp. 334-338

Lown, J.W., Joshua, A.V. & McLaughlin, L.W. (1980) Novel antitumour nitrosoureas and related compounds and their reactions with DNA. *J. med. Chem.*, 23, 798-805

Meijers, A.P. & van der Leer, R.C. (1976) The occurrence of organic micropollutants in the river Rhine and the river Maas in 1974. *Water Res.*, 10, 597-604

Morton Thiokol/Alfa Products Division (1981) *Material Safety Data Sheet: 10142 ($ClCH_2CH_2O)_3P(O)$)*, Danvers, MA

Nakamura, A., Tateno, N., Kojima, S., Kaniwa, M.-A. & Kawamura, T. (1979) The mutagenicity of halogenated alkanols and their phosphoric acid esters for *Salmonella typhimurium*. *Mutat. Res.*, 66, 373-380

Pouchert, C.J., ed. (1981) *The Aldrich Library of Infrared Spectra*, 3rd ed., Milwaukee, WI, Aldrich Chemical Co., p. 556

Pouchert, C.J., ed. (1983) *The Aldrich Library of NMR Spectra*, 2nd ed., Vol. 2, Milwaukee, WI, Aldrich Chemical Co., p. 876

Pouchert, C.J., ed. (1985) *The Aldrich Library of FT-IR Spectra*, Vol. 1, Milwaukee, WI, Aldrich Chemical Co., p. 926

Prival, M.J., McCoy, E.C., Gutter, B. & Rosenkranz, H.S. (1977) Tris(2,3-dibromopropyl)phosphate: mutagenicity of a widely used flame retardant. *Science*, 195, 76-78

Sadtler Research Laboratories (1980) *Standard Spectra Collection, 1980 Cumulative Index*, Philadelphia, PA

Sala, M., Gu, Z.G., Meons, G. & Chouroulinkov, I. (1982) In vivo and in vitro biological effects of the flame retardants tris(2,3-dibromopropyl)phosphate and tris(2-chloroethyl)orthophosphate. *Eur. J. Cancer*, 18, 1337-1344

Shepel'skaia, N.R. & Dyshginevich, N.E. (1981) Experimental study of the gonadotoxic effect of tris(chloroethyl) phosphate (Russ.). *Gig. Sanit.*, 6, 20-21

Smith, M.I. (1936) II. The pharmacologic action of some alcoholic phosphoric esters. *Natl Inst. Health Bull.*, 165, 11-25

Sprague, G.L., Sandvik, L.L., Brookins-Hendricks, M.J. & Bickford, A.A. (1981) Neurotoxicity of two organophosphorus ester flame retardants in hens. *J. Toxicol. environ. Health*, 8, 507-518

Ulsamer, A.G., Osterberg, R.E. & McLaughlin, J., Jr (1980) Flame-retardant chemicals in textiles. *Clin. Toxicol.*, 17, 101-131

US Environmental Protection Agency (1988) Twenty-third report of the Interagency Testing Committee to the administrator; receipt of report and request for comments regarding priority list of chemicals. *Fed. Regist.*, 53, 46262-46282

Weil, E.D. (1980) Flame retardants (phosphorus compounds). In: Mark, H.F., Othmer, D.F., Overberger, C.G., Seaborg, G.T. & Grayson, M., eds, *Kirk-Othmer Encyclopedia of Chemical Technology*, 3rd ed., Vol. 10, New York, John Wiley & Sons, pp. 401-402

Williams, D.T. & LeBel, G.L. (1981) A national survey of tri(haloalkyl)-, trialkyl-, and triarylphosphates in Canadian drinking water. *Bull. environ. Contam. Toxicol.*, 27, 450-457

Williams, D.T., Nestmann, E.R., LeBel, G.L., Benoit, F.M., Otson, R. & Lee, E.G.H. (1982) Determination of mutagenic potential and organic contaminants of Great Lakes drinking water. *Chemosphere*, 11, 263-276

Zoeteman, B.C.J., Harmsen, K., Linders, J.B.H.J., Morra, C.F.H. & Slooff, W. (1980) Persistent organic pollutants in river water and ground water of the Netherlands. *Chemosphere*, 9, 231-249

# TEXTILE DYES

# *para*-CHLORO-*ortho*-TOLUIDINE AND ITS STRONG ACID SALTS

This monograph covers *para*-chloro-*ortho*-toluidine and its strong acid salts; data on chemistry, production and use and occurrence are presented only for *para*-chloro-*ortho*-toluidine and its hydrochloride salt, which are the major commercial products and the only forms for which biological data were available.

*para*-Chloro-*ortho*-toluidine (hydrochloride) was considered by a previous working group (IARC, 1978). Since that time, new data have become available and these have been incorporated into the monograph and taken into consideration in the present evaluation.

## 1. Chemical and Physical Data

### 1.1 Synonyms

*para*-Chloro-*ortho*-toluidine

> *Chem. Abstr. Services Reg. No.*: 95-69-2
> *Chem. Abstr. Name*: Benzenamine, 4-chloro-2-methyl-
> *IUPAC Systematic Name*: 4-Chloro-*ortho*-toluidine
> *Colour Index No.*: 37085
> *Synonyms*: 2-Amino-5-chlorotoluene; 3-chloro-6-aminotoluene; 5-chloro-2-aminotoluene; 4-chloro-2-methylaniline; 4-chloro-6-methylaniline; 4-chloro-2-toluidine; 2-methyl-4-chloroaniline

*para*-Chloro-*ortho*-toluidine hydrochloride

> *Chem. Abstr. Services Reg. No.*: 3165-93-3
> *Chem. Abstr. Name*: Benzenamine, 4-chloro-2-methyl-, hydrochloride
> *IUPAC Systematic Name*: 4-Chloro-*ortho*-toluidine hydrochloride
> *Colour Index No.*: 37085
> *Synonyms*: 4-Chloro-2-methylaniline hydrochloride; C.I. Azoic Diazo Component 11; 2-methyl-4-chloroaniline hydrochloride

## 1.2 Structural and molecular formulae and molecular weight

[Chemical structure: benzene ring with NH₂, CH₃ (ortho), and Cl (para) substituents]

$C_7H_8ClN$  Mol. wt: 141.61

Hydrochloride: $C_7H_8ClN·HCl$  Mol. wt: 178.07

## 1.3 Chemical and physical properties of the pure substance

From Weast (1985), unless otherwise specified

### para-Chloro-ortho-toluidine

- (a) *Description*: Leaflets (from ethanol)
- (b) *Boiling-point*: 241°C
- (c) *Melting-point*: 29-30°C
- (d) *Spectroscopy data*: Infrared (grating [669]; prism [730H] [17155]; prism-FT [1219B]), ultraviolet [5411] and nuclear magnetic resonance ([558]; [1027B]) spectral data have been reported (Sadtler Research Laboratories, 1980; Pouchert, 1981, 1983, 1985).
- (e) *Solubility*: Soluble in ethanol

### para-Chloro-ortho-toluidine hydrochloride

*Description*: Buff-coloured powder (Currie, 1933); light-pink powder (National Cancer Institute, 1979)

## 1.4 Technical products and impurities

### para-Chloro-ortho-toluidine

*Trade Names*: Daito Red Base TR; Fast Red Base TR; Fast Red 5CT Base; Fast Red TR Base; Fast Red TRO Base; Fast Red TR-T Base; Kako Red TR Base; Mitsui Red TR Base; Red Base NTR; Red TR Base; Sanyo Fast Red TR Base

### para-Chloro-ortho-toluidine hydrochloride

*Trade Names*: Azogene Fast Red TR; Devol Red K; Devol Red TR; Echtrot TR Base; Neutrosel Red TRVA

No other data were available to the Working Group.

## 2. Production, Use, Occurrence and Analysis

### 2.1 Production and use

*(a) Production*

*para*-Chloro-*ortho*-toluidine was first synthesized in 1870 by Beilstein and Kuhlberg by the reduction of 2-nitrotoluene with tin and hydrochloric acid (Prager *et al.*, 1929). It has also been produced by the direct chlorination of *ortho*-toluidine (Schimelpfenig, 1975) and by the chlorination of 2-formylaminotoluene (Grieder, 1977) or 2-acetylaminotoluene followed by hydrolysis or alcoholysis (Society of Dyers and Colourists, 1971). *para*-Chloro-*ortho*-toluidine has been sold commercially both as the free amine and its hydrochloride salt (US Tariff Commission, 1940, 1945). Commercial production of *para*-chloro-*ortho*-toluidine began in Germany in 1924 (Uebelin & Pletscher, 1954) and was first reported in the USA in 1939 (US Tariff Commission, 1940). In Switzerland, *para*-chloro-*ortho*-toluidine and its salts were produced from 1956 through to 1976; production in 1976 was estimated at 100-200 thousand kg (IARC, 1978).

Production of *para*-chloro-*ortho*-toluidine in the USA ceased in 1979, and all importation and distribution of the substance was discontinued in 1986 (US Environmental Protection Agency, 1988); production and distribution in the Federal Republic of Germany were stopped in 1986 (Stasik, 1988). *para*-Chloro-*ortho*-toluidine and its hydrochloride were produced in the UK in 1930 (Currie, 1933); it is not known if they are still produced there. *para*-Chloro-*ortho*-toluidine has not been produced commercially in Japan (IARC, 1978).

*(b) Use*

*para*-Chloro-*ortho*-toluidine and its hydrochloride salt have been used to produce azo dyes for cotton, silk, acetate and nylon and as intermediates in the production of Pigment Red 7 and Pigment Yellow 49 (Society of Dyers and Colourists, 1971; US Environmental Protection Agency, 1988). As an azoic diazo component, *para*-chloro-*ortho*-toluidine is used with naphthol derivatives to form azo dyes *in situ* on fabric and yarns. Dyeing with naphthol dyes takes place in two phases: the textile is first immersed in a solution of azoic coupling component, naphthol, and then allowed to react with azoic diazonium component consisting of an aromatic amine first converted to a diazonium derivative (Priha *et al.*, 1988).

*para*-Chloro-*ortho*-toluidine has also been used since the 1960s in the manufacture of chlordimeform [N'-(4-chloro-2-methylphenyl)-*N,N*-dimethylformamidine; see IARC, 1983], an acaricide and insecticide (Kossmann *et al.*, 1971; Sittig, 1980).

*(c) Regulatory status and guidelines*

No regulatory standard or guideline has been established for *para*-chloro-*ortho*-toluidine.

## 2.2 Occurrence

*(a) Natural occurrence*

*para*-Chloro-*ortho*-toluidine and its hydrochloride salt are not known to occur as natural products.

*(b) Occupational exposure*

Exposures were reported to occur during the charging of mixing vats and the basification stage at a *para*-chloro-*ortho*-toluidine purification plant in the UK (Currie, 1933). Workers in a batch-operated chemical processing plant (at a bromindigo and thioindigo production area) in the USA were reported to be exposed by inhalation and dermal contact to *para*-chloro-*ortho*-toluidine (Ott & Langner, 1983). Workers were also reported to be exposed to this compound during its production and processing at a plant in the Federal Republic of Germany (Stasik, 1988). In none of these studies were data provided on exposure levels.

*para*-Chloro-*ortho*-toluidine has been detected in the urine of workers exposed to chlordimeform (Folland *et al.*, 1978; Geyer & Fattal, 1987). It is a major metabolite of chlordimeform in dogs, rats and goats (Knowles, 1970; Watanabe & Matsumura, 1987).

*(c) Food*

*para*-Chloro-*ortho*-toluidine has been isolated and identified in field samples of different plant materials treated with chlordimeform, at concentrations of less than 0.1 to 0.2 ppm (mg/kg) in young bean leaves, 0.02-0.3 ppm (mg/kg) in grape stems, 0.02-0.05 ppm (mg/kg) in a mixture of grape stems and berries, and less than 0.04 ppm (mg/kg) in prunes and apples (Kossmann *et al.*, 1971). *para*-Chloro-*ortho*-toluidine can also be formed from chlordimeform by enzymes present in the leaves of apple seedlings (Gupta & Knowles, 1969) and in cotton plants (Bull, 1973).

Residues of chlordimeform and its metabolites were measured in rice plants and paddy soil following experimental field application (one to three treatments, with harvesting 42 days after the last treatment). Residue concentrations of *para*-chloro-*ortho*-toluidine were 3-61 ppb ($\mu$g/kg) in rice grains, 80-7200 ppb ($\mu$g/kg) in straw parts, 2-68 ppb ($\mu$g/kg) in the upper layer of soil (0-5 cm) and from trace to 20 ppb ($\mu$g/kg) in the lower layer of soil (5-10 cm; Iizuka & Masuda, 1979). In another experimental field application of chlordimeform (one to three treatments, either sprayed or applied to the soil, with analysis 20-55 days after treatment), no residue of *para*-chloro-*ortho*-toluidine (< 0.02 ppm [mg/kg]) was found in rice grains or husks (Fan & Ge, 1982).

## 2.3 Analysis

Selected methods for the analysis of *para*-chloro-*ortho*-toluidine are given in Table 1.

## Table 1. Methods for the analysis of *para*-chloro-*ortho*-toluidine

| Sample matrix | Sample preparation[a] | Assay procedure[a] | Limit of detection | Reference |
|---|---|---|---|---|
| Air | Extract from filter with dichloromethane; evaporate | GC/MS | Not reported | Hunt & Hoyt (1982) |
| | Collect on membrane filter; desorb with water | HPLC/UV | 3 µg/sample | Eller (1985) |
| Plants, soil | Extract with methanol/hydrochloric acid and methanol/dichloromethane; separate by TLC; treat eluate with acetic acid and sodium hydroxide; diazotize and couple with N-ethylnaphthylamine | Colorimetric | 0.02-0.03 ppm (mg/kg) | Kossmann et al. (1971) |
| | Steam distill; extract into isooctane; diazotize and couple with N-ethyl-1-naphthylamine; clean up by column chromatography | Colorimetric | 0.05 ppm (mg/kg) | Geissbühler et al. (1971) |
| Soil | Extract with ethanol; purify by TLC; extract with diethyl ether or dichloromethane | GC/FID and GC/MS | Not reported | Bollag et al. (1978) |
| Rice | Extract with ethanol; clean up on neutral alumina column; elute with ethanol | GC/FID | 0.02 ppm (mg/kg) | Fan & Ge (1982) |
| Solid waste | Extract with dichloromethane; dry with anhydrous sodium sulfate and sonicate | GC/MS | 1 ppm (mg/kg) | Warner et al. (1983) |
| Urine, faeces | Add sodium bicarbonate and hexane; shake and centrifuge; add sulfuric acid to organic layer; shake, centrifuge and separate layers; inject aqueous phase | HPLC | 5 ng/ml | Holdiness & Morgan (1983) |
| Urine | Buffer with ammonia/ammonium chloride; extract with toluene; analyse organic layer by high-performance TLC; visualize by coupling with N-ethyl-1-naphthylamine | TLC | 6 ng/ml | Sistovaris & Bartsch (1984) |
| | Extract an alkaline hydrolysate with hexane; evaporate off the solvent; reconstitute residue with an aqueous acetonitrile | HPLC/UV | 0.2 mg/l | Geyer & Fattal (1987) |

[a]Abbreviations: GC/MS, gas chromatography/mass spectrometry; HPLC/UV, high-performance liquid chromatography/ultraviolet detection; TLC, thin-layer chromatography; GC/FID, gas chromatography/flame ionization detection; HPLC, high-performance liquid chromatography

# 3. Biological Data Relevant to the Evaluation of Carcinogenic Risk to Humans

## 3.1 Carcinogenicity studies in animals

*Oral administration*

*Mouse*: As part of a larger carcinogenicity study of several compounds, groups of 25 male and 25 female random-bred CD-1 albino mice (derived from HaM/ICR mice), six to eight weeks of age, were fed dietary levels of 0, 750 or 1500 (males) and 0, 2000 or 4000 (females) mg/kg of diet *para*-chloro-*ortho*-toluidine hydrochloride (97-99% pure) for 18 months and were observed for an additional three months. Haemangiosarcomas or haemangiomas were observed in 13/20 high-dose males, 12/20 low-dose males, 12/16 high-dose females and 18/19 low-dose females, mainly in the spleen and subcutaneous and retroperitoneal adipose tissues. Tumours of these types were not seen in the simultaneous controls but were found in 5/99 male and 9/102 female pooled controls from the larger study (Weisburger *et al.*, 1978).

Groups of 50 male and 50 female B6C3F$_1$ mice, six weeks old, were fed *ad libitum* diets containing 3750 or 15 000 (males) and 1250 or 5000 (females) mg/kg of diet *para*-chloro-*ortho*-toluidine hydrochloride (purity, 99%) for 92 (high-dose females) and 99 weeks, when survivors were killed. A group of 20 male and 20 female untreated mice served as controls. The mean body weights of treated mice were lower than those of the corresponding controls. All males survived beyond 52 weeks; of the females, 49/50 high-dose, 48/50 low-dose and 19/20 controls were still alive at that time, but all high-dose females had died by 92 weeks. Haemangiosarcomas occurred in 3/50 low-dose males, 37/50 high-dose males, 40/49 low-dose females and 39/50 high-dose females, mainly in the fatty tissue adjacent to the genital organs. No such tumour occurred in the untreated controls (National Cancer Institute, 1979).

*Rat*: Groups of 25 male Charles River CD Sprague-Dawley-derived rats, six to eight weeks of age, were fed 2000 or 4000 mg/kg of diet *para*-chloro-*ortho*-toluidine hydrochloride (97-99% pure) for three months, after which time the doses were reduced to 500 and 1000 mg/kg of diet, respectively, for 15 months. A group of 25 untreated males served as controls. All animals were killed after 24 months. No statistically significant difference in the incidence of tumours was found between treated and control groups (Fisher exact test; Weisburger *et al.*, 1978). [The Working Group noted the small number of rats tested, the low doses used after three months and the relatively short duration of treatment.]

Groups of 50 male and 50 female Fischer 344 rats, six weeks of age, were fed diets containing 1250 or 5000 mg/kg of diet *para*-chloro-*ortho*-toluidine hydrochloride (purity, 99%) for 107 weeks, at which time all surviving animals were killed. A group of 20 male and 20 female untreated rats served as controls. The mean body weights of the high-dose male and female rats were lower than those of the corresponding controls. Treated animals of each sex lived longer than controls. Chromophobe adenomas of the pituitary gland were observed in 1/19 control, 13/48 low-dose and 15/48 high-dose females [$p = 0.025$; one-sided Cochran-Armitage test for trend], and 2/19 control, 6/48 low-dose and 15/47 high-dose males ($p = 0.006$; Cochran-Armitage test for trend). In historical controls, pituitary adenomas were observed in 18% of male and 21% of female rats. Adrenal phaeochromocytomas were observed in 0/20 control, 0/49 low-dose and 4/49 high-dose males ($p = 0.014$; Cochran-Armitage test for trend) (National Cancer Institute, 1979). [The Working Group noted the small number and low survival of the controls.]

### 3.2 Other relevant data

(a) *Experimental systems*

(i) *Absorption, distribution, excretion and metabolism*

Following oral administration of [$^{14}$C-methyl]-*para*-chloro-*ortho*-toluidine to male and female white rats, 71% of the administered radioactivity was eliminated in the urine and 24.5% in the faeces within 72 h (Knowles & Gupta, 1970).

After intraperitoneal administration of 14 mg/kg bw [$^{14}$C-methyl]-*para*-chloro-*ortho*-toluidine hydrochloride to Osborne-Mendel rats, radiolabel was bound to DNA, RNA and protein of liver; in other tissues, these macromolecules contained little radioactivity. *In vitro*, a phenobarbital-inducible liver microsomal enzyme converted *para*-chloro-*ortho*-toluidine to a reactive metabolite, 5-chloro-2-hydroxyaminotoluene (Hill *et al.*, 1979).

After a single oral administration of 25 mg/kg bw [$^{14}$C-ring]-labelled *para*-chloro-*ortho*-toluidine hydrochloride to male mice and male Sprague-Dawley rats, the extent of binding to hepatic DNA in mice was about twice as high as that in rats at 6, 12 and 20 h. Two major DNA adducts were formed in both species, but one of these adducts was formed to a much greater extent (six to 30 fold) in mice than in rats. Binding to proteins was more pronounced in rats. Preliminary analysis of metabolite patterns in the urine indicated that *para*-chloro-*ortho*-toluidine was metabolized differently in the two species (Bentley *et al.*, 1986).

Binding of *para*-chloro-*ortho*-toluidine to haemoglobin was observed after oral administration of 85 mg/kg bw to female Wistar rats (Neumann, 1988).

*para*-Chloro-*ortho*-toluidine inhibited RNA synthesis in HeLa cells (Murakami & Fukami, 1974). It also inhibited thymidine incorporation in mouse testicular DNA *in vivo* (Seiler, 1977).

(ii) *Toxic effects*

The intraperitoneal $LD_{50}$ of *para*-chloro-*ortho*-toluidine hydrochloride was 720 mg/kg bw in male and 680 mg/kg bw in female CD-1 albino mice and 560 mg/kg bw in male and 700 mg/kg bw in female Charles River CD (Sprague-Dawley derived) rats (Weisburger *et al.*, 1978).

Skin applications of 4 g *para*-chloro-*ortho*-toluidine in lard caused haematuria in cats (Lehmann, 1933). [The Working Group noted that the compound now known as *para*-chloro-*ortho*-toluidine was called 5-chloro-*ortho*-toluidine by Lehmann (1933), but that the chemical structures of the two are identical.] Application of 50 mg/kg bw to cats caused mild oedema and congestion of the bladder mucosa in cats; none of the cats, however, showed the severe haemorrhagic cystitis reported by Lehman (1933) in workers exposed to *para*-chloro-*ortho*-toluidine (Kimbrough, 1980).

In male Sprague-Dawley rats, intraperitoneal injection of *para*-chloro-*ortho*-toluidine increased hepatic cytochrome P450, ethoxyresorufin-*O*-deethylase, ethoxycoumarin-*O*-deethylase, glutathione *S*-transferase and epoxide hydrolase activities. The activities of the 7α, 6β and 16β androstenedione hydroxylase pathways were also increased (Leslie *et al.*, 1988).

(iii) *Effects on reproduction and prenatal toxicity*
No data were available to the Working Group.

(iv) *Genetic and related effects* (see Appendix 1)

*para*-Chloro-*ortho*-toluidine was assayed in indirect tests for DNA repair using as an indicator the diameter of zones of growth inhibition in DNA repair-proficient and -deficient strains of bacteria. At doses at or above 1000 mg per disc, differential killing was observed in tests with *Salmonella typhimurium* TA1538 and TA1978 and with *Escherichia coli* WP2, WP2*uvr*A, WP67, CM611 and CM571, in the absence of an exogenous metabolic system (Rashid *et al.*, 1984). [The Working Group noted the extremely high doses required to elicit a positive response.]

Conflicting results have been reported with regard to the mutagenicity of *para*-chloro-*ortho*-toluidine to bacteria. It was mutagenic to *S. typhimurium* TA100 in the presence of an exogenous metabolic system from Aroclor 1254-induced rat liver and mouse liver. Liquid pre-incubation assays were less effective in demonstrating the mutagenicity of *para*-chloro-*ortho*-toluidine than standard pour-plate assays. In other studies, it was not mutagenic to strains TA1537 and TA98 in the presence or absence of exogenous metabolic systems (Zimmer *et al.*, 1980), nor to strains TA1535, TA1537, TA98 and TA100, in the presence or absence of an exogenous metabolic system from livers of rats or Syrian hamsters treated with Aroclor 1254 (Haworth *et al.*, 1983), nor to strains TA1537, TA1538, TA98 and TA100 in the absence of an exogenous metabolic system from Aroclor 1254-induced rat liver. The compound did not induce mutagenicity in *E. coli* WP2, WP2*uvr*A, WP67, CM611 or CM571, in the presence or absence of an exogenous metabolic system from Aroclor 1254-induced rat liver (Rashid *et al.*, 1984).

*para*-Chloro-*ortho*-toluidine caused DNA strand breaks in Chinese hamster V79 cells at 3 mM (Zimmer *et al.*, 1980). It induced sister chromatid exchange in the Chinese hamster CHO cell line *in vitro*, in the presence and absence of an exogenous metabolic system from Aroclor 1254-induced rat liver, but with a greater effect in the absence of activation. The compound induced chromosomal aberrations *in vitro* in CHO cells in the presence of metabolic activation, only at 400 μg/ml (Galloway *et al.*, 1987). It did not induce heritable translocations in SPF NMRI mice at toxic oral doses of 200 mg/kg bw (Lang & Adler, 1982). It was reported not to induce dominant lethal mutations or micronuclei in mice *in vivo* [details not given]. It induced mutations in female C57Bl/6J mice after oral administration to the dams of 100 mg/kg bw (Lang, 1984).

## (b) Humans

*(i) Absorption, distribution, excretion and metabolism*

No data were available to the Working Group.

*(ii) Toxic effects*

Chloroaniline derivatives have been reported to cause haematuria and to affect the bladder mucosa in humans (Currie, 1933; Lehmann, 1933; Folland *et al.*, 1978; Kimbrough, 1980); and haematuria and severe haemorrhagic cystitis have been reported in workers exposed to *para*-chloro-*ortho*-toluidine (Lehmann, 1933). [The Working Group noted that the compound now known as *para*-chloro-*ortho*-toluidine was called 5-chloro-*ortho*-toluidine by Currie (1933) and Lehmann (1933) but that the chemical structures of the two are identical.] Gross haematuria and strangury were observed among workers exposed to *para*-chloro-*ortho*-toluidine in a chemical plant in the UK; most of the 11 patients had suprapubic pain, and all developed symptoms within days after the first exposure. Follow-up examination of three patients within three years of their illness showed that one had had no subsequent bladder trouble, one had had slight cystitis and urethritis and one had a carcinoma of the bladder (Currie, 1933).

*(iii) Effects on reproduction and prenatal toxicity*

No data were available to the Working Group.

*(iv) Genetic and related effects*

No data were available to the Working Group.

## 3.3 Case reports and epidemiological studies of carcinogenicity to humans

Investigations of the occurrence of bladder tumours among small groups of men exposed to *para*-chloro-*ortho*-toluidine were reported by Currie (1933) and Uebelin and Pletscher (1954); one case of bladder carcinoma was found (Currie, 1933).

Ott and Langner (1983) reported a cohort study of 342 men engaged in the manufacture of organic dyes in the USA between 1914 and 1958. In one area of the plant, involving 117 men in five processes in the production of brom- and thioindigos, there was potential exposure to *para*-chloro-*ortho*-toluidine and other raw materials and intermediates, including *ortho*-toluidine. During follow-up of this subcohort from 1940 to 1975, a nonsignificant excess of cancer deaths occurred (12 observed, 8.0 expected from age-specific US white male mortality rates), and no bladder cancer was observed [expected figure unspecified but estimated to be about 0.5]. [The Working Group noted that the study involved mixed exposures.]

Stasik (1988) re-examined a cohort of 335 male workers in *para*-chloro-*ortho*-toluidine production and processing plants in the Federal Republic of Germany who had been followed up for mortality from 1929 to 1982. No death from bladder cancer was found [expected figure unspecified but estimated to be less than 0.5] (Stasik *et al.*, 1985). The second study was limited to a subcohort of 116 men who had been exposed before 1970 (when improvements in industrial hygiene were introduced) to levels of *para*-chloro-*ortho*-toluidine that were probably high, and was prompted by the occurrence of two urinary bladder carcinomas among the current work force. Excluding these two cases, six cases of bladder carcinoma were found between January 1983 and June 1986 through hospital and other institutions. These were compared with cancer registration rates for a different region of the Federal Republic of Germany from that in which the plant was located, as there was no cancer registry in the latter area. The expected number was 0.11 based on sex- and age-specific cancer registration rates. The latent periods of the eight tumours ranged from 17 to 38 years. Two of the patients had had haemorrhagic cystitis thought to be due to massive exposure to *para*-chloro-*ortho*-toluidine prior to diagnosis. Cigarette smoking was not thought to be a confounding variable on the basis of the smoking histories of the patients, three of whom were nonsmokers. No quantitative measure of exposure was available, but the predominant exposure was to *para*-chloro-*ortho*-toluidine; exposure to other amines was also possible. [The Working Group noted that the way in which the cases were ascertained and compared could have introduced bias.]

## 4. Summary of Data Reported and Evaluation

### 4.1 Exposure data

*para*-Chloro-*ortho*-toluidine and its hydrochloride have been produced since the 1920s and have been used as chemical intermediates in the manufacture of azo dyes for textiles and pigments and, since the 1960s, in the manufacture of chlordimeform, an insecticide. Occupational exposure can occur during production and use of *para*-chloro-*ortho*-toluidine; however, no data on levels were available. *para*-Chloro-*ortho*-toluidine has been detected as a metabolite of chlordimeform in plants and in humans.

### 4.2 Experimental carcinogenicity data

*para*-Chloro-*ortho*-toluidine hydrochloride was tested for carcinogenicity by administration in the diet in two strains of mice and in two strains of rats. It produced haemangiomas and haemangiosarcomas in one strain of mice and haemangiosarcomas in the other. In one study in rats, an increase in the incidence of adrenal phaeochromocytomas was seen in male animals given the high dose.

### 4.3 Human carcinogenicity data

A mortality study of workers in the manufacture of organic dyes with mixed exposures, including potential exposure to *para*-chloro-*ortho*-toluidine, showed a small, nonsignificant excess of cancers at all sites. Following two reported cases of bladder cancer among workers exposed before 1970 in the production and processing of *para*-chloro-*ortho*-toluidine, who were probably exposed to higher levels than in the previous study, a large excess of bladder carcinoma was found on further follow-up.

## 4.4 Other relevant data

*para*-Chloro-*ortho*-toluidine caused bladder irritation and haematuria in men exposed occupationally. It formed DNA adducts in rats and mice and bound to haemoglobin in rats treated *in vivo*.

In a single study, *para*-chloro-*ortho*-toluidine did not induce heritable translocations in mice *in vivo*; in another study, it induced somatic specific locus mutations in mice *in vivo*. In single studies in rodent cells in culture, it caused DNA strand breaks, sister chromatid exchange and chromosomal aberrations. It was mutagenic to bacteria in one study in the presence of an exogenous metabolic system.

## 4.5 Evaluation[1]

There is *sufficient evidence* for the carcinogenicity of *para*-chloro-*ortho*-toluidine hydrochloride in experimental animals.

There is *limited evidence* for the carcinogenicity of *para*-chloro-*ortho*-toluidine in humans.

In formulating the overall evaluation, the Working Group took note of the fact that any salt of *para*-chloro-*ortho*-toluidine with a strong acid can be expected to behave chemically in a manner similar to the hydrochloride salt in solution and *in vivo*.

### Overall evaluation

*para*-Chloro-*ortho*-toluidine and its strong acid salts *are probably carcinogenic to humans (Group 2A)*.

# 5. References

Bentley, P., Waechter, F., Bieri, F., Staübli, W. & Muecke, W. (1986) Species differences in the covalent binding of *p*-chloro-*o*-toluidine to DNA. *Arch. Toxicol., Suppl. 9*, 163-166

Bollag, J.-M., Blattmann, P. & Laanio, T. (1978) Adsorption and transformation of four substituted anilines in soil. *J. agric. Food Chem., 26*, 1302-1306

Bull, D.L. (1973) Metabolism of chlordimeform in cotton plants. *Environ. Entomol., 2*, 869-871

Currie, A.N. (1933) Chemical haematuria from handling 5-chloro-*ortho*-toluidine. *J. ind. Hyg., 15*, 205-213

Eller, P.M. (1985) *NIOSH Manual of Analytical Methods*, 3rd ed. (*DHHS (NIOSH) Publ. No. 84-1000*), Washington DC, US Government Printing Office, pp. 5013-1-5013-5

Fan, D.-F. & Ge, S.-D. (1982) Gas-liquid chromatographic determination of chlordimeform and its metabolites in cargo rice and husk. *J. Assoc. off. anal. Chem., 65*, 1517-1520

---

[1]For description of the italicized terms and criteria for making the evaluation, see Preamble, pp. 25-29.

## Summary table of genetic and related effects of *para*-chloro-*ortho*-toluidine

| Nonmammalian systems | | | | | | | | | | | | Mammalian systems | | | | | | | | | | | | | | | | | | |
|---|---|---|---|---|---|---|---|---|---|---|---|---|---|---|---|---|---|---|---|---|---|---|---|---|---|---|---|---|---|---|
| Proka-ryotes | | Lower eukaryotes | | | | Plants | | | | Insects | | In vitro | | | | | | | | | | | | | In vivo | | | | | |
| | | | | | | | | | | | | Animal cells | | | | | | | Human cells | | | | | | Animals | | | | | Humans | | |
| D | G | D | R | G | A | D | G | C | R | G | C | A | D | G | S | M | C | A | T | I | D | G | S | M | C | A | T | I | D | G | S | M | C | DL | A | D | S | M | C | A |
| + | | | | | | | | | | | | | +¹ | | +¹ | +¹ | | | | | | | | | | | | | +¹ | ? | | | | | | | | | | |

A, aneuploidy; C, chromosomal aberrations; D, DNA damage; DL, dominant lethal mutation; G, gene mutation; I, inhibition of intercellular communication; M, micronuclei; R, mitotic recombination and gene conversion; S, sister chromatid exchange; T, cell transformation

*In completing the tables, the following symbols indicate the consensus of the Working Group with regard to the results for each endpoint:*

+    considered to be positive for the specific endpoint and level of biological complexity
+¹   considered to be positive, but only one valid study was available to the Working Group
?    considered to be equivocal or inconclusive (e.g., there were contradictory results from different laboratories; there were confounding exposures; the results were equivocal)

Folland, D.S., Kimbrough, R.D., Cline, R.E., Swiggart, R.C. & Schaffner, W. (1978) Acute hemorrhagic cystitis. Industrial exposure to the pesticide chlordimeform. *J. Am. med. Assoc.*, 239, 1052-1055

Galloway, S.M., Armstrong, M.J., Reuben, C., Colman, S., Brown, B., Cannon, C., Bloom, A.D., Nakamura, F., Ahmed, M., Duk, S., Rimpo, J., Margolin, B.H., Resnick, M.A., Anderson, B. & Zeiger, E. (1987) Chromosome aberrations and sister chromatid exchanges in Chinese hamster ovary cells: evaluations of 108 chemicals. *Environ. mol. Mutagenesis*, 10 (Suppl. 10), 1-175

Geissbühler, H., Kossmann, K., Baunok, I. & Boyd, V.F. (1971) Determination of total residues of chlorphenamidine [$N'$-(4-chloro-o-tolyl)-$N,N$-dimethylformamine] in plant and soil material by colorimetry and thin-layer and electron capture gas chromatography. *J. agric. Food Chem.*, 19, 365-371

Geyer, R. & Fattal, F. (1987) HPLC determination of the metabolite 4-chloro-o-toluidine in the urine of workers occupationally exposed to chlordimeform. *J. anal. Toxicol.*, 11, 24-26

Grieder, A. (1977) *Alcoholic Hydrolysis of 2-Formylaminochlorotoluene* (US Patent 4,034,043 (to Ciba-Geigy Corp.))

Gupta, A.K.S. & Knowles, C.O. (1969) Metabolism of $N'$-(4-chloro-o-tolyl)-$N,N$-dimethylformamidine by apple seedlings. *J. agric. Food Chem.*, 17, 595-600

Haworth, S., Lawlor, T., Mortelmans, K., Speck, W. & Zeiger, E. (1983) *Salmonella* mutagenicity test results for 250 chemicals. *Environ. Mutagenesis*, 5 (Suppl. 1), 3-142

Hill, D.L., Shih, T.-W. & Struck, R.F. (1979) Macromolecular binding and metabolism of the carcinogen 4-chloro-2-methylaniline. *Cancer Res.*, 39, 2528-2531

Holdiness, M.R. & Morgan, L.R., Jr (1983) High-performance liquid chromatographic analysis of 5-chloroaminotoluene in rats. *J. Chromatogr.*, 278, 193-198

Hunt, G.T. & Hoyt, M.P. (1982) General applications of fused silica capillary column (FSCC) chromatography to the analysis of non-priority pollutant organics in environmental samples. *J. high Resolut. Chromatogr. Chromatogr. Commun.*, 5, 291-298

IARC (1978) *IARC Monographs on the Evaluation of the Carcinogenic Risk of Chemicals to Man*, Vol 16, *Some Aromatic Amines and Related Nitro Compounds — Hair Dyes, Colouring Agents and Miscellaneous Industrial Chemicals*, Lyon, pp. 277-285

IARC (1983) *IARC Monographs on the Evaluation of the Carcinogenic Risk of Chemicals to Humans*, Vol. 30, *Miscellaneous Pesticides*, Lyon, pp. 61-72

Iizuka, H. & Masuda, T. (1979) Residual fate of chlorphenamidine in rice plant and paddy soil. *Bull. environ. Contam. Toxicol.*, 22, 745-749

Kimbrough, R.D. (1980) Human health effects of selected pesticides. Chloroaniline derivatives. *J. environ. Sci. Health*, B15, 977-992

Knowles, C.O. (1970) Metabolism of two acaricidal chemicals, $N'$-(4-chloro-o-tolyl)-$N,N$-dimethylformamidine (chlorphenamidine) and $m$-{[(dimethylamino)methylene]-amino}phenyl methylcarbamate hydrochloride (formetanate). *J. agric. Food Chem.*, 18, 1038-1047

Knowles, C.O. & Gupta, A.K.S. (1970) $N'$-(4-Chloro-o-tolyl)-$N,N$-dimethylformamide-$^{14}$C (Galecron) and 4-chloro-o-toluidine-$^{14}$C metabolism in the white rat. *J. Econ. Entomol.*, 63, 856-859

Kossmann, K., Geissbühler, H. & Boyd, V.F. (1971) Specific determination of chlorphenamidine [$N'$-(4-chloro-o-tolyl)-$N,N$-dimethylformamidine] in plants and soil material by colorimetry and thin-layer and electron capture gas chromatography. *J. agric. Food Chem.*, 19, 360-364

Lang, R. (1984) The mammalian spot test and its use for testing of mutagenic and carcinogenic potential: experience with the pesticide chlordimeform, its principal metabolites and the drug lisuride hydrogen maleate. *Mutat. Res.*, 135, 219-224

Lang, R. & Adler, I.-D. (1982) Studies on the mutagenic potential of the pesticide chlordimeform and its principal metabolites in the mouse heritable translocation assay. *Mutat. Res.*, *92*, 243-248

Lehmann, K.B. (1933) Studies on the action of chloroaniline and chlorotoluidine and of 5-chloro-2-toluidine hydrochloride (Ger.). *Arch. Hyg. Bakteriol.*, *110*, 12-32

Leslie, C., Reidy, G.F., Murray, M. & Stacey, N.H. (1988) Induction of xenobiotic biotransformation by the insecticide chlordimeform, a metabolite of 4-chloro-o-toluidine and a structurally related chemical o-toluidine. *Biochem. Pharmacol.*, *37*, 2529-2535

Murakami, M. & Fukami, J.-I. (1974) Effects of chlorphenamidine and its metabolites on HeLa cells. *Bull. environ. Contam. Toxicol.*, *11*, 184-188

National Cancer Institute (1979) *Bioassay of 4-Chloro-o-toluidine Hydrochloride for Possible Carcinogenicity (Tech. Rep. Ser. No. 165; DHEW Publ. No. (NIH) 79-1721)*, Washington DC, US Government Printing Office

Neumann, H.-G. (1988) Haemoglobin binding in control of exposure to and risk assessment of aromatic amines. In: Bartsch, H., Hemminki, K. & O'Neill, I.K., eds, *Methods for Detecting DNA Damaging Agents in Humans: Applications in Cancer Epidemiology and Prevention (IARC Scientific Publications No. 89)*, Lyon, IARC, pp. 157-165

Ott, M.G. & Langner, R.R. (1983) A mortality study of men engaged in the manufacture of organic dyes. *J. occup. Med.*, *25*, 763-768

Pouchert, C.J., ed. (1981) *The Aldrich Library of Infrared Spectra*, 3rd ed., Milwaukee, WI, Aldrich Chemical Co., p. 730

Pouchert, C.J., ed. (1983) *The Aldrich Library of NMR Spectra*, 2rd ed., Vol. 1, Milwaukee, WI, Aldrich Chemical Co., p. 1027

Pouchert, C.J., ed. (1985) *The Aldrich Library of FT-IR Spectra*, Vol. 1, Milwaukee, WI, Aldrich Chemical Co., p. 1219

Prager, B., Jacobson, P., Schmidt, P. & Stern, D., eds (1929) *Beilsteins Handbuch der Organischen Chemie*, 4th ed., Vol. 12, Syst. No. 1680-1681, Berlin (West), Springer-Verlag, p. 835

Priha, E., Vuorinen, R., Schimberg, R. & Ahonen, I. (1988) *Tekstiilien Viimeistysaineet* (Textile Finishing Agents) (*Series on Working Conditions No. 65*), Helsinki, Institute of Occupational Health

Rashid, K.A., Ercegovich, C.D. & Mumma, R.O. (1984) Evaluation of chlordimeform and degradation products for mutagenic and DNA-damaging activity in *Salmonella typhimurium* and *Escherichia coli*. *J. environ. Sci. Health*, *B19*, 95-110

Sadtler Research Laboratories (1980) *The Sadtler Standard Spectra, Cumulative Index*, Philadelphia, PA

Schimelpfenig, C.W. (1975) *Ring Chlorination of o-Toluidine (US Patent 3,890,388 (to E.I. du Pont de Nemours & Co.))*

Seiler, J.P. (1977) Inhibition of testicular DNA synthesis by chemical mutagens and carcinogens. Preliminary results in the validation of a novel short-term test. *Mutat. Res.*, *46*, 305-310

Sistovaris, N. & Bartsch, W. (1984) Quantitative thin-layer chromatography for cost-effective, sensitive and selective assaying of aromatic amines in urine. *Fresenius Z. anal. Chem.*, *318*, 271-272

Sittig, M., ed. (1980) *Pesticide Manufacturing and Toxic Materials Control Encyclopedia*, Park Ridge, NJ, Noyes Data Corp., pp. 174-175

Society of Dyers and Colourists (1971) *Colour Index*, 3rd ed., Vol. 4, Bradford, Yorkshire, pp. 4025, 4037, 4042, 4348

Stasik, M.J. (1988) Carcinomas of the urinary bladder in a 4-chloro-o-toluidine cohort. *Int. Arch. occup. environ. Health*, *60*, 21-24

Stasik, M.J., Lange, H.-J., Ulm, K. & Schukmann, F. (1985) A historic cohort study of 4-chloro-2-methylaniline workers. In: *Proceedings of the MEDICHEM Meeting, Bahia, Brazil, 1985*, London, ICI plc, pp. 2-11

Uebelin, F. & Pletscher, A. (1954) Aetiology and prophylaxis of industrial tumours in the dye industry (Ger.). *Schweiz. med. Wochenschr.*, 84, 917-928

US Environmental Protection Agency (1988) Benzenamine, 4-chloro-2-methyl-; benzenamine, 4-chloro-2-methyl-, hydrochloride; benzenamine, 2-chloro-6-methyl-; proposed significant new use of chemical substances. *Fed. Regist.*, 53, 36076-36080

US Tariff Commission (1940) *Synthetic Organic Chemicals, US Production and Sales, 1939 (Report No. 140, Second Series)*, Washington DC, US Government Printing Office, p. 9

US Tariff Commission (1945) *Synthetic Organic Chemicals, US Production and Sales, 1941-43 (Report No. 153, Second Series)*, Washington DC, US Government Printing Office, p. 73

Warner, J.S., Landes, M.C. & Slivon, L.E. (1983) Development of a solvent extraction method for determining semivolatile organic compounds in solid wastes. In: Conway, R.A. & Gulledge, W.P., eds, *Hazardous and Industrial Solid Waste Testing: Second Symposium (ASTM 805)*, Philadelphia, PA, American Society for Testing and Materials, pp. 203-213

Watanabe, Y. & Matsumura, F. (1987) Comparative metabolism of sulfamidine and chlordimeform in rats. *J. agric. Food Chem.*, 35, 379-384

Weast, R.C., ed. (1985) *CRC Handbook of Chemistry and Physics*, 66th ed., Boca Raton, FL, CRC Press, p. C-526

Weisburger, E.K., Russfield, A.B., Homburger, F., Weisburger, J.H., Boger, E., Van Dongen, C.G. & Chu, K.C. (1978) Testing of twenty-one environmental aromatic amines or derivatives for long-term toxicity or carcinogenicity. *J. environ. Pathol. Toxicol.*, 2, 325-356

Zimmer, D., Mazurek, J., Petzold, G. & Bhuyan, B.K. (1980) Bacterial mutagenicity and mammalian cell DNA damage by several substituted anilines. *Mutat. Res.*, 77, 317-326

# DISPERSE BLUE 1

## 1. Chemical and Physical Data

Disperse Blue 1 is produced and used as a mixture of chemicals (see section 1.4). Sections 1.1-1.3 give the chemical and physical characteristics of the principal colour component or of the dye.

### 1.1 Synonyms

*Chem. Abstr. Services Reg. No.*: 2475-45-8
*Chem. Abstr. Name*: 9,10-Anthracenedione, 1,4,5,8-tetraamino-
*IUPAC Systematic Name*: 1,4,5,8-Tetraaminoanthraquinone
*Colour Index No.*: 64500
*Synonyms*: CI Disperse Blue 1; CI Solvent Blue 18; 1,4,5,8-tetraaminoanthraquinone

### 1.2 Structural and molecular formulae and molecular weight of 1,4,5,8-tetraaminoanthraquinone

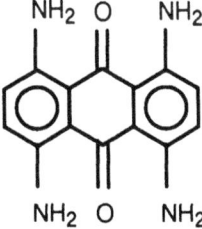

$C_{14}H_{12}N_4O_2$             Mol. wt: 268.28

### 1.3 Chemical and physical properties of Disperse Blue 1

(a) *Description*: Blue-black microcrystalline powder (National Toxicology Program, 1986)

(b) *Melting-point*: 332°C (National Toxicology Program, 1986); >285°C (Nishida *et al.*, 1977)

(c) *Spectroscopy data*: Infrared, ultraviolet and nuclear magnetic resonance spectral data have been reported (National Toxicology Program, 1986); infrared (prism [1477B]; prism-FT [1018A]) spectral data have also been reported by Pouchert (1981, 1985).

(d) *Solubility*: Very slightly soluble in water (30 μg/l at 25°C; Kuroiwa & Ogasawara, 1973); soluble in acetone, ethanol and cellosolve; slightly soluble in benzene and linseed oil (Enviro Control, 1981)

(e) *Volatility*: Vapour pressure, $1.37 \times 10^{-5}$ mm Hg [calculated by the Working Group] (Nishida *et al.*, 1977)

(f) *Stability*: Degrades at > −20°C (National Toxicology Program, 1986)

(g) *Octanol/water partition coefficient (P)*: log P = −0.96 (Baughman & Perenich, 1988)

### 1.4 Technical products and impurities

*Trade Names*: Acetate Blue G; Acetoquinone Blue L; Acetoquinone Blue R; Acetylon Fast Blue G; Amacel Blue GG; Amacel Pure Blue B; Artisil Blue SAP; Artisil Blue SAP Conc; Brasilazet Blue GR; Celanthrene Pure Blue BRS; Celliton Blue BB; Celliton Blue BB-CF; Celliton Blue Extra; Celliton Blue G; Celliton Blue GA; Celliton Blue GA-CF; Cibacet Blue 2GS; Cibacet Sapphire Blue G; Cilla Blue Extra; Diacelliton Fast Blue R; Dianix Blue QTA; Disperse Fast Blue BR; Duranol Brilliant Blue CB; Durosperse Blue CTP; Fenacet Blue G; Fenacet Blue GE; Grasol Blue 2GS; Hisperse Blue PRB; Intrasperse Printing Blue 2B; Intrasperse Sapphire Blue G; Kayalon Fast Blue BR; Microsetile Blue EB; Miketon Fast Blue; Miketon Fast Blue B; Nacelan Blue G; Navicet Blue Extra; Neosetile Blue EB; Nyloquinone Blue 2J; Oracet Sapphire Blue G; Palacet Blue Extra; Pamacel Pure Blue B-I; Perliton Blue B; Serinyl Blue 2G; Serinyl Blue 3G; Serinyl Blue 3GN; Setacyl Blue 2GS; Setacyl Blue 2GS II; Solvent Blue 18; Supracet Brilliant Blue 2GN; Supracet Deep Blue R

Commercial preparations of Disperse Blue 1 (approximately 50% 1,4,5,8-tetraaminoanthraquinone, 30% structurally related compounds and 20% water) contain approximately equal amounts of dyestuff and lignosulfonate dispersants (Burnett & Squire, 1986; National Toxicology Program, 1986). One US distributor markets Disperse Blue 1 with a dye content of approximately 30% (Aldrich Chemical Co., 1988).

## 2. Production, Use, Occurrence and Analysis

### 2.1 Production and use

(a) *Production*

Disperse Blue 1 has been prepared by acylation of 1,5-diaminoanthraquinone with oxalic acid, then nitration in sulfuric acid, followed by hydrolysis and reduction to the tetraamino compound; and by the reduction of mixed 1,5- and 1,8-dinitroanthraquinone to the corresponding diamino compounds, followed by acetylation, nitration, reduction and hydrolysis (Society of Dyers and Colourists, 1971).

US production of Disperse Blue 1 was reported to be 159 tonnes in 1972 (US Tariff Commission, 1974). Separate figures were not reported after 1972, but production of all Disperse Blue dyes was approximately 6030, 9940 and 5740 tonnes in 1975, 1980 and 1985, respectively (US International Trade Commission, 1977, 1981, 1986). Disperse Blue 1 is no longer produced in the USA, but approximately 4-6 tonnes of the material are imported annually (National Toxicology Program, 1986).

No information on production of this dye in other countries was available to the Working Group.

*(b) Use*

Disperse Blue 1 is used in the USA in semipermanent hair colour formulations (see IARC, 1982) at concentrations of less than 1%. The solubility of the material in these preparations (approximately 500 ppm [mg/l]) is considerably greater than its solubility in water (National Toxicology Program, 1986).

Disperse Blue 1 has been used as a fabric dye for nylon, cellulose acetate and triacetate, polyester and acrylate fibres. It has also been used for surface dyeing of thermoplastics and as a solvent dye in cellulose acetate plastics (Enviro Control, 1981).

*(c) Regulatory status and guidelines*

No regulatory standard or guideline has been established for Disperse Blue 1.

## 2.2 Occurrence

*(a) Natural occurrence*

Disperse Blue 1 is not known to occur as a natural product.

*(b) Occupational exposure*

No data were available to the Working Group on exposure levels in the workplace; however, since Disperse Blue 1 is used in hair dyes, dermal and inhalation exposures may occur among people producing and applying such products.

## 2.3 Analysis

A method has been described for the spectrophotometric determination of Disperse Blue 1 sorbed on polyethylene terephthalate fibres by dye extraction in mixed solvent systems (Madan & Khan, 1978). A polarographic method for the determination of aminoanthraquinones, including 1,4,5,8-tetraaminoanthraquinone, in environmental and biological samples can be used to determine concentrations as low as 0.1-0.5 mg/ml (Popescu & Barbacaru, 1985).

# 3. Biological Data Relevant to the Evaluation of Carcinogenic Risk to Humans

## 3.1 Carcinogenicity studies in animals

*Oral administration*

*Mouse*: Groups of 50 male and 50 female B6C3F$_1$ mice, seven weeks of age, were fed diets containing 0, 600, 1200 or 2500 ppm (mg/kg) diet Disperse Blue 1 (commercial grade without lignosulfonate dispersants, containing approximately 50% 1,4,5,8-tetraaminoanthraquinone, 19.5% water and ~30% other impurities, mainly an isomer of tetraaminoanthraquinone and a nitrotriaminoanthraquinone isomer) for 104 weeks to give doses in mg/kg bw per day of 0, 112, 239 and 540 in males and 0, 108, 235 and 520 in females. All animals were killed at 112-113 weeks of age. A significant trend to lower survival in higher dose males was observed when early deaths were excluded. The combined incidences of hepatocellular adenomas and carcinomas were increased in treated males (control, 9/50; low-dose, 21/50; mid-dose, 20/50; high dose, 16/50) and in low-dose females (control, 3/50; low-dose, 13/49; mid-dose, 3/50; high-dose, 4/50). Group incidences did not indicate a dose-response effect, and survival-adjusted trends were not significant. The observed incidences of alveolar/bronchiolar adenomas and carcinomas in male mice were 4/50 in controls, 9/49 in low-dose animals, 5/50 in mid-dose animals and 11/50 in high-dose animals. When adjusted for survival, the increase was dose-related ($p = 0.018$, incidental tumour test for trend; adjusted rates, 15.0, 27.2, 13.9 and 49.3%, respectively). A high incidence of urinary bladder calculi was observed in mice of each sex. High-dose males and females also had a high incidence of transitional-cell hyperplasia of the bladder (National Toxicology Program, 1986).

*Rat*: Groups of 50 male and 50 female Fischer 344/N rats, seven weeks of age, were fed diets containing 0, 1250, 2500 or 5000 ppm (mg/kg) diet Disperse Blue 1 (same grade as above) for 103 weeks to give doses in mg/kg bw per day of 0, 45, 95 and 217 in males and 0, 56, 111 and 240 in females. All animals were killed at 111-112 weeks of age. Survival in high-dose males and females and in mid-dose males was significantly reduced. Dose-related increases in the combined incidences of squamous-cell papillomas and carcinomas, transitional-cell papillomas and carcinomas, and leiomyomas and leiomyosarcomas of the bladder were observed in males and females. In addition, urinary bladder calculi were observed in the groups of rats in which the incidence of bladder tumours was increased (see Table 1). A dose-related increase in the incidence of pancreatic islet-cell adenomas and carcinomas combined was seen in males: control, 1/49; low-dose, 2/50; mid-dose, 5/50; high-dose, 3/50 ($p = 0.042$, incidental tumour test for trend; National Toxicology Program, 1986).

Table 1. Incidence of urinary bladder lesions in rats fed Disperse Blue 1[a]

| Urinary bladder lesion | Dose group | | | | Incidental tumour test for trend |
|---|---|---|---|---|---|
| | Control | 1250 ppm | 2500 ppm | 5000 ppm | |
| **Males** | | | | | |
| Squamous–cell papillomas and carcinomas | 0/49 | 0/50 | 2/50 | 4/49 | $p = 0.02$ |
| Transitional–cell papillomas and carcinomas | 0/49 | 0/50 | 10/50 | 11/49 | $p = 0.001$ |
| Leiomyomas and leiomyosarcomas | 0/49 | 0/50 | 7/50 | 41/49 | $p < 0.001$ |
| Calculi (gross) | 0/49 | 0/50 | 16/50 | 21/49 | |
| **Females** | | | | | |
| Squamous–cell papillomas and carcinomas | 0/48 | 0/50 | 1/50 | 11/48 | $p < 0.001$ |
| Transitional–cell papillomas and carcinomas | 0/48 | 0/50 | 15/50 | 21/48 | $p < 0.001$ |
| Leiomyomas and leiomyosarcomas | 0/48 | 0/50 | 3/50 | 26/48 | $p < 0.001$ |
| Calculi (gross) | 0/48 | 0/50 | 12/50 | 37/48 | |

[a]From National Toxicology Program (1986)

### 3.2 Other relevant biological data

(a) *Experimental systems*

(i) *Absorption, distribution, excretion and metabolism*

No data were available to the Working Group.

(ii) *Toxic effects*

The oral $LD_{50}$ value for various dyes, including Disperse Blue 1, in rats ranged from 1.2 to >6.3 g/kg bw (Wernick *et al.*, 1975).

Disperse Blue 1 (containing 50% lignosulfonate dispersants) was administered to Fischer 344 rats in two short-term and one long-term studies. In one short-term study, it was given either by gavage at 1 g/kg bw for one to three days or in the diet at 1% for four days, and rats were killed the following day. In the second short-term study, it was given for four days, both orally by gavage at 1 g/kg bw and at dietary levels of 0.5% commercial dye or 0.25% and 0.5% dye without dispersants. In the long-term study, the dye was administered to rats at dietary levels of 0, 0.01, 0.10 and 1.0% for up to 19 months; interim sacrifices were made for tritiated thymidine autoradiography of the bladder and examination of the principal body organs. Administration by gavage resulted in accumulation of the dye within the renal tubules and nephropathy within three days. Dietary dosing with 1% resulted in low-grade hyperplasia of the bladder urothelium, epithelial erosion, with adhesion of dye particles, and submucosal oedema after four days. At weeks 5, 9 and 17, there was increased DNA synthesis in the urothelium of high-dose rats but no increased labelling in any other group. Bladder lesions were seen only at the 1% level; epithelial erosion with adhering dye particles was seen by day 4, calculi and hyperplasia by week 5 and squamous metaplasia by week 9. The calculi contained more dye in males than in females and more calcium in females than in males. By month 6, dye particles were embedded in the bladder wall, with some evidence of histiocyte accumulation in their vicinity (Burnett & Squire, 1986).

Disperse Blue 1 was administered to Fischer 344/N rats and B6C3F$_1$ mice by oral administration in the diet for 14 days, 13 weeks or two years. In the 14-day studies, 2/5 female rats died after receiving 50 000 ppm [mg/kg], and all mice receiving 25 000 ppm or more died. In the 13-week studies, diets containing concentrations up to 20 000 and 10 000 ppm were fed to rats and mice, respectively. No compound-related death occurred in rats, but deaths occurred with 10 000 ppm in mice of each sex. Pathological changes that occurred in rats and mice given diets containing 2500 ppm or more included urinary tract calculi, urinary bladder inflammation, hyperplasia of the urinary bladder transitional epithelium and nephrosis. In the two-year studies (see also section 3.1), lesions related to treatment in rats included renal and urinary bladder calculi, renal casts, hydronephrosis and renal degeneration, renal and urinary bladder epithelial hyperplasia, urinary bladder squamous metaplasia and pigmentation of the urinary bladder and kidney. Lesions in mice that were considered to be related to treatment were inflammation, epithelial hyperplasia, calculi and fibrosis in the urinary bladder, casts in the renal tubular lumina and renal tubular degeneration (National Toxicology Program, 1986).

(iii) *Effects on reproduction and prenatal toxicity*

Oral administration of a commercial product (a composite of dyes and base components found in semipermanent hair dyes) containing 0.61% Disperse Blue 1 among other dyes had no effect on fertility, gestation, lactation or viability indices in rats and induced no teratogenicity in rats or rabbits (Wernick *et al.*, 1975).

(iv) *Genetic and related effects*

Disperse Blue was weakly mutagenic to *Salmonella typhimurium* TA1537, in the presence and absence of an exogenous metabolic system from Aroclor 1254-induced rat liver; it was not mutagenic to several other strains (Brown & Brown, 1976). In liquid preincubation asssays, it was mutagenic to TA1535, TA97 and TA98 (National Toxicology Program, 1986).

(b) *Humans*

No data were available to the Working Group.

### 3.3 Case reports and epidemiological studies of carcinogenicity to humans

No data were available to the Working Group.

## 4. Summary of Data Reported and Evaluation

### 4.1 Exposure data

Disperse Blue 1 is an aminoanthraquinone-based dyestuff used in hair colour formulations and in colouring fabrics and plastics. No data on occupational exposure levels were available.

### 4.2 Experimental carcinogenicity data

Disperse Blue 1 was tested for carcinogenicity by oral administration in one strain of mice and in one strain of rats. In mice, it produced an increase in the incidence of alveolar/bronchiolar adenomas and carcinomas (combined) and a marginal increase in the incidence of hepatocellular tumours in treated males. In rats of each sex, it produced transitional-cell papillomas and carcinomas, squamous-cell papillomas and carcinomas, and leiomyomas and leiomyosarcomas of the urinary bladder; in addition, urinary bladder calculi were observed in the groups of rats in which the incidence of urinary bladder neoplasms was increased. In male rats, the incidence of islet-cell adenomas and carcinomas of the pancreas was marginally increased.

### 4.3 Human carcinogenicity data

No data were available to the Working Group.

### 4.4 Other relevant data

Calculi were observed in the urinary tract of rats and mice given Disperse Blue 1 in the diet. Urinary bladder lesions included epithelial hyperplasia in rats and mice and squamous metaplasia in rats. Hyperplasia of the transitional epithelium of the renal pelvis occurred in rats.

Disperse Blue 1 was mutagenic to bacteria in the presence and absence of an exogenous metabolic system.

### 4.5 Evaluation[1]

There is *sufficient evidence* for the carcinogenicity of Disperse Blue 1 in experimental animals.

No data were available from studies in humans on the carcinogenicity of Disperse Blue 1.

---

[1]For description of the italicized terms and criteria for making the evaluation, see Preamble, pp. 25-29.

## Summary table of genetic and related effects of Disperse Blue 1

| Nonmammalian systems | | | | | | | | | | | | | Mammalian systems | | | | | | | | | | | | | | | | |
|---|---|---|---|---|---|---|---|---|---|---|---|---|---|---|---|---|---|---|---|---|---|---|---|---|---|---|---|---|---|
| Proka- ryotes | Lower eukaryotes | | | | Plants | | | Insects | | | In vitro | | | | | | | | | | | | | In vivo | | | | | |
| | | | | | | | | | | | Animal cells | | | | | | | Human cells | | | | | | Animals | | | | Humans | | |
| D | D | G | R | G | A | D | G | C | R | G | C | A | D | G | S | M | C | A | T | I | D | G | S | M | C | A | T | I | D | G | S | M | C | DL | A | D | S | M | C | A |
| | + | | | | | | | | | | | | | | | | | | | | | | | | | | | | | | | | | | | | | | | |

A, aneuploidy; C, chromosomal aberrations; D, DNA damage; DL, dominant lethal mutation; G, gene mutation; I, inhibition of intercellular communication; M, micronuclei; R, mitotic recombination and gene conversion; S, sister chromatid exchange; T, cell transformation

*In completing the table, the following symbol indicates the consensus of the Working Group with regard to the results for each endpoint:*
+ considered to be positive for the specific endpoint and level of biological complexity

**Overall evaluation**

Disperse Blue 1 is *possibly carcinogenic to humans (Group 2B)*.

# 5. References

Aldrich Chemical Co. (1988) *1988-1989 Aldrich Catalog/Handbook of Fine Chemicals*, Milwaukee, WI, p. 653

Baughman, G.L. & Perenich, T.A. (1988) Fate of dyes in aquatic systems: I. Solubility and partitioning of some hydrophobic dyes and related compounds. *Environ. Toxicol. Chem.*, 7, 183-199

Brown, J.P. & Brown, R.J. (1976) Mutagenesis by 9,10-anthraquinone derivatives and related compounds in *Salmonella typhimurium*. *Mutat. Res.*, 40, 203-224

Burnett, C.M. & Squire, R.A. (1986) The effect of dietary administration of Disperse Blue 1 on the urinary system of the Fischer 344 rat. *Food chem. Toxicol.*, 24, 269-276

Enviro Control (1981) *Anthraquinone Dye Toxicological Profiles (CSPC-Mono-82-2; US NTIS PB83-166033)*, Rockville, MD

IARC (1982) *IARC Monographs on the Evaluation of the Carcinogenic Risk of Chemicals to Humans*, Vol. 27, *Some Aromatic Amines, Anthraquinones and Nitroso Compounds, and Inorganic Fluorides Used in Drinking-water and Dental Preparations*, Lyon, pp. 307-318

Kuroiwa, S. & Ogasawara, S. (1973) Studies on the dispersed state of dyes and their dyeing properties. VIII. Solubilities of disperse dyes in water (Jpn.). *Nippon Kagaku Kaishi*, 9, 1738-1743

Madan, G.L. & Khan, A.H. (1978) Determination of dye on textile fibers. I. Disperse dyes on polyethylene terephthalate. *Text. Res. J.*, 48, 481-486

National Toxicology Program (1986) *Toxicology and Carcinogenesis Studies of C.I. Disperse Blue 1 (A Commercial Dye Containing Approximately 50% 1,4,5,8-Tetraaminoanthraquinone, 30% Other Compounds Structurally Related to 1,4,5,8-Tetraaminoanthraquinone, and 20% Water) (CAS No. 2475-45-8) in F344/N Rats and B6C3F$_1$ Mice (Feed Studies) (Technical Report No. 299)*, Research Triangle Park, NC, US Department of Health and Human Services

Nishida, K., Ishihara, E., Osaka, T. & Koukitu, M. (1977) Vapour pressures and heats of sublimation of some disperse dyes. *J. Soc. Dyers Colour.*, 93, 52-54

Popescu, S.D. & Barbacaru, E. (1985) A polarographic study of some aminoanthraquinones. *Anal. Lett.*, 18, 947-956

Pouchert, C.J., ed. (1981) *The Aldrich Library of Infrared Spectra*, 3rd ed., Milwaukee, WI, Aldrich Chemical Co., p. 1477

Pouchert, C.J., ed. (1985) *The Aldrich Library of FT-IR Spectra*, Vol. 2, Milwaukee, WI, Aldrich Chemical Co., p. 1018

Society of Dyers and Colourists (1971) *Colour Index*, 3rd. ed., Vol. 4, Bradford, Yorkshire, p. 4557

US International Trade Commission (1977) *Synthetic Organic Chemicals, US Production and Sales, 1975 (USITC Publication 804)*, Washington DC, US Government Printing Office, p. 51

US International Trade Commission (1981) *Synthetic Organic Chemicals, US Production and Sales, 1980 (USITC Publication 1183)*, Washington DC, US Government Printing Office, p. 68

US International Trade Commission (1986) *Synthetic Organic Chemicals, US Production and Sales, 1985 (USITC Publication 1892)*, Washington DC, US Government Printing Office, p. 59

US Tariff Commission (1974) *Synthetic Organic Chemicals, US Production and Sales, 1972 (TC Publication 681)*, Washington DC, US Government Printing Office, p. 62

Wernick, T., Lanman, B.M. & Fraux, J.L. (1975) Chronic toxicity, teratologic and reproduction studies with hair dyes. *Toxicol. appl. Pharmacol.*, *32*, 450-460

# DISPERSE YELLOW 3

Disperse Yellow 3 was evaluated by a previous working group (IARC, 1975)[1]. Since that time, new data have become available, and these have been incorporated into the monograph and taken into consideration in the present evaluation.

## 1. Chemical and Physical Data

Disperse Yellow 3 is produced and used as a mixture of chemicals (see section 1.4). Sections 1.1-1.3 give the chemical and physical characteristics of the principal colour component or of the dye.

### 1.1 Synonyms

*Chem. Abstr. Services Reg. No.*: 2832-40-8
(Replaced CAS Reg. Nos 12227-01-9, 12238-70-9 and 66057-65-6)
*Chem. Abstr. Name*: Acetamide, N-{4-[(2-hydroxy-5-methylphenyl)azo]phenyl}-
*IUPAC Systematic Names*: 4'-[(6-Hydroxy-*meta*-tolyl)azo]acetanilide; CI Disperse Yellow 3
*Colour Index No.*: 11855
*Synonyms*: 4-Acetamido-2'-hydroxy-5'-methylazobenzene; CI Solvent Yellow 77; CI Solvent Yellow 92; CI Solvent Yellow 99; 4'-[(2-hydroxy-5-methylphenyl)azo]acetanilide; 4'-(6-hydroxy-*meta*-tolylazo)acetanilide

---

[1]The earlier evaluation of the carcinogenicity of this compound was based on the results of a study in experimental animals by Boyland *et al.* (1964), which was subsequently found to concern an isomer of Disperse Yellow 3.

## 1.2 Structural and molecular formulae and molecular weight of the principal component

$$\text{HO-C}_6\text{H}_2(\text{CH}_3)\text{-N=N-C}_6\text{H}_4\text{-NH-CO-CH}_3$$

$C_{15}H_{15}N_3O_2$    Mol. wt: 269.30

## 1.3 Chemical and physical properties of Disperse Yellow 3

(a) *Melting-point*: Decomposes at 192-195°C (National Toxicology Program, 1982); 195°C (Patterson & Sheldon, 1960)

(b) *Spectroscopy data*: Infrared (prism [1452A]; prism-FT [969A]) and ultraviolet spectral data have been reported (Pouchert, 1981; National Toxicology Program, 1982; Pouchert, 1985).

(c) *Solubility*: Soluble in acetone, ethanol and benzene (Society of Dyers and Colourists, 1971a); soluble in water at 1.5-6.1 mg/l at 60°C (Patterson & Sheldon, 1960)

## 1.4 Technical products and impurities

*Trade Names*: Acetamine Yellow CG; Acetate Fast Yellow G; Acetoquinone Light Yellow 4JLZ; Altco Sperse Fast Yellow GFN New; Amacel Yellow G; Atrisil Direct Yellow G; Atrisil Yellow G; Atrisil Yellow 2GN; Calcosyn Yellow GCN; Celliton Discharge Yellow GL; Celliton Fast Yellow G; Celliton Fast Yellow GA; Celliton Fast Yellow GA-CF; Celliton Yellow G; Celutate Yellow GH; Cibacet Yellow GBA; Cibacet Yellow 2GC; Cilla Fast Yellow G; Diacelliton Fast Yellow G; Disperse Yellow G; Disperse Yellow Z; Dispersol Fast Yellow G; Dispersol Printing Yellow G; Dispersol Yellow A-G; Dispersyl Fast Yellow J; Durgacet Yellow G; Dursperse Yellow G; Eastone Yellow GN; Esteroquinone Light Yellow 4JL; Fenacet Fast Yellow G; Hispacet Fast Yellow G; Hisperse Yellow G; Interchem Acetate Yellow G; Interchem Hisperse Yellow GH; Intrasperse Yellow GBA; Intrasperse Yellow GBA Extra; Kayalon Fast Yellow G; Kayaset Yellow G; KCA Acetate Fast Yellow G; Lurafix Yellow 142; Microsetile Yellow GR; Miketon Fast Yellow G; Nacelan Fast Yellow CG; Navicet Yellow G; Navilene Yellow G; Novalon Yellow 2GN; Nyloquinone Yellow 4J; Ostacet Yellow P2G; Palacet Yellow GN; Palanil Yellow G; Pamacel Yellow G-3; Perliton Yellow G; Reliton Yellow C; Resiren Yellow TG; Safaritone Yellow G; Serinyl Hosiery Yellow GD; Seriplas Yellow GD; Serisol Fast Yellow GD; Setacyl Yellow G; Setacyl Yellow 2GN; Setacyl Yellow P 2GL; Silotras Yellow TSG; Sumiplast Yellow FC; Supracet Fast Yellow G; Synten Yellow 2G; Terasil Yellow GBA Extra; Terasil Yellow 2GC; Tertranese Yellow N-2GL; Transetile Yellow P-GR; Tuladisperse Fast Yellow 2G; Vonteryl Yellow G; Vonteryl Yellow R; Yellow Reliton G; Yellow Z

Analysis of a commercial batch of Disperse Yellow 3 before formulation indicated approximately 87.6% dyestuff, 7% water, 4% sodium chloride and 1% sodium carbonate. Several impurities were detected but were not identified (National Toxicology Program, 1982). In commercial formulations, the dyestuff content is approximately 42-44%.

## 2. Production, Use, Occurrence and Analysis

### 2.1 Production and use

*(a) Production*

Disperse Yellow 3 was first prepared by Fischer and Müller (1926) by coupling diazotized 4-acetamidoaniline with *para*-cresol, but it is not known whether this is the method used for commercial production.

Large-scale production of Disperse Yellow 3 in the USA was first reported in 1941 (US Tariff Commission, 1945). US production of Disperse Yellow 3 in 1972, 1975, 1979 and 1980 was 1280, 1420, 1460 and 930 tonnes, respectively (US Tariff Commission, 1974; US International Trade Commission, 1977, 1980, 1981). Separate figures were not reported after 1980. Production of all Disperse Yellow dyes ranged from a low of approximately 760 tonnes in 1985 to a high of approximately 1490 tonnes in 1983 (US International Trade Commission, 1983-1988).

As many as 11 companies may manufacture this dye in western Europe, with an estimated annual total production of 1 million kg. Production of Disperse Yellow 3 by three Japanese manufacturers was 82 tonnes 1972 and 44 tonnes in 1973 (IARC, 1975). This dye is also manufactured in India.

*(b) Use*

Disperse Yellow 3 is a monoazo pigment dye of low aqueous solubility, used to colour nylon, polyvinyl chloride and acrylic fibres, wools and furs, cellulose acetate, polystyrene and other thermoplastics. Finished products containing this material include clothing, hosiery and carpeting (Society of Dyers and Colourists, 1971b; Foussereau *et al.*, 1972; National Toxicology Program, 1982).

*(c) Regulatory status and guidelines*

No regulatory standard or guideline has been established for Disperse Yellow 3.

### 2.2 Occurrence

*(a) Natural occurrence*

Disperse Yellow 3 is not known to occur as a natural product.

*(b) Occupational exposure*

Approximately 17 000 workers were estimated to be potentially exposed to Disperse Yellow 3 in the USA in 1972-74 (National Institute for Occupational Safety and Health, 1977).

(c) *Water and sediments*

Disperse Yellow 3 was identified in wastewater and mud samples from the Coosa River Basin, Atlanta, GA, USA. The Coosa River Basin and its tributaries carry approximately 50% of all carpet dyeing wastewater in the USA. Concentrations of Disperse Yellow 3 in samples of waste treatment plant influents and effluents ranged from none detected to 436 ppb (µg/l). Concentrations in mud samples ranged from 140 to 455 ppb (µg/kg; Tincher & Robertson, 1982).

(d) *Other*

Disperse Yellow 3 was identified in dichloromethane extracts of 51 out of 52 beige stockings and pantihose collected in Belgium, France, the Federal Republic of Germany, Italy, Portugal, Romania and the UK (Berger *et al.*, 1984).

## 2.3 Analysis

Selected methods for the analysis of Disperse Yellow 3 are given in Table 1.

**Table 1. Methods for the analysis of Disperse Yellow 3**

| Sample matrix | Sample preparation[a] | Assay procedure[a] | Limit of detection | Reference |
|---|---|---|---|---|
| Air | Collect on filter; extract with solvent; separate by TLC | Spectrophotometry | 0.5 mg/m$^3$ | Zenina *et al.* (1986) |
| Wastewater | Adsorb on macroreticular resin; recover by backwashing with solvents | HPLC | 0.1 ppm (mg/l) | Tincher & Robertson (1982) |
| Hosiery | Extract with dichloromethane; evaporate; dissolve in dichloromethane | TLC | Not reported | Berger *et al.* (1984) |
| Dye lots | Extract with hexane/-ethanol; evaporate; dissolve in dichloromethane | TLC | Not reported | Foussereau & Dallara (1986) |
| Hand skin wash-off samples | Extract with ethanol/water; concentrate; resuspend with solvent; separate by TLC | Spectrophotometry | Not reported | Zenina *et al.* (1986) |
| Dyestuffs | Extract with solvent | TLC | Not reported | Foussereau *et al.* (1972) |

[a]Abbreviations: TLC, thin-layer chromatography; HPLC, high-performance liquid chromatography

# 3. Biological Data Relevant to the Evaluation of Carcinogenic Risk to Humans

## 3.1 Carcinogenicity studies in animals

*Oral administration*

*Mouse*: Groups of 50 male and 50 female B6C3F$_1$ mice, six weeks of age, were fed diets containing 2500 or 5000 mg/kg Disperse Yellow 3 (87.6% dye [impurities unspecified]) for 103 weeks and were observed for two additional weeks. Groups of 50 male and 50 female mice served as untreated controls. All animals were killed at 111 weeks of age. Mean body weights of mice of each sex tended to be lower those of than controls; survival was comparable in all groups. The incidence of hepatocellular adenomas was significantly ($p < 0.001$, Cochran-Armitage test) increased in treated females: controls, 0/50; low-dose, 6/50; high-dose, 12/50. The incidence of hepatocellular carcinomas was also increased in treated females, but not significantly (control, 2/50; low-dose, 4/50; high-dose, 5/50). A significantly ($p = 0.019$, Cochran-Armitage test) increased incidence of alveolar/bronchiolar adenomas was observed in male mice: control, 2/50; low-dose, 6/49; high-dose, 9/49; and a significant ($p = 0.032$, Cochran-Armitage test) increase in the incidence of malignant lymphomas was observed in female mice (control, 10/50; low-dose, 16/50; high-dose, 19/50; National Toxicology Program, 1982).

*Rat*: Groups of 50 male and 50 female Fischer 344/N rats, six weeks of age, were fed diets containing 5000 or 10 000 mg/kg of diet Disperse Yellow 3 (87.6% dye [impurities unspecified]) for 103 weeks and were observed for one additional week. Groups of 50 male and 50 female rats served as untreated controls. All animals were killed at 111 weeks of age. Mean body weights of treated rats of each sex were lower than those of controls; survival in male and female treated rats was significantly longer than that in corresponding controls. A significant ($p = 0.014$, Cochran-Armitage test) increase in the incidence of neoplastic nodules in the liver [adenomas (Maronpot *et al.*, 1986)] was observed in treated males: controls, 1/49; low-dose, 15/50; high-dose, 10/50. The incidence of foci of altered hepatocytes in males, predominantly composed of vacuolated, clear and eosinophilic cells, was dose-related (controls, 1/49; low-dose, 4/50; high-dose, 17/50). Stomach tumours were also observed in treated males, with one adenocarcinoma and a sarcoma in a high-dose male and one squamous-cell papilloma, one fibrosarcoma, one adenoma and one mucinous adenocarcinoma in animals in the low-dose group. This incidence was not significantly higher than that in controls. Analysis by a survival-adjusted test did not change the results (National Toxicology Program, 1982).

## 3.2 Other relevant biological data

(a) *Experimental systems*

(i) *Absorption, distribution, excretion and metabolism*

No data were available to the Working Group.

(ii) *Toxic effects*

In 14-day studies in which Disperse Yellow 3 was incorporated into the diet of Fischer 344 rats and B6C3F$_1$ mice, rats died at concentrations of 50 000 ppm (mg/kg) and higher, and mice at a concentration of 100 000 ppm. Splenic enlargement was noted in mice given 25 000 ppm and more (National Toxicology Program, 1982).

Of Fischer 344 rats and B6C3F$_1$ mice fed Disperse Yellow 3 (1250 to 20 000 ppm) in the diet for 13 weeks and then killed, 1/10 high-dose female rats died; no other death appeared to be related to treatment. Weight gains were depressed in rats and mice receiving diets containing 10 000 ppm or more. In rats, proliferative lesions of the thyroid follicular cells were observed as well as vacuolar degeneration of the pars distalis of the pituitary gland, haemosiderosis in the spleen and pigment deposition in the kidney. In mice, haemosiderosis of the renal tubular epithelium and spleen and cytoplasmic swelling of centrilobular hepatocytes were related to treatment (National Toxicology Program, 1982).

(iii) *Effects on reproduction and prenatal toxicity*

No data were available to the Working Group.

(iv) *Genetic and related effects*

Disperse Yellow 3 was mutagenic to several frame-shift mutants of *Salmonella typhimurium* in the presence and absence of an exogenous metabolic system from Aroclor 1254-induced rat liver or Syrian hamster liver; however, it was not mutagenic to strain TA1535 (Cameron *et al.*, 1987; Zeiger *et al.*, 1988). In one of the studies, it was mutagenic to TA100 only in the presence of a metabolic system from Syrian hamsters (Cameron *et al.*, 1987).

Disperse Yellow 3 was reported to cause unscheduled DNA synthesis in primary cultures of rat hepatocytes [details not given] (Tennant *et al.*, 1987a). In one study, it was weakly mutagenic at the TK locus in mouse lymphoma cells in culture in the absence of an exogenous metabolic system (Cameron *et al.*, 1987); in another, it was mutagenic in the presence of an exogenous metabolic system (McGregor *et al.*, 1988). It induced sister chromatid exchanges, but not chromosomal aberrations in the Chinese hamster CHO cell line in the absence of an exogenous metabolic system from Aroclor 1254-induced rat liver (Tennant *et al.*, 1987b).

(b) *Humans*

(i) *Absorption, distribution, excretion and metabolism*

No data were available to the Working Group.

(ii) *Toxic effects*

Textiles coloured with dyes containing Disperse Yellow 3 caused allergic, contact-type dermatitis (Dobkevitch & Baer, 1947; Cronin, 1968; Foussereau *et al.*, 1971, 1972; Conde-Salazar *et al.*, 1984). Skin tests with isolated dyes indicated that Disperse Yellow 3 is a contact allergen (Cronin, 1968; Kousa & Soini, 1980; Hausen & Schulz, 1984).

(iii) *Effects on reproduction and prenatal toxicity*

No data were available to the Working Group.

(iv) *Genetic and related effects*

No data were available to the Working Group.

## 3.3 Case reports and epidemiological studies of carcinogenicity to humans

No data were available to the Working Group.

# 4. Summary of Data Reported and Evaluation

## 4.1 Exposure data

Disperse Yellow 3 is a monoazo pigment dye which has been produced in significant quantities since the 1940s to colour fabrics and plastics. There is potentially widespread exposure to Disperse Yellow 3 because of its use in clothing, hosiery and carpets. No data on occupational exposure levels were available.

## 4.2 Experimental carcinogenicity data

Disperse Yellow 3 was tested for carcinogenicity by oral administration in one strain of mice and in one strain of rats. In female mice, it produced increases in the incidences of hepatocellular tumours and malignant lymphomas; in male mice, the incidence of alveolar/bronchiolar adenomas was increased. In rats, it produced an increase in the incidence of hepatocellular adenomas in males.

## 4.3 Human carcinogenicity data

No data were available to the Working Group.

## 4.4 Other relevant data

In a single study, Disperse Yellow 3 induced sister chromatid exchange but not chromosomal aberrations in Chinese hamster cells in culture. It was mutagenic to mouse cells in culture. Disperse Yellow 3 was mutagenic to bacteria in the presence and absence of an exogenous metabolic system.

## Summary table of genetic and related effects of Disperse Yellow 3

| Nonmammalian systems | | | | | | | | | | | | | Mammalian systems | | | | | | | | | | | | | | | | | | | |
|---|---|---|---|---|---|---|---|---|---|---|---|---|---|---|---|---|---|---|---|---|---|---|---|---|---|---|---|---|---|---|---|---|
| Proka-ryotes | | Lower eukaryotes | | | | Plants | | | | Insects | | | | In vitro | | | | | | | | | | | | | In vivo | | | | | |
| | | | | | | | | | | | | | | Animal cells | | | | | | | | Human cells | | | | | | Animals | | | | | Humans | | |
| D | G | D | R | G | A | D | G | C | A | R | G | C | A | D | G | S | M | C | A | T | I | D | G | S | M | C | A | T | I | D | G | S | M | C | DL | A | D | S | M | C | A |
| | + | | | | | | | | | | | | | | | +¹ | | | | -¹ | | | | | | | | | | | | | | | | | | | | | |

A, aneuploidy; C, chromosomal aberrations; D, DNA damage; DL, dominant lethal mutation; G, gene mutation; I, inhibition of intercellular communication; M, micronuclei; R, mitotic recombination and gene conversion; S, sister chromatid exchange; T, cell transformation

*In completing the table, the following symbols indicate the consensus of the Working Group with regard to the results for each endpoint:*

+ considered to be positive for the specific endpoint and level of biological complexity
+¹ considered to be positive, but only one valid study was available to the Working Group
-  considered to be negative, but only one valid study was available to the Working Group

### 4.5 Evaluation[1]

There is *limited evidence* for the carcinogenicity of Disperse Yellow 3 in experimental animals.

No data were available from studies in humans on the carcinogenicity of Disperse Yellow 3.

**Overall evaluation**

Disperse Yellow 3 is *not classifiable as to its carcinogenicity to humans (Group 3)*.

## 5. References

Berger, C., Muslmani, M., Menezes Brandao, F. & Foussereau, J. (1984) Thin-layer chromatography search for Disperse Yellow 3 and Disperse Orange 3 in 52 stockings and pantyhose. *Contact Derm.*, 10, 154-157

Boyland, E., Busby, E.R., Dukes, C.E., Grover, P.L. & Manson, D. (1964) Further experiments on implantation of materials into the urinary bladder of mice. *Br. J. Cancer*, 18, 575-581

Cameron, T.P., Hughes, T.J., Kirby, P.E., Fung, V.A. & Dunkel, V.C. (1987) Mutagenic activity of 27 dyes and related chemicals in the *Salmonella*/microsome and mouse lymphoma TK$^{+/-}$ assays. *Mutat. Res.*, 189, 223-261

Conde-Salazar, L., Guimeraens, D., Domero, L. & Harto, A. (1984) Contact dermatis after azo dyes (Sp.). *Med. Segur. Trab.*, 31, 29-34

Cronin, E. (1968) Studies in contact dermatitis. XVIII. Dyes in clothing. XIX. Nylon stocking dyes. *Trans. St John's Hosp. Dermatol. Soc.*, 54, 156-169

Dobkevitch, S. & Baer, R.L. (1947) Eczematous cross-hypersensitivity to azodyes in nylon stockings and to *para*-phenylenediamine. *J. invest. Dermatol.*, 9, 203-211

Fischer, E. & Müller, E. (1926) *Dyeing and Printing Cellulose Esters or Ethers. German Patent 469,514* (24 April to I. Farbernind, A.-G.)

Foussereau, J. & Dallara, J.M. (1986) Purity of standardized textile dye allergens: a thin layer chromatography study. *Contact Derm.*, 14, 303-306

Foussereau, J., Sengel, D., Tanahashi, Y., Limam-Mestiri, S. & Malaville, J. (1971) Allergy due to Disperse Yellow 3 of clothing dyes (stockings and socks). Detection of this dye in commercial products (Fr.). *Bull. Soc. fr. Derm. Syphiligr.*, 78, 70-73

Foussereau, J., Tanahashi, Y., Grosshans, E., Liman-Mestiri, S. & Khochnevis, A. (1972) Allergic eczema from Disperse Yellow 3 in nylon stockings and socks. *Trans. St John's Hosp. Dermatol. Soc.*, 58, 75-80

---

[1]For description of the italicized terms and criteria for making the evaluation, see Preamble, pp. 25-29.

Hausen, B.M. & Schulz, K.H. (1984) Allergy to stocking dyes (Ger.). *Dtsch. med. Wochenschr.*, *109*, 1469-1475

IARC (1975) *IARC Monographs on the Evaluation of Carcinogenic Risk of Chemicals to Man*, Vol. 8, *Some Aromatic Azo Compounds*, Lyon, pp. 97-100

Kousa, M. & Soini, M. (1980) Contact allergy to a stocking dye. *Contact Derm.*, *6*, 472-476

Maronpot, R.R., Montgomery, C.A., Jr, Boorman, G.A. & McConnell, E.E. (1986) National Toxicology Program nomenclature for hepatoproliferative lesions of rats. *Toxicol. Pathol.*, *14*, 263-273

McGregor, D.B., Brown, A., Cattanach, P., Edwards, I., McBride, D., Riach, C. & Caspary, W.J. (1988) Responses of the L5178Y $tk^+/tk^-$ mouse lymphoma cell forward mutation assay. III. 72 coded chemicals. *Environ. mol. Mutagenesis*, *12*, 85-154

National Institute for Occupational Safety and Health (1977) *National Occupational Hazard Survey (1972-74)*, Cincinnati, OH

National Toxicology Program (1982) *Carcinogenesis Bioassay of C.I. Disperse Yellow 3 (CAS No. 2832-40-8) in F344 Rats and $B6C3F_1$ Mice (Feed Study)* (Technical Report No. 222), Research Triangle Park, NC, US Department of Health and Human Services

Patterson, D. & Sheldon, R.P. (1960) The solubilities and heats of solution of disperse dyes in water. *J. Soc. Dyers Colour.*, *76*, 178-181

Pouchert, C.J., ed. (1981) *The Aldrich Library of Infrared Spectra*, 3rd ed., Milwaukee, WI, Aldrich Chemical Co., p. 1452

Pouchert, C.J., ed. (1985) *The Aldrich Library of FT-IR Spectra*, Vol. 2, Milwaukee, WI, Aldrich Chemical Co., p. 969

Society of Dyers and Colourists (1971a) *Colour Index*, 3rd. ed., Vol. 4, Bradford, Yorkshire, p. 4027

Society of Dyers and Colourists (1971b) *Colour Index*, 3rd. ed., Vol. 2, Bradford, Yorkshire, p. 2484

Tennant, R.W., Spalding, J.W., Stasiewicz, S., Caspary, W.D., Mason, J.M. & Resnick, M.A. (1987a) Comparative evaluation of genetic toxicity patterns of carcinogens and non-carcinogens: strategies for predictive use of short-term assay. *Environ. Health Perspect.*, *75*, 87-95

Tennant, R.W., Margolin, B.H., Shelby, M.D., Zeiger, E., Haseman, J.K., Spalding, J., Caspary, W., Resnick, M., Stasiewicz, S., Anderson, B. & Minor, R. (1987b) Prediction of chemical carcinogenicity in rodents from *in vitro* genetic toxicity assays. *Science*, *236*, 933-941

Tincher, W.C. & Robertson, J.R. (1982) Analysis of dyes in textile dyeing wastewater. *Text. Chem. Color.*, *14*, 269-275

US International Trade Commission (1977) *Synthetic Organic Chemicals, US Production and Sales, 1975* (*USITC Publication 804*), Washington DC, US Government Printing Office, p. 51

US International Trade Commission (1980) *Synthetic Organic Chemicals, US Production and Sales, 1979* (*USITC Publication 1099*), Washington DC, US Government Printing Office, p. 67

US International Trade Commission (1981) *Synthetic Organic Chemicals, US Production and Sales, 1980* (*USITC Publication 1183*), Washington DC, US Government Printing Office, p. 67

US International Trade Commission (1983) *Synthetic Organic Chemicals, US Production and Sales, 1982* (*USITC Publication 1422*), Washington DC, US Government Printing Office, p. 61

US International Trade Commission (1984) *Synthetic Organic Chemicals, US Production and Sales, 1983* (*USITC Publication 1588*), Washington DC, US Government Printing Office, p. 61

US International Trade Commission (1985) *Synthetic Organic Chemicals, US Production and Sales, 1984* (*USITC Publication 1745*), Washington DC, US Government Printing Office, p. 55

US International Trade Commission (1986) *Synthetic Organic Chemicals, US Production and Sales, 1985* (*USITC Publication 1892*), Washington DC, US Government Printing Office, p. 59

US International Trade Commission (1987) *Synthetic Organic Chemicals, US Production and Sales, 1986 (USITC Publication 2009)*, Washington DC, US Government Printing Office, p. 48

US International Trade Commission (1988) *Synthetic Organic Chemicals, US Production and Sales, 1987 (USITC Publication 2118)*, Washington DC, US Government Printing Office, p. 4-3

US Tariff Commission (1945) *Synthetic Organic Chemicals, US Production and Sales, 1941-43 (Report No. 153)*, Washington DC, US Government Printing Office, p. 81

US Tariff Commission (1974) *Synthetic Organic Chemicals, US Production and Sales, 1972 (TC Publication 681)*, Washington DC, US Government Printing Office, p. 62

Zeiger, E., Anderson, B., Haworth, S., Lawlor, T. & Mortelmans, K. (1988) *Salmonella* mutagenicity tests: IV. Results from the testing of 300 chemicals. *Environ. mol. Mutagenesis, 11 (Suppl. 12)*, 1-158

Zenina, G.A., Gubernatorova, V.V. & Voronin, A.P. (1986) Chromatography analysis of some dyes in air of workplace of textile industry and in hand skin washing-off samples of workers (Russ.). *Gig. Sanit., 4*, 76-77

# VAT YELLOW 4

## 1. Chemical and Physical Data

Vat Yellow 4 is produced and used as a mixture of chemicals (see section 1.4). Sections 1.1-1.3 give the chemical and physical characteristics of the principal colour component or of the dye.

### 1.1 Synonyms

*Chem. Abstr. Services Reg. No.*: 128-66-5
(Replaced CAS Reg. Nos 12772-52-0, 39280-74-5 and 115685-46-6)
*Chem. Abstr. Name*: Dibenzo[*b,def*]chrysene-7,14-dione
*IUPAC Systematic Name*: Dibenzo[*b,def*]chrysene-7,14-dione
*Colour Index No.*: 59100
*Synonyms*: CI Vat Yellow 4; dibenzochrysenedione; dibenzo[*a,h*]pyrene-7,14-dione; 3,4:8,9-dibenzopyrene-5,10-dione; dibenzpyrenequinone

### 1.2 Structural and molecular formulae and molecular weight of dibenzo[*b,def*]chrysene-7,14-dione

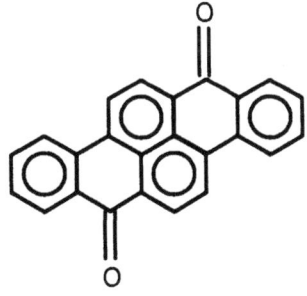

$C_{24}H_{12}O_2$            Mol. wt: 332.36

### 1.3 Chemical and physical properties of the dye or quinone

(a) *Melting-point*: 390°C (Pierce & Katz, 1976) [quinone]; 385°C (Dacre *et al.*, 1979) [dye]

(b) *Solubility*: Soluble in nitrobenzene, sulfuric acid, tetrahydronaphthalene and xylene; slightly soluble in acetone, benzene, chloroform, ethanol, pyridine and toluene; insoluble in water (Dacre *et al.*, 1979; Enviro Control, 1981) [dye]

(c) *Spectroscopy data*: Ultraviolet, infrared, proton and C-13 nuclear magnetic resonance and mass spectral data have been reported (Pierce & Katz, 1976; Rubin & Buchanan, 1983) [quinone].

## 1.4 Technical products and impurities

*Trade Names*: Ahcovat Printing Golden Yellow GK; Amanthrene Golden Yellow GK; Anthravat Golden Yellow GK; Arlanthrene Golden Yellow GK; Benzadone Gold Yellow GK; Calcoloid Golden Yellow GKWP; Caledon Golden Yellow GK; Caledon Printing Yellow GK; Caledon Yellow GK; Carbanthrene Golden Yellow GK; Cibanone Golden Yellow FGK; Cibanone Golden Yellow GK; Fenanthren Golden Yellow GK; Golden Yellow ZhKh; Helanthrene Yellow GOK; Hostavat Golden Yellow GK; Indanthrene Golden Yellow GK; Indanthren Golden Yellow GK; Indanthren Printing Yellow GOK; Kambanthrene Golden Yellow GK; Leucosol Golden Yellow GK; Mayvat Golden Yellow GK; Mikethrene Gold Yellow GK; Nihonthrene Golden Yellow GK; Novatic Golden Yellow GK; Nyanthrene Golden Yellow GK; Palanthrene Golden Yellow GK; Paradone Golden Yellow GK; Pharmanthrene Golden Yellow GK; Romantrene Golden Yellow FGK; Romantrene Golden Yellow GOK; Sandothrene Golden Yellow GK; Sandothrene Printing Yellow NH; Solanthrene Brilliant Yellow J; Tinon Golden Yellow GK; Tyrian Yellow I-GOK; Vat Golden Yellow ZhKh; Vat Golden Yellow ZhKhD; Yellow GK base

Vat Yellow 4 is available in a commercial grade, with the following specifications: approximately 18% dibenzo[*b,def*]chrysene-7,14-dione, 31% sorbitol, 6% dispersant, 3% glycerine and 43% water (National Cancer Institute, 1979). A commercial sample of Vat Yellow 4 analysed in the 1960s was found to contain 0.1% dibenzochrysene (3,4:8,9-dibenzpyrene; Dacre *et al.*, 1979). A US military specification (Anon., 1977) limits the content of dibenzochrysene in Vat Yellow 4 used for smoke screen formulations to a maximum of 0.1%.

Analysis of a Vat Yellow 4 standard revealed the presence of at least six compounds: dibenzochrysenedione, benzanthrone (a starting material in the manufacture of Vat Yellow 4), three diketones (possibly 3-benzoylbenzanthrone and 1,5-dibenzoylnaphthalene, both of which may be intermediates in the manufacture of Vat Yellow 4) and an unknown (Rubin & Buchanan, 1982).

Analysis of a yellow smoke screen formulation for military use showed the presence of dibenzochrysenedione, benzanthrone, some hydrocarbon impurities (possibly the antidusting agent), anthraquinone and an unspecified diketone. Analysis of a green smoke screen formulation showed the presence of dibenzochrysenedione, 1,4-di-*para*-toluidinoanthraquinone, benzanthrone, some hydrocarbon impurities (possibly the antidusting agent) and several unidentified impurities (Rubin & Buchanan, 1982).

## 2. Production, Use, Occurrence and Analysis

### 2.1 Production and use

(a) *Production*

Vat Yellow 4 was reportedly first synthesized by Kränzlein and co-workers in 1922 (Society of Dyers and Colourists, 1971). It has been prepared by the following methods: benzoylation of benzanthrone (the original synthetic route) and ring closure of 3-benzoylbenzanthrone with aluminium chloride and an oxidizing agent; ring closure of 1,5-dibenzoylnaphthalene in the presence of aluminium chlorides; benzoylation of 1-benzoylnaphthalene, followed by ring closure; and direct condensation of naphthalene with benzoyl chloride (see IARC, 1987a) in aluminium chloride at 160°C (Society of Dyers and Colourists, 1971; Savoca, 1974; Dacre *et al.*, 1979).

US production of Vat Yellow 4 was reported to be 161 tonnes in 1972 (US Tariff Commission, 1974). Separate figures were not reported after 1972. Production of all Vat Yellow dyes was approximately 880 tonnes in 1975 and 5 tonnes in 1987 (US International Trade Commission, 1977, 1988).

(b) *Use*

Vat Yellow 4 has an anthraquinoid structure. In the dye process, the keto groups are first reduced to hydroxyls to facilitate penetration of the fibre by the dye; the dye is then fixed by oxidation back to the keto form. Vat Yellow 4 is used to dye cellulose fibres, some cellulose synthetics (e.g., cellulose acetate, cellulose polyester), wool, silk and paper (National Cancer Institute, 1979; Enviro Control, 1981).

Vat Yellow 4 has also been used to manufacture Vat Orange 1, another commercial vat dye (Savoca, 1974).

The dye has been used by the US and other armed services to colour smoke screens and as a signalling agent (National Cancer Institute, 1979; Enviro Control, 1981). The dye mixture is approximately 40-50% of the total pyrotechnic composition, which also includes an oxidizer (potassium chlorate), a fuel (sugar), a coolant (sodium bicarbonate) and a binder (diatomaceous earth; see IARC, 1987b). For example, a typical green-coloured smoke contains 44% green dye mix (benzanthrone, Solvent Green 3 and Vat Yellow 4), 28.5% potassium chlorate, 23% sugar, 2.5% sodium bicarbonate and 2.0% diatomaceous earth (Chin & Borer, 1982; Smith & Stewart, 1982).

(c) *Regulatory status and guidelines*

No regulatory standard or guideline has been established for Vat Yellow 4.

### 2.2 Occurrence

(a) *Natural occurrence*

Vat Yellow 4 is not known to occur as a natural product.

*(b) Occupational exposure*

During the 1940s and 1950s, soldiers were exposed to chemical smoke screens that contained Vat Yellow 4, sometimes for several months. No data on exposure levels were available (National Cancer Institute, 1979).

Swedish workers were reported to be exposed to Vat Yellow 4 contained in a paste used to polish steel; no data were provided on exposure levels (Järvholm *et al.*, 1982).

*(c) Air*

Vat Yellow 4 has been identified in particulate matter from air samples collected in Toronto, Ontario, Canada (Pierce & Katz, 1976).

## 2.3 Analysis

One method for the analysis of polycyclic quinones, including Vat Yellow 4, involves isolation by column and thin-layer chromatography and spectral analysis by ultraviolet, visible and fluorescence spectrophotometry and mass spectrometry (Pierce & Katz, 1976).

Vat Yellow 4 is a component in two coloured smoke mixes — yellow and green. Vat Yellow 4 was separated from the yellow smoke mix by vacuum sublimation, Soxhlet extraction and differential solubility. For the green smoke mix, Vat Yellow 4 was separated by chromatography on a basic alumina column and vacuum sublimation (Rubin & Buchanan, 1982).

# 3. Biological Data Relevant to the Evaluation of Carcinogenic Risk to Humans

## 3.1 Carcinogenicity studies in animals

*Oral administration*

*Mouse*: Groups of 50 male and 50 female B6C3F$_1$ mice, six weeks of age, were fed 25 000 or 50 000 (males) and 12 500 and 25 000 (females) mg/kg of diet (ppm) Vat Yellow 4 (commercial formulation containing approximately 18% of the dyestuff dibenzo[*b,def*]chrysene-7,14-dione) for 106 weeks. Groups of 20 males and 20 females served as untreated controls. Neither survival nor body weight gain was affected by the treatment. A significant increase ($p = 0.002$, Cochran-Armitage test) in the incidence of lymphomas was observed in male mice (control, 3/20; low-dose, 7/47; high-dose, 22/50). The incidences of hepatic tumours (all considered to be hepatocellular carcinomas) in treated mice were: 3/20 in male controls, 22/47 in low-dose males ($p = 0.012$; Fisher exact test), 21/50 in high-dose males ($p = 0.027$; Fisher exact test), 2/19 in control females, 6/48 in low-dose females and 9/50 in high-dose females. The trend was not significant for either sex (National Cancer Institute, 1979).

*Rat*: Groups of 50 male and 50 female Fischer 344 rats, six weeks of age, were fed 3500 or 7000 mg/kg of diet Vat Yellow 4 (commercial formulation containing approximately 18%

dibenzo[*b*,*def*]chrysene-7,14-dione) for 104 weeks. Groups of 20 males and 20 females served as untreated controls. Mean body weights of the treated rats were lower than those of the corresponding controls; survival was not affected by the treatment. The incidences of tumours were not significantly higher in treated groups than in controls (National Cancer Institute, 1979). [The Working Group noted the small number of control animals used.]

## 3.2 Other relevant biological data

(a) *Experimental systems*

(i) *Absorption, distribution, excretion and metabolism*

No data were available to the Working Group.

(ii) *Toxic effects*

No data relevant to an evaluation of carcinogenicity were available to the Working Group.

(iii) *Effects on reproduction and prenatal toxicity*

No data were available to the Working Group.

(iv) *Genetic and related effects* (see Appendix 1)

Vat Yellow was not mutagenic to several strains of *Salmonella typhimurium* in the presence or absence of an exogenous metabolic system from Aroclor 1254-induced rat or Syrian hamster liver (Zeiger *et al.*, 1987).

(b) *Humans*

No data were available to the Working Group.

## 3.3 Case reports and epidemiological studies of carcinogenicity to humans

No data were available to the Working Group.

# 4. Summary of Data Reported and Evaluation

## 4.1 Exposure data

Vat Yellow 4 is an anthraquinone-type dyestuff which is used to colour fabrics and paper and in smoke-screen formulations for military use. No data on occupational exposure levels were available.

## 4.2 Experimental carcinogenicity data

Vat Yellow 4 was tested for carcinogenicity by oral administration in one strain of mice and in one strain of rats, producing an increased incidence of lymphomas and hepatocellular tumours in male mice.

### 4.3 Human carcinogenicity data

No data were available to the Working Group.

### 4.4 Other relevant data

In a single study, Vat Yellow 4 was not mutagenic to bacteria in the presence or absence of an exogenous metabolic system.

### 4.5 Evaluation[1]

There is *limited evidence* for the carcinogenicity of Vat Yellow 4 in experimental animals.

No data were available from studies in humans on the carcinogenicity of Vat Yellow 4.

**Overall evaluation**

Vat Yellow 4 is *not classifiable as to its carcinogenicity to humans (Group 3)*.

## 5. References

Anon. (1977) *Military Specification, Dye, Vat Yellow 14 (MIL-D-0050029D (MA))*, Fort Detrick, Frederick, MD, US Army Medical Research and Development Command

Chin, A. & Borer, L. (1982) Investigations of the effluents produced during the functioning of Navy colored smoke devices. *Proc. Int. Pyrotech. Semin.*, 8, 129-148

Dacre, J.C., Burrows, W.D., Wade, C.W.R., Hegyeli, A.F., Miller, T.A. & Cogley, D.R., eds (1979) *Problem Definition Studies on Potential Environmental Pollutants. V. Physical, Chemical, Toxicological, and Biological Properties of Seven Chemicals used in Pyrotechnic Compositions (Technical Report 7704; US NTIS AD-A090631)*, Fort Detrick, Frederick, MD, US Army Medical Research and Development Command, pp. 66-73

Enviro Control (1981) *Anthraquinone Dye Toxicological Profiles (CSPC-Mono-82-2; US NTIS PB83-166033)*, Rockville, MD

IARC (1987a) *IARC Monographs on the Evaluation of Carcinogenic Risks to Humans*, Suppl. 7, *Overall Evaluations of Carcinogenicity: An Updating of* IARC Monographs *Volumes 1 to 42*, Lyon, pp. 126-127

IARC (1987b) *IARC Monographs on the Evaluation of the Carcinogenic Risk of Chemicals to Humans*, Vol. 42, *Silica and Some Silicates*, Lyon, pp. 39-143

---

[1]For description of the italicized terms and criteria for making the evaluation, see Preamble, pp. 25-29.

# Summary table of genetic and related effects of Vat Yellow 4

| Nonmammalian systems | | | | | | | | | | | | | Mammalian systems | | | | | | | | | | | | | | | | | | | | |
|---|---|---|---|---|---|---|---|---|---|---|---|---|---|---|---|---|---|---|---|---|---|---|---|---|---|---|---|---|---|---|---|---|---|
| Proka-ryotes | | Lower eukaryotes | | | Plants | | | Insects | | | | | In vitro | | | | | | | | | | | | | In vivo | | | | | | | |
| | | | | | | | | | | | | | Animal cells | | | | | | | Human cells | | | | | | | Animals | | | | | Humans | | |
| D | G | D | R | G | A | D | G | C | R | G | C | A | D | G | S | M | C | A | T | I | D | G | S | M | C | A | T | I | D | G | S | M | C | DL | A | D | S | M | C | A |
| | | −¹ | | | | | | | | | | | | | | | | | | | | | | | | | | | | | | | | | | | | | | |

A, aneuploidy; C, chromosomal aberrations; D, DNA damage; DL, dominant lethal mutation; G, gene mutation; I, inhibition of intercellular communication; M, micronuclei; R, mitotic recombination and gene conversion; S, sister chromatid exchange; T, cell transformation

*In completing the table, the following symbol indicates the consensus of the Working Group with regard to the results for each endpoint:*

¹ considered to be negative, but only one valid study was available to the Working Group

Järvholm, B., Thiringer, G. & Axelson, O. (1982) Cancer morbidity among polishers. *Br. J. ind. Med., 39*, 196-197

National Cancer Institute (1979) *Bioassay of C.I. Vat Yellow 4 for Possible Carcinogenicity (CAS No. 128-66-5) (Technical Report No. 134; DHEW Publ. No. (NIH) 79-1389)*, Bethesda, MD, US Department of Health, Education, and Welfare

Pierce, R.C. & Katz, M. (1976) Chromatographic isolation and spectral analysis of polycyclic quinones. Application to air pollution analysis. *Environ. Sci. Technol., 10*, 45-51

Rubin, I.B. & Buchanan, M.V. (1982) The preparative scale separation and the identification of constituents of anthraquinone-derived dye mixtures. Part 2. Benzanthrone, dibenzochrysenedione, and 1,4-di-*p*-toluidino-anthraquinone. *Anal. chim. Acta, 135*, 121-128

Rubin, I.B. & Buchanan, M.V. (1983) *Chemical Characterization and Toxicologic Evaluation of Airborne Mixtures. Chemical Characterization of Army Colored Smokes: Inventory Smoke Mixes (Red, Violet, Yellow, and Green). Final Report (Report No. ORNL/TM-8956; US NTIS AD-A134777)*, Fort Detrick, Frederick, MD, US Army Medical Research and Development Command

Savoca, J.P. (1974) *Process for Manufacturing Dibenzo(a,h)pyrene-7,14-dione (US Patent 3,796,733 (to American Cyanamid Co.))*

Smith, M.D. & Stewart, F.M. (1982) Environmentally acceptable smoke munitions. *Proc. int. Pyrotech. Semin., 8*, 623-635

Society of Dyers and Colourists (1971) *Colour Index*, 3rd ed., Vol 4, Bradford, Yorkshire, p. 4524

US International Trade Commission (1977) *Synthetic Organic Chemicals, US Production and Sales, 1975 (USITC Publication 804)*, Washington DC, US Government Printing Office, p. 53

US International Trade Commission (1988) *Synthetic Organic Chemicals, US Production and Sales, 1987 (USITC Publication 2118)*, Washington DC, US Government Printing Office, p. 4-5

US Tariff Commission (1974) *Synthetic Organic Chemicals, US Production and Sales, 1972 (TC Publication 681)*, Washington DC, US Government Printing Office, p. 64

Zeiger, E., Anderson, B., Haworth, S., Lawlor, T., Mortelmans, K. & Speck, K. (1987) *Salmonella* mutagenicity tests. III. Results from the testing of 255 chemicals. *Environ. Mutagenesis, 9* (Suppl. 9), 1-110

# 5-NITRO-*ortho*-TOLUIDINE

## 1. Chemical and Physical Data

### 1.1 Synonyms

*Chem. Abstr. Services Reg. No.*: 99-55-8
*Chem. Abstr. Name*: Benzenamine, 2-methyl-5-nitro-
*IUPAC Systematic Name*: 5-Nitro-*ortho*-toluidine
*Colour Index No.*: 37105
*Synonyms*: 1-Amino-2-methyl-5-nitrobenzene; 2-amino-4-nitrotoluene; azoic diazo component 12; 2-methyl-5-nitroaniline; 6-methyl-3-nitroaniline; 4-nitro-2-aminotoluene; 3-nitro-6-methylaniline; 5-nitro-2-methylaniline; 5-nitro-2-toluidine; PNOT

### 1.2 Structural and molecular formulae and molecular weight

$C_7H_8N_2O_2$  Mol. wt: 152.16

### 1.3 Chemical and physical properties of the pure substance

From Weast (1985), unless otherwise specified
(a) *Description*: Yellow monoclinic prisms (from ethanol)
(b) *Melting-point*: 107-108°C
(c) *Spectroscopy data*: Infrared, ultraviolet, nuclear magnetic resonance and mass spectral data have been reported (Sadtler Research Laboratories, 1980; Pouchert, 1981, 1983, 1985; Weast & Astle, 1985).
(d) *Solubility*: Soluble in acetone, benzene, chloroform, diethyl ether and ethanol

### 1.4 Technical products and impurities

*Trade Names*: Amarthol Fast Scarlet G Base; Amarthol Fast Scarlet G Salt; Azoene Fast Scarlet GC Base; Azoene Fast Scarlet GC Salt; Azofix Scarlet G Salt; Azogene Fast Scarlet G; Dainichi Fast Scarlet G Base; Daito Scarlet Base G; Devol Scarlet B; Devol Scarlet G Salt; Diabase Scarlet G; Diazo Fast Scarlet G; Fast Red SG Base; Fast Scarlet G; Fast Scarlet G Base; Fast Scarlet GC Base; Fast Scarlet G Salt; Fast Scarlet J Base; Fast Scarlet J Salt; Fast Scarlet M 4NT Base; Fast Scarlet T Base; Hiltonil Fast Scarlet G Base; Hiltonil Fast Scarlet GC Base; Hiltonil Fast Scarlet G Salt; Kayaku Scarlet G Base; Lake Scarlet G Base; Lithosol Orange R Base; Mitsui Scarlet G Base; Naphthanil Scarlet G Base; Naphtoelan Fast Scarlet G Base; Naphtoelan Fast Scarlet G Salt; Scarlet Base Ciba II; Scarlet Base Irga II; Scarlet Base NSP; Scarlet G Base; Sugai Fast Scarlet G Base; Symulon Scarlet G Base

5-Nitro-*ortho*-toluidine is available commercially with a purity of 99% (Aldrich Chemical Co., 1988).

## 2. Production, Use, Occurrence and Analysis

### 2.1 Production and use

*(a) Production*

Several processes have been reported for the preparation of nitrotoluidines, including 5-nitro-*ortho*-toluidine. These include the reaction of nitrocresol with aqueous ammonia, the catalytic hydrogenation of aromatic nitro compounds in the presence of Raney copper, reacting aromatic nitro compounds with hydrogen sulfide in the presence of ammonia dissolved in dioxane, reacting 2,4-dinitrotoluene with hydrogen sulfide in a pyridine solution, and reacting 2,4-dinitrotoluene with carbon monoxide in the presence of cupric oxide and manganese dioxide (Scott, 1971).

5-Nitro-*ortho*-toluidine has also been synthesized by the nitration of *ortho*-toluidine and the monoreduction of 2,4-dinitrotoluene with alcoholic ammonium sulfide (Glinsukon *et al.*, 1975). It can be prepared by the electrolytic reduction of *ortho*-nitrotoluene to *ortho*-toluidine sulfate and subsequent nitration (Udupa *et al.*, 1984).

US production of 5-nitro-*ortho*-toluidine was reported to be 180 tonnes in 1972, with an additional 190 tonnes reported as azoic diazo component 12, salt (US Tariff Commission, 1974). US production of 5-nitro-*ortho*-toluidine in 1975 was reported to be 57 tonnes (US International Trade Commission, 1977).

No data were available on production elsewhere.

*(b) Use*

5-Nitro-*ortho*-toluidine has been used as an intermediate in the synthesis of Pigment Red 17 and Pigment Red 22. It has also been used as a precursor in the synthesis of a wide assortment of azo dyes of various red, yellow, orange, violet and brown hues (National Cancer Institute, 1978).

As an azoic diazo component, 5-nitro-*ortho*-toluidine is used with naphthol derivatives to form azo dyes *in situ* on fabric and yarns. Dyeing with naphthol dyes takes place in two phases: the textile is first immersed in a solution of azoic coupling component, naphthol, and then allowed to react with an azoic diazonium component consisting of an aromatic amine converted first to a diazonium derivative (Priha et al., 1988).

(c) *Regulatory status and guidelines*

No regulatory standard or guideline has been established for 5-nitro-*ortho*-toluidine.

## 2.2 Occurrence

(a) *Natural occurrence*

5-Nitro-*ortho*-toluidine is not known to occur as a natural product.

(b) *Occupational exposure*

No data were available to the Working Group.

(c) *Water and sediments*

5-Nitro-*ortho*-toluidine was identified as a product of the microbial transformation by *Mucrosporium* sp. of 2,4-dinitrotoluene, a compound common in water discharges and effluents from ammunition plants, ammunition loading facilities and sites for the destruction of stockpiled weapons (McCormick et al., 1978). 5-Nitro-*ortho*-toluidine was identified as an intermediate in the anaerobic biotransformation of 2,4-dinitrotoluene added to a sample of municipal activated sludge (Liu et al., 1984).

This compound was identified in samples of water effluent resulting from the continuous 2,4,6-trinitrotoluene manufacturing process. The concentration of 5-nitro-*ortho*-toluidine in samples collected over a one-year period from an effluent pipe ranged from 0.002-0.10 mg/l, with an occurrence rate of 7.6% (Spanggord et al., 1982a).

(d) *Animals*

5-Nitro-*ortho*-toluidine is formed enzymatically from 2,4-dinitrotoluene by liver and lung microsomal fractions from mice (Schut et al., 1985), by liver microsomal and cytosolic fractions from rats (Decad et al., 1982; Mori et al., 1984a) and by intestinal microorganisms from rats and mice (Guest et al., 1982; Mori et al., 1985).

5-Nitro-*ortho*-toluidine and its *N*-acetyl derivative were identified as minor metabolites of 2,4-$^{14}$C-dinitrotoluene when this compound was administered orally to male and female Fischer 344 rats at doses of 35, 63 or 100 mg/kg bw (Medinsky & Dent, 1983).

(e) *Humans*

Human intestinal microflora catalyse the reductive metabolism of 2,4-dinitrotoluene to 5-nitro-*ortho*-toluidine and 4-amino-2-nitrotoluene *via* nitroso intermediates (Guest et al., 1982; Mori et al., 1984b).

## 2.3 Analysis

A diazotization-coupling spectrophotometric technique has been applied to the determination of diverse aromatic amines, including 5-nitro-*ortho*-toluidine, using 8-amino-1-hydroxynaphthalene-3,6-disulfonic acid or *N*-(1-naphthyl)ethylenediamine as the coupling agent (Norwitz & Keliher, 1982).

A method for quantifying 5-nitro-*ortho*-toluidine in effluents from the production and purification of 2,4,6-trinitrotoluene involves gas chromatography with flame ionization for detection and gas chromatography with mass spectrometry for confirmation of identity (Spanggord *et al.*, 1982a).

The principal hazardous organic constituents in various streams from an incinerator facility, including 5-nitro-*ortho*-toluidine, can be detected by high-performance liquid chromatography with reverse-phase columns and ultraviolet spectrophotometric detection, with a detection limit of 1 ng (James *et al.*, 1983).

A method for the determination of 5-nitro-*ortho*-toluidine in activated sludge involves extraction of a broth sample with dichloromethane, transfer of the extract into hexane, evaporation and analysis by gas chromatography with flame ionization and electron capture detection (Liu *et al.*, 1984).

5-Nitro-*ortho*-toluidine in air has been collected on a membrane filter, desorbed with water and analysed by high-performance liquid chromatography with ultraviolet detection, with a detection limit of 3 µg/sample (Eller, 1985).

# 3. Biological Data Relevant to the Evaluation of Carcinogenic Risk to Humans

## 3.1 Carcinogenicity studies in animals

*(a) Oral administration*

*Mouse*: Groups of 49 or 50 male and 50 female B6C3F$_1$ mice, six weeks old, were fed 0.12% or 0.23% (time-weighted average concentration) 5-nitro-*ortho*-toluidine (considered to be of high purity) in the diet for 78 weeks and observed for up to 19-20 additional weeks. Groups of 50 males and 50 females served as untreated controls. Mean body weight depression was observed in treated mice of each sex; there was no significant difference in survival between treated and control animals. A significant increase in the incidence of hepatic tumours (all considered to be hepatocellular carcinomas; $p < 0.001$, Cochran-Armitage test) was observed in treated groups of each sex: in 12/50 control males, 12/44 low-dose males and 29/45 high-dose males; and in 2/47 control females, 7/46 low-dose females and 20/45 high-dose females (National Cancer Institute, 1978).

*Rat*: Groups of 50 male and 50 female Fischer 344 rats, six weeks of age, were fed 0.005% or 0.01% (time-weighted average concentration) 5-nitro-*ortho*-toluidine (considered to be of high purity) in the diet for 78 weeks and observed for up to 30 or 31 additional weeks.

Groups of 50 males and 50 females served as untreated controls. A slight depression in mean body weight was observed in high-dose males and in both high- and low-dose females; there was no significant difference in survival between the treated and control groups. A positive trend ($p = 0.039$, Cochran-Armitage test) in the incidence of hepatocellular carcinomas was observed in male rats (control, 0/47; low-dose, 0/41; high-dose, 3/46) (National Cancer Institute, 1978).

*(b) Intraperitoneal injection*

*Mouse*: In a screening study in strain A mice, based on the induction of lung tumours, groups of 20 female A/St mice, six to eight weeks of age, received intraperitoneal injections of 25, 50 or 100 mg/kg bw 5-nitro-*ortho*-toluidine [purity unspecified] in tricaprylin three times a week for eight weeks. A control group of 80 female mice was untreated and a group of 60 females received intraperitoneal injections of tricaprylin alone. All surviving animals were killed at 16 weeks, when lung adenomas were found in 8% of untreated controls, 11% of tricaprylin-treated controls, 18% of low-dose animals, 30% of mid-dose animals and 6% of high-dose animals (Maronpot *et al.*, 1986).

In a similar screening study, groups of 30 male A/J mice, six to eight weeks of age, received intraperitoneal injections of 40, 100 or 200 mg/kg bw 5-nitro-*ortho*-toluidine [purity unspecified] in corn oil three times a week for eight weeks. A control group of 20 male mice was untreated and a group of 30 males received intraperitoneal injections of corn oil alone. All surviving animals were killed at 16 weeks. No significant difference in the percentage of survivors with lung adenomas was observed compared to vehicle controls (Maronpot *et al.*, 1986).

### 3.2 Other relevant biological data

(a) *Experimental systems*

(i) *Absorption, distribution, excretion and metabolism*

No data were available to the Working Group.

(ii) *Toxic effects*

Methaemoglobin was detected in guinea-pigs and cats after intraperitoneal injection of 0.6-0.7 g/kg bw and 5-10 mg/kg bw 5-nitro-*ortho*-toluidine in vegetable oil, respectively (Reiter, 1948).

(iii) *Effects on reproduction and prenatal toxicity*

No data were available to the Working Group.

(iv) *Genetic and related effects* (see Appendix 1)

5-Nitro-*ortho*-toluidine was mutagenic to several strains of *Salmonella typhimurium* in the presence and absence of an exogenous metabolic system from Aroclor 1254-induced rat liver (Spanggord *et al.*, 1982b; Dunkel *et al.*, 1985; Couch *et al.*, 1987), mouse liver or Syrian hamster liver (Dunkel *et al.*, 1985). In one of the studies (Spanggord *et al.*, 1982b), positive results were obtained in TA1535 only in the absence of an exogenous metabolic system.

5-Nitro-*ortho*-toluidine was not mutagenic to *Escherichia coli* WP2*uvr*A in the presence or absence of an exogenous metabolic system (Dunkel *et al.*, 1985).

(*b*) *Humans*

No data were available to the Working Group.

### 3.3 Case reports and epidemiological studies of carcinogenicity to humans

No data were available to the Working Group.

## 4. Summary of Data Reported and Evaluation

### 4.1 Exposure data

5-Nitro-*ortho*-toluidine is used as an intermediate in the production of a wide assortment of pigments and azo dyes. No data on occupational exposure levels were available.

### 4.2 Experimental carcinogenicity data

5-Nitro-*ortho*-toluidine was tested for carcinogenicity by oral administration in one strain of mice and in one strain of rats. It produced an increase in the incidence of hepatocellular tumours in mice of each sex and a marginal increase in the incidence of hepatocellular carcinomas in male rats.

### 4.3 Human carcinogenicity data

No data were available to the Working Group.

### 4.4 Other relevant data

5-Nitro-*ortho*-toluidine was mutagenic to bacteria in the presence and absence of an exogenous metabolic system.

### 4.5 Evaluation[1]

There is *limited evidence* for the carcinogenicity of 5-nitro-*ortho*-toluidine in experimental animals.

---

[1] For descriptions of the italicized terms and criteria for making the evaluation, see Preamble, pp. 25-29.

## Summary table of genetic and related effects of 5-nitro-*ortho*-toluidine

| Nonmammalian systems | | | | | | | | | | | | | Mammalian systems | | | | | | | | | | | | | | | | | | |
|---|---|---|---|---|---|---|---|---|---|---|---|---|---|---|---|---|---|---|---|---|---|---|---|---|---|---|---|---|---|---|---|
| Proka-ryotes | | Lower eukaryotes | | | | Plants | | | | Insects | | | | *In vitro* | | | | | | | | | | | | | *In vivo* | | | | |
| | | | | | | | | | | | | | | Animal cells | | | | | | | Human cells | | | | | | Animals | | | | Humans |
| D | G | D | R | G | A | A | D | G | C | R | G | C | A | D | G | S | M | C | A | T | I | D | G | S | M | C | A | T | I | D | G | S | M | C | DL | A | D | S | M | C | A |
|  | + | | | | | | | | | | | | | | | | | | | | | | | | | | | | | | | | | | | | | | | | |

A, aneuploidy; C, chromosomal aberrations; D, DNA damage; DL, dominant lethal mutation; G, gene mutation; I, inhibition of intercellular communication; M, micronuclei; R, mitotic recombination and gene conversion; S, sister chromatid exchange; T, cell transformation

*In completing the table, the following symbol indicates the consensus of the Working Group with regard to the results for each endpoint:*

+ considered to be positive for the specific endpoint and level of biological complexity

No data were available from studies in humans on the carcinogenicity of 5-nitro-*ortho*-toluidine.

**Overall evaluation**

5-Nitro-*ortho*-toluidine is *not classifiable as to its carcinogenicity to humans (Group 3)*.

# 5. References

Aldrich Chemical Co. (1988) *1988-1989 Aldrich Catalog/Handbook of Fine Chemicals*, Milwaukee, WI, p. 1033

Couch, D.B., Abernethy, D.J. & Allen, P.F. (1987) The effect of biotransformation of 2,4-dinitrotoluene on its mutagenic potential. *Mutagenesis, 2*, 415-418

Decad, G.M., Graichen, M.E. & Dent, J.G. (1982) Hepatic microsomal metabolism and covalent binding of 2,4-dinitrotoluene. *Toxicol. appl. Pharmacol., 62*, 325-334

Dunkel, V.C., Zeiger, E., Brusick, D., McCoy, E., McGregor, D., Mortelmans, K., Rosenkranz, H.S. & Simmon, V.F. (1985) Reproducibility of microbial mutagenicity assays: II. Testing of carcinogens and noncarcinogens in *Salmonella typhimurium* and *Escherichia coli*. *Environ. Mutagenesis, 7 (Suppl. 5)*, 1-248

Eller, P.M. (1985) *NIOSH Manual of Analytical Methods*, 3rd ed. (*DHHS (NIOSH) Publ. No. 84-1000*), Washington DC, US Government Printing Office, pp. 5013-1-5013-5

Glinsukon, T., Weisburger, E.K., Benjamin, T. & Roller, P.P. (1975) Preparation and spectra of some acetyl derivatives of 2,4-toluenediamine. *J. chem. Eng. Data, 20*, 207-209

Guest, D., Schnell, S.R., Rickert, D.E. & Dent, J.G. (1982) Metabolism of 2,4-dinitrotoluene by intestinal microorganisms from rat, mouse and man. *Toxicol. appl. Pharmacol., 64*, 160-168

James, R.H., Dillon, H.K. & Miller, H.C. (1983) Survey methods for the determination of principal organic hazardous constituents (POHCs). In: Schultz, D.W., ed., *Incineration and Treatment of Hazardous Waste: Proceedings of the Eighth Annual Research Symposium, Ft Mitchell, KY, 1982 (US EPA Report No. EPA-600/9-83-003; US NTIS PB83-210450)*, Cincinnati, OH, US Environmental Protection Agency, pp. 159-173

Liu, D., Thomson, K. & Anderson, A.C. (1984) Identification of nitroso compounds from biotransformation of 2,4-dinitrotoluene. *Appl. environ. Microbiol., 47*, 1295-1298

Maronpot, R.R., Shimkin, M.B., Witschi, H.P., Smith, L.H. & Cline, J.M. (1986) Strain A mouse pulmonary tumor test results for chemicals previously tested in the National Cancer Institute carcinogenicity tests. *J. natl Cancer Inst., 76*, 1101-1112

McCormick, N.G., Cornell, J.H. & Kaplan, A.M. (1978) Identification of biotransformation products from 2,4-dinitrotoluene. *Appl. environ. Microbiol., 35*, 945-948

Medinsky, M.A. & Dent, J.G. (1983) Biliary excretion and enterohepatic circulation of 2,4-dinitrotoluene metabolites in Fischer-344 rats. *Toxicol. appl. Pharmacol., 68*, 359-366

Mori, M.-A., Matsuhashi, T., Miyahara, T., Shibata, S., Izima, C. & Kozuka, H. (1984a) Reduction of 2,4-dinitrotoluene by Wistar rat liver microsomal and cytosol fractions. *Toxicol. appl. Pharmacol., 76*, 105-112

Mori, M.-A., Miyahara, T., Hasegawa, Y., Kudo, Y. & Kozuka, H. (1984b) Metabolism of dinitrotoluene isomers by *Escherichia coli* isolated from human intestine. *Chem. pharm. Bull. (Tokyo), 32*, 4070-4075

Mori, M.-A., Kudo, Y., Nunozawa, T., Miyahara, T. & Kozuka, H. (1985) Intestinal metabolism of 2,4-dinitrotoluene in rats. *Chem. pharm. Bull. (Tokyo), 33*, 327-332

National Cancer Institute (1978) *Bioassay of 5-Nitro-o-toluidine for Possible Carcinogenicity (CAS No. 99-55-8) (Technical Report No. 107; DHEW Publ. No. (NIH) 78-1357)*, Bethesda, MD, US Department of Health, Education, and Welfare

Norwitz, G. & Keliher, P.N. (1982) Spectrophotometric determination of aromatic amines by the diazotization-coupling technique with 8-amino-1-hydroxynaphthalene-3,6-disulfonic acid and *N*-(1-naphthyl)ethylenediamine as the coupling agents. *Anal. Chem., 54*, 807-809

Pouchert, C.J., ed. (1981) *The Aldrich Library of Infrared Spectra*, 3rd ed., Milwaukee, WI, Aldrich Chemical Co., p. 824

Pouchert, C.J., ed. (1983) *The Aldrich Library of NMR Spectra*, 2nd ed., Vol. 1, Milwaukee, WI, Aldrich Chemical Co., p. 1167

Pouchert, C.J., ed. (1985) *The Aldrich Library of FT-IR Spectra*, Vol. 1, Milwaukee, WI, Aldrich Chemical Co., p. 1365

Priha, E., Vuorinen, R., Schimberg, R. & Ahonen, I. (1988) *Tekstiilien Viimeistysaineet* (Textile Finishing Agents) *(Series on Working Conditions No. 65)*, Helsinki, Institute of Occupational Health

Reiter, M. (1948) Methaemoglobin due to *p*-nitro-*o*-toluidine (Ger.). *Arch. exp. Pathol. Pharmakol., 205*, 327-331

Sadtler Research Laboratories (1980) *Standard Spectra Collection, 1980 Cumulative Index*, Philadelphia, PA

Schut, H.A.J., Dixit, R., Loeb, T.R. & Stoner, G.D. (1985) In vivo and in vitro metabolism of 2,4-dinitrotoluene in strain A mice. *Biochem. Pharmacol., 34*, 969-976

Scott, J.A. (1971) *Process for Preparing Toluidines (US Patent 3,578,713 (to Olin Corp.))*

Spanggord, R.J., Gibson, B.W., Keck, R.G., Thomas, D.W. & Barkley, J.J., Jr (1982a) Effluent analysis of wastewater generated in the manufacture of 2,4,6-trinitrotoluene. 1. Characterization study. *Environ. Sci. Technol., 16*, 229-232

Spanggord, R.J., Mortelmans, K.E., Griffin, A.F. & Simmon, V.F. (1982b) Mutagenicity in *Salmonella typhimurium* and structure-activity relationships of wastewater components emanating from the manufacture of trinitrotoluene. *Environ. Mutagenesis, 4*, 163-179

Udupa, H.V., Venkatachalapathy, M.S., Chidambaram, S.I., Srinivasan, R.K. & Balasubramanian, L. (1984) *An Electrochemical Process for the Production of 2-Amino 4-Nitro Toluene from o-Nitro Toluene (Indian Patent 154,403)*

US International Trade Commission (1977) *Synthetic Organic Chemicals, US Production and Sales, 1975 (USITC Publication 804)*, Washington DC, US Government Printing Office, p. 49

US Tariff Commission (1974) *Synthetic Organic Chemicals, US Production and Sales, 1972 (TC Publication 681)*, Washington DC, US Government Printing Office, pp. 21, 59

Weast, R.C., ed. (1985) *CRC Handbook of Chemistry and Physics*, 66th ed., Boca Raton, FL, CRC Press, p. C-526

Weast, R.C. & Astle, M.J. (1985) *Handbook of Data on Organic Compounds*, Boca Raton, FL, CRC Press, p. 380

# OTHER TEXTILE CHEMICALS

# NITRILOTRIACETIC ACID AND ITS SALTS

## 1. Chemical and Physical Data

### 1.1 Synonyms

**Nitrilotriacetic acid (NTA)**

*Chem. Abstr. Services Reg. No.*: 139-13-9
(Replaced CAS Reg. Nos 26627-44-1, 26627-45-2 and 80751-51-5)
*Chem. Abstr. Name*: Glycine, *N,N*-bis(carboxymethyl)-
*IUPAC Systematic Name*: Nitrilotriacetic acid
*Synonyms*: Nitrilo-2,2′,2″-triacetic acid; triglycine; triglycollamic acid; $\alpha,\alpha',\alpha''$-trimethylaminetricarboxylic acid

**Nitrilotriacetic acid, sodium salt (unspecified)**

*Chem. Abstr. Services Reg. No.*: 10042-84-9
*Chem. Abstr. Name*: Glycine, *N,N*-bis(carboxymethyl)-, sodium salt
*IUPAC Systematic Name*: Nitrilotriacetic acid, sodium salt
*Synonyms*: Sodium aminotriacetate; sodium nitriloacetate; sodium nitrilotriacetate; sodium NTA

**Nitrilotriacetic acid, monosodium salt (NTA, monosodium salt)**

*Chem. Abstr. Services Reg. No*: 18994-66-6
*Chem. Abstr. Name*: Glycine, *N,N*-bis(carboxymethyl)-, monosodium salt
*IUPAC Systematic Name*: Sodium dihydrogen nitrilotriacetate
*Synonyms*: Monosodium nitriloacetate; monosodium nitrilotriacetate; NaNTA

**Nitrilotriacetic acid, disodium salt (NTA, disodium salt)**

*Chem. Abstr. Services Reg. No.*: 15467-20-6
*Chem. Abstr. Name*: Glycine, *N,N*-bis(carboxymethyl)-, disodium salt
*IUPAC Systematic Name*: Disodium hydrogen nitrilotriacetate
*Synonyms*: Disodium nitrilotriacetate; Na$_2$NTA

**Nitrilotriacetic acid, disodium salt, monohydrate (NTA disodium salt, monohydrate)**

*Chem. Abstr. Services Reg. No.*: 23255-03-0
*Chem. Abstr. Name*: Glycine, *N,N*-bis(carboxymethyl)-, disodium salt, monohydrate
*IUPAC Systematic Name*: Disodium hydrogen nitrilotriacetate, monohydrate
*Synonyms*: Acetic acid, nitrilotri-, disodium salt, monohydrate; disodium nitrilotriacetic acid monohydrate; Na$_2$NTA.H$_2$O

**Nitrilotriacetic acid, trisodium salt (NTA, trisodium salt)**

*Chem. Abstr. Services Reg. No.*: 5064-31-3
(Replaced CAS Reg. No. 37291-81-9)
*Chem. Abstr. Name*: Glycine, *N,N*-bis(carboxymethyl)-, trisodium salt
*IUPAC Systematic Name*: Trisodium nitrilotriacetate
*Synonym*: Na$_3$NTA

**Nitrilotriacetic acid, trisodium salt, monohydrate (NTA, trisodium salt, monohydrate)**

*Chem. Abstr. Services Reg. No.*: 18662-53-8
*Chem. Abstr. Name*: Glycine, *N,N*-bis(carboxymethyl)-, trisodium salt, monohydrate
*IUPAC Systematic Name*: Trisodium nitrilotriacetate, monohydrate
*Synonyms*: Na$_3$NTA.H$_2$O; trisodium salt of nitrilotriacetic acid, monohydrate

Many other salts of NTA have been reported, and selected examples are listed in Table 1. Chemical and physical properties have not been reported for most of these.

### 1.2 Structural and molecular formulae and molecular weights

**NTA**

$$HOOC-CH_2-N(-CH_2-COOH)-CH_2-COOH$$

C$_6$H$_9$NO$_6$      Mol. wt: 191.14

**NTA, monosodium salt**

C$_6$H$_8$NO$_6$·Na      Mol. wt: 213.14

**NTA, disodium salt**

C$_6$H$_7$NO$_6$·2Na      Mol. wt: 235.13

**NTA, disodium salt, monohydrate**

C$_6$H$_7$NO$_6$·2Na·H$_2$O      Mol. wt: 253.11

**NTA, trisodium salt**

C$_6$H$_6$NO$_6$·3Na      Mol. wt: 257.13

**NTA, trisodium salt, monohydrate**

C$_6$H$_6$NO$_6$·3Na·H$_2$O      Mol. wt: 275.11

Table 1. Examples of nitrilotriacetic acid salts and complexes

| CAS No. | Common name |
|---|---|
| 1188-47-2 | NTA, copper(2+) salt (1:1) |
| 1188-48-3 | NTA, magnesium salt (1:1) |
| 2399-81-7 | NTA, beryllium salt (1:1) |
| 2399-83-9 | NTA, barium salt (1:1) |
| 2399-85-1 | NTA, tripotassium salt |
| 2399-86-2 | NTA, dipotassium salt |
| 2399-88-4 | NTA, potassium magnesium salt (1:1:1) |
| 2399-89-5 | NTA, potassium strontium salt (1:1:1) |
| 2399-94-2 | NTA, calcium salt (1:1) |
| 2455-08-5 | NTA, calcium potassium salt (1:1:1) |
| 3130-95-8 | NTA, scandium (3+) salt (1:1) |
| 5798-43-6 | NTA, disodium salt, compound with oxo(dihydrogen nitriloacetato)bismuth sodium salt (3:1) |
| 10413-71-5 | NTA, erbium(3+) salt (3:1) |
| 14695-88-6 | NTA, compound with iron chloride (FeCl3) |
| 14981-08-9 | NTA, calcium salt |
| 15414-25-2 | NTA, yttrium (3+) salt (1:1) |
| 15844-52-7 | NTA, copper(2+) complex |
| 15934-02-8 | NTA, monoammonium salt |
| 16448-54-7 | NTA, iron(3+) complex [replaced: 5905-54-4; 107288-49-3] |
| 18105-03-8 | NTA, mercury(2+) salt (2:3) |
| 18432-54-7 | NTA, cadmium(2+) complex |
| 18946-94-6 | NTA, neodymium(3+) salt (1:1) [alternative: 3438-06-0] |
| 18983-72-7 | NTA, beryllium potassium salt (1:1) [alternative: 2399-87-3] |
| 19010-73-2 | NTA, aluminium(3+) complex |
| 19456-58-7 | NTA, indium(3+) complex |
| 22965-60-2 | NTA, nickel(3+) complex |
| 23319-51-9 | NTA, cobalt(3+) complex |
| 23555-96-6 | NTA, potassium strontium salt (2:4:1) |
| 23555-98-8 | NTA, calcium potassium salt (2:1:4) |
| 25817-24-7 | NTA, potassium salt |
| 28444-53-3 | NTA, monopotassium salt |
| 28927-38-0 | NTA, holmium salt |
| 29027-90-5 | NTA, cerium salt |
| 29507-58-2 | NTA, zinc(3+) complex sodium salt [replaced: 26856-43-9] |
| 32685-17-9 | NTA, triammonium salt |
| 34831-02-2 | NTA, copper(2+) hydrogen complex |
| 34831-03-3 | NTA, nickel(2+) hydrogen complex |
| 36711-58-7 | NTA, manganese salt |
| 46242-44-8 | NTA, antimony(3+) complex |
| 50648-02-7 | NTA, tricadmium(2+) complex |

**Table 1 (contd)**

| CAS No. | Common name |
|---|---|
| 53108-47-7 | NTA, copper(2+) complex sodium salt |
| 53108-50-2 | NTA, cobalt(3+) hydrogen complex |
| 53818-84-1 | NTA, tin(2+) salt |
| 60034-45-9 | NTA, calcium sodium salt (1:1:1) |
| 61017-62-7 | NTA, iron(2+) complex sodium salt (1:1:1) |
| 62979-89-6 | NTA, calcium salt (2:3) |
| 71264-32-9 | NTA, diammonium salt |
| 71484-80-5 | NTA, copper(2+) complex ammonium salt |
| 72629-49-3 | NTA, dilithium salt |
| 73772-91-5 | NTA, magnesium salt |
| 79849-02-8 | NTA, lead(2+) salt (1:1) |
| 79915-08-5 | NTA, lead(2+) potassium salt (1:1:1) |
| 79915-09-6 | NTA, lead(2+) salt (2:3) |
| 86892-89-9 | NTA, disodium ammonium salt |
| 92474-39-0 | NTA, trisilver salt |
| 92988-11-9 | NTA, strontium sodium salt |

### 1.3 Chemical and physical properties of the pure substance

**NTA**

(a) *Description*: White crystalline powder (Anderson *et al.*, 1985; W.R. Grace & Co., 1985)

(b) *Melting-point*: Decomposes at 246°C (Sadtler Research Laboratories, 1980; Aldrich Chemical Co., 1988)

(c) *Spectroscopy data*: Infrared (prism [5940, 13213]; grating [18901]) and nuclear magnetic resonance spectral data have been reported (Sadtler Research Laboratories, 1980; Pouchert, 1981, 1983, 1985).

(d) *Solubility*: 1.5 g/l water at 25°C (Anderson *et al.*, 1985; W.R. Grace & Co., 1985)

(e) *pH of saturated aqueous solution*: 2-3 (W.R. Grace & Co., 1985)

(f) *Reactivity*: Forms water-soluble complexes with many metal ions (chelates); reacts with strong oxidizing agents such as hypochlorite, chlorine and ozone (Anderson *et al.*, 1985)

**NTA, disodium salt**

(a) *Melting-point*: >300°C (Aldrich Chemical Co., 1988)

(b) *Spectroscopy data*: Infrared (prism-FT [566B]) spectral data have been reported (Pouchert, 1985).

(c) *Reactivity*: Forms water-soluble complexes with many metal ions (chelates); reacts with strong oxidizing agents such as hypochlorite, chlorine and ozone (Anderson et al., 1985)

**NTA, trisodium salt, monohydrate**

(a) *Description*: White crystalline powder (Anderson et al., 1985; Monsanto Co., 1985)

(b) *Melting-point*: Decomposes at 340°C (Monsanto Co., 1985)

(c) *Spectroscopy data*: Infrared and nuclear magnetic resonance spectral data have been reported (Pouchert, 1981, 1983, 1985).

(d) *Density*: 1.782 g/cm³ (Monsanto Co., 1985)

(e) *Solubility*: 50 g/100 g water at 25°C (Anderson et al., 1985; Monsanto Co., 1985)

(f) *pH of 1% solution at 25°C*: 10.6-11.0 (Monsanto Co., 1985)

(g) *Reactivity*: Forms water-soluble complexes with many metal ions (chelates); reacts with strong oxidizing agents such as hypochlorite, chlorine and ozone (Anderson et al., 1985)

*Salt and complex formation*

As a carboxylic acid, NTA forms simple salts with some metal ions (e.g., sodium, potassium), but the association between NTA and other metals ions that have available additional coordination sites for binding may involve more than one of the NTA functional groups. NTA in its fully ionized form [$N(CH_2CO_2^-)_3$; $NTA^{3-}$] has four functional groups—the three carboxylates and one amine group—that are available for complexing with a metal ion. This phenomenon, in which more than one of the NTA functional groups is involved in binding with a metal ion, is known as chelation. For example, the structure of the $Fe^{3+}$/$NTA^{3-}$ complex involves simultaneous binding of the three carboxylate groups and the amine group to the $Fe^{3+}$ ion. Other metal ions show intermediate degrees of complexation with NTA in its ionized (salt) form in solution.

Complexes are formed between metal ions and NTA when metal salts and NTA salts are combined in aqueous solutions. The proportion of metal ions complexed in a given solution depends on a number of factors, and the complex is always in equilibrium with uncomplexed metal ion and NTA. In aqueous solution, the extent of protonation of the NTA carboxylate groups varies with pH ($pKA_1 = 1.89$, $pKA_2 = 2.49$, $pKA_3 = 9.73$); protonation competes with metal ion complexation. The extent of metal complex formation in solution depends on the concentrations of the ionized forms of NTA and the metal ion, and on the formation constant (inverse of dissociation constant) of the complex. Table 2 gives the formation constants for several common metal ions. As can be seen, the weakest NTA/metal ion complexes are formed with the alkaline earth ions, $Mg^{2+}$ and $Ca^{2+}$, and the strongest complexes are formed with $Hg^{2+}$ and $Fe^{3+}$ (Martell & Smith, 1974; Anderson et al., 1985).

Table 2. Metal ion/NTA$^{3-}$ formation constants at 25°C$^a$

| Metal | log K |
|---|---|
| $Mg^{2+}$ | 5.47 |
| $Ca^{2+}$ | 6.39 |
| $Mn^{2+}$ | 7.46 |
| $Fe^{2+}$ | 8.33$^b$ |
| $Cd^{2+}$ | 9.78 |
| $Co^{2+}$ | 10.38 |
| $Zn^{2+}$ | 10.66 |
| $Pb^{2+}$ | 11.34 |
| $Ni^{2+}$ | 11.50 |
| $Cu^{2+}$ | 12.94 |
| $Hg^{2+}$ | 14.6 |
| $Fe^{3+}$ | 15.9 |

$^a$From Martell & Smith (1974)
$^b$At 20°C

### 1.4 Technical products and impurities

*Trade Names*:

**NTA**: Chel 300; Complexon I; Hampshire® NTA acid; IDRANAL® I; Titriplex I; Versene NTA acid

**NTA, sodium salt**: Chelest NTA

**NTA, disodium salt**: Chelest NTB

**NTA, trisodium salt**: Chemcolox 365 Powder; Hampshire® NTA 150; Masquol NP 140; Syntron A; Trilon A; Trilon A 50; Versene NTA 150; Versene NTA 335

**NTA, trisodium salt, monohydrate**: Hampshire® NTA Na3 Crystals; NTA Powder; Trilon® A92

NTA and its sodium salts are commercially available in several products with the following specifications: (i) crystals (white granular powder) of NTA, trisodium salt, monohydrate; purity, 98.5% min (W.R. Grace & Co., 1985) and 99% (Aldrich Chemical Co., 1988); (ii) aqueous solution (clear, pale straw-coloured liquid) of NTA, trisodium salt, 40% min); specific gravity, 1.30-1.33 at 25°C; and (iii) crystalline form (free-flowing, white, crystalline powder) of NTA; purity, 99% (W.R. Grace & Co., 1985). Another manufacturer markets NTA, trisodium salt, monohydrate with a reported purity of 100%; density, 1.782 g/cm$^3$ (Monsanto Co., 1985). Reagent-grade NTA, disodium salt is commercially available with a purity of >99% (Aldrich Chemical Co., 1988). Reagent-grade NTA is also available with the following specifications: purity, 99.5% min; calcium, 0.002% max; iron, 0.0005% max; potassium, 0.001% max; magnesium, 0.001% max; sodium, 0.02% max; chloride, 0.02% max; and sulfate, 0.01% max (Riedel-de Haen, 1984).

Analysis of commercial NTA, trisodium salt, monohydrate has shown the following impurities: sodium cyanide, 4 ppm (mg/kg); sodium hydroxide, 0.3%; sodium carbonate, 0.4%; primary and secondary amines, approximately 0.2%; iminodiacetic acid, 0.2%; potassium, 6 ppm; zinc, 2 ppm; copper, 1 ppm; iron, < 10 ppm; and lead (see IARC, 1987a), 1-2 ppm (Anderson et al., 1985). The typical composition of another commercial product (also NTA trisodium salt, monohydrate) was given as: NTA, trisodium salt, monohydrate, 99%; iminodiacetic acid, disodium salt, < 0.2%; sodium hydroxide, < 0.5%; sodium carbonate, < 0.5%; ammonia, < 70 ppm; formaldehyde (see IARC, 1987b), < 5 ppm; and sodium cyanide, < 5 ppm (Gesellschaft Deutscher Chemiker, 1987).

## 2. Production, Use, Occurrence and Analysis

### 2.1 Production and use

*(a) Production*

NTA was first synthesized by Heintz in 1862, and its properties and chemistry were described in 1865 (Anderson et al., 1985).

First commercial production of NTA occurred in Europe in the 1930s. Subsequently, it was found that ethylenediaminetetraacetate (EDTA) could be synthesized at a lower cost, and, in a relatively short period of time, EDTA replaced NTA in most commercial applications. With the later development of an efficient, low-cost process for manufacturing highly pure NTA products, NTA has again become competitive for many applications (W.R. Grace & Co., 1985).

NTA, trisodium salt, monohydrate is synthesized commercially by the reaction of formaldehyde, hydrocyanic acid and sodium hydroxide in water (Anderson et al., 1985). The trisodium salt, isolated from aqueous solution as the monohydrate, can be converted to other forms by dehydration or acidification.

Combined European production capacity for NTA in the early 1980s was estimated at 50 000 tonnes, and overall annual consumption of NTA and its salts estimated at about 20 000 tonnes. About 8000 tonnes of NTA and its salts were produced in the Federal Republic of Germany in 1984 (Gesellschaft Deutscher Chemiker, 1987). They have also been manufactured in France, the Netherlands, Spain, Sweden and the UK. US production in the early 1980s was about 30 000 tonnes per year, most of which was exported. In that period, Japan produced less than 1000 tonnes per year and imported 1000-2000 tonnes. Canada imported 7400 tonnes in 1984 but only 420 tonnes in 1987 due to increased use of zeolite in detergent formulations; NTA is also produced in Canada, but production figures were not available (Universities Associated for Research and Education in Pathology, 1985).

*(b) Use*

NTA has numerous commercial applications as a metal ion chelator, including principally its use in cleaning products, industrial water treatment, textile preparation and metal finishing. It has also been used to a lesser extent in the pulp and paper industry, in rubber processing, in photographic products, in the electrochemical industry, in the tanning of leather, and in cosmetics (Anderson *et al.*, 1985; Universities Associated for Research and Education in Pathology, 1985).

The major use of NTA, as the trisodium salt, has been in detergent systems as a chelating agent and as a laundry detergent builder. NTA was originally proposed as a substitute for phosphates in detergents, when the eutrophic effect of phosphates on the aquatic environment was recognized. It has been accepted for use as an ingredient in domestic detergent products in at least 16 countries and has actually been used in detergents in Canada and several European countries since the early 1970s. NTA is also used to reduce fabric yellowing by hypochlorite bleach and to increase the effectiveness in hard water of liquid detergent-sanitizer formulations based on quaternary ammonium germicides (Universities Associated for Research and Education in Pathology, 1985; W.R. Grace & Co., 1985; Wendt *et al.*, 1988).

NTA can chelate metal ions that commonly cause water 'hardness' ($Ca^{2+}$ and $Mg^{2+}$) and is widely used to control precipitation and scaling of salts of these ions, for example, in boiler feedwater. Various salts of NTA have been used to remove scale. Since the sodium-calcium NTA complex is relatively insoluble, it can form a coating on the scale and retard further scale formation. Iron oxide deposits such as mill scale are removed with NTA, ammonium salts in the alkaline pH range, resulting in a degreased and cleaned surface (Anderson *et al.*, 1985; W.R. Grace & Co., 1985).

Trace metals in dye processing are often responsible for uneven dyeing of stock, piece and continuous goods by forming interfering metal lakes, which result in streaking and dulling of shades. Hardness can be controlled and heavy metals eliminated by incorporating NTA in the processing. NTA is also used in scouring and fulling operations, in peroxide bleaching and in desizing operations (Anderson *et al.*, 1985; W.R. Grace & Co., 1985).

The addition of NTA to conventional alkaline metal cleaners assists in dissolving water-insoluble metal oxides and hydroxides which are formed when metals corrode (Anderson *et al.*, 1985; W.R. Grace & Co., 1985).

*(c) Regulatory status and guidelines*

The US Food and Drug Administration (1987) has approved the use of NTA, trisodium salt as an additive to boiler water used in the preparation of steam that will come into contact with food. It may not exceed 5 ppm (mg/l) in boiler feedwater and may not be used when steam will be in contact with milk and milk products.

One US manufacturer has adopted for their operations a workplace exposure limit to NTA powder (as total dust) of 1 mg/m$^3$ as an 8-h time-weighted average and 2 mg/m$^3$ as a short-term exposure level (Monsanto Co., 1985).

## 2.2 Occurrence

### (a) Natural occurrence

NTA, its salts and its complexes are not known to occur as natural products.

### (b) Occupational exposure

About 2600 workers in the USA may be potentially exposed to NTA salts during their production or during the formulation of detergents. In the production of NTA, people loading hopper cars have the highest potential exposure. In one study, mean airborne levels of NTA in the workplace during the production of NTA were 0.033 mg/m$^3$ in the normal line area (US Environmental Protection Agency, 1979; Universities Associated for Research and Education in Pathology, 1985), but 0.82 mg/m$^3$ in the hopper-car loader area (US Environmental Protection Agency, 1979).

Increases recorded in the concentrations of NTA in influent sewage in several countries imply that the potential exposure of sewage treatment workers to this compound has risen steadily since the early 1970s (Anderson et al., 1985).

### (c) Water and sediments

#### (i) Sewage treatment systems

In an environmental monitoring programme carried out in 1971-75, concentrations of NTA and certain metals were measured in Canadian wastewaters and streams. During 1971 and 1972, the average level of NTA in detergents in Canada was 6%; between 1973 and 1975, it had increased to 15%. The levels of NTA that were found in sewage influents and effluents during the two periods are shown in Table 3. In 13 cities, the levels of NTA that were found in receiving streams above the sewage outfall ranged from 0 to 190 µg/l during 1971-72 and 0 to 283 µg/l during 1973-75; the levels below the sewage outfall ranged from 0 to 340 and from 0 to 3364 µg/l in the two periods, respectively (Woodiwiss et al., 1979).

Table 3. Mean concentrations (mg/l) of NTA in 13 Canadian sewage influents and effluents[a]

| Treatment | 1971-72 | | 1973-75 | |
|---|---|---|---|---|
| | Influent | Effluent | Influent | Effluent |
| Activated sludge | 2.14 | 0.40 | 3.80 | 0.60 |
| Trickling filter | 1.76 | 1.27 | 5.16 | 3.22 |
| Primary | 1.14 | 0.75 | 3.19 | 2.98 |
| No treatment | 1.09 | NA | 1.75 | NA |
| Total geometric mean | 1.73 | | 3.62 | |

[a]From Woodiwiss et al. (1979)
NA, not applicable

Concentrations of NTA in 1980 at four sewage treatment plants in the Netherlands ranged from 37 to 113 µg/l in influent samples and from 6 to 21 µg/l in effluent samples (Games et al., 1981). In a later environmental monitoring programme conducted at the same four treatment plants, NTA concentrations ranged from 80 to 254 µg/l in influent samples and from 4 to 48 µg/l in effluent samples (Anderson et al., 1985).

In an environmental monitoring programme conducted in Indiana, USA, in 1979-83, the concentrations of NTA were measured before and after NTA was incorporated into laundry detergents at five types of site: in wastewaters before and after treatment, in river water above and below wastewater outfalls, and in finished drinking-water drawn from rivers receiving large amounts of NTA (Table 4). Concentrations of metals were also measured, in order to determine whether NTA used in laundry detergents affected metal concentrations in wastewater, river water or drinking-water; no effect was observed (Wendt et al., 1988).

Table 4. Concentrations (mg/l) of NTA in wastewaters, river waters and drinking-water in Indiana, USA[a]

| Water type | No. of samples | Before NTA use | | During NTA use | |
|---|---|---|---|---|---|
| | | Mean | Range | Mean | Range |
| Wastewaters | | | | | |
| Influent | 4 | 0.025 | 0.010-0.069 | 0.789 | 0.385-2.314 |
| Effluent | 4 | 0.013 | 0.003-0.036 | 0.137 | 0.021-0.639 |
| River waters | 9 | 0.002 | <0.001-0.006 | 0.008 | 0.003-0.031 |
| Below wastewater outfall | - | | | 0.012 | |
| Drinking-water | 4 | 0.001 | <0.001-0.003 | 0.004 | 0.002-0.008 |

[a]From Wendt et al. (1988)
-, not measured

(ii) *Drinking-water*

Concentrations of NTA in domestic drinking-water supplies have been monitored in several studies; the results are summarized in Table 5.

### 2.3 Analysis

Methods for the analysis of NTA in the environment have been reviewed (Kirk & Lester, 1981; Kirk et al., 1982). Selected methods are presented in Table 6.

Table 5. Concentrations of NTA in domestic water supplies[a]

| Area | Date | Drinking-water | | No. of samples | Concentration (μg/l) | Reference |
|---|---|---|---|---|---|---|
| | | Type | Source | | | |
| USA | | | | | | |
| New York (Upstate) | 1981–83 | Municipal | Surface or groundwater | 46<br>24 | ND<br><5 | Procter & Gamble Co. (1983a) |
| Indiana | 1981–83 | Municipal | Surface water | 152 | Average, 4 | Procter & Gamble Co. (1981, 1982, 1983b) |
| Canada | | | | | | |
| Nationwide | 1972–75 | Municipal | Surface water | 650<br>51 | ND<br>10–80 | Matheson (1977) |
| | 1972–75 | Municipal | Groundwater | 77<br>1 | ND<br>Detected, no level reported | Matheson (1977) |
| | 1976–77 | Municipal | Surface water | | National average, 2.8 | Malaiyandi et al. (1979) |
| Ottawa–Carleton, Ontario | 1976–77 | Private | Groundwater | 20<br>1 | ND<br>16.9 | Malaiyandi et al. (1979) |
| | 1983 | Private | Groundwater | 18<br>1 | ND<br>2.7 | Procter & Gamble Co. (1983c) |

**Table 5 (contd)**

| Area | Date | Drinking-water | | No. of samples | Concentration (µg/l) | Reference |
|---|---|---|---|---|---|---|
| | | Type | Source | | | |
| Finch, Ontario | 1972 | Private | Groundwater | 47<br>21 | <10<br>15–250 | Matheson (1977) |
| | 1972–73 | Private | Groundwater | 68<br>4 | <10<br>70 | Matheson (1977) |
| | 1973 | Private | Groundwater | 5<br>1 | <10<br>3900 | Matheson (1977) |
| | 1983 | Private | Groundwater | 13<br>7<br>2 | ND<br><5<br>5.2 and 14 | Procter & Gamble Co. (1983c) |
| Port Kells, British Columbia | 1983 | Private | Groundwater | 18<br>2 | ND<br>2.5 and 2.6 | Procter & Gamble Co. (1983c) |

[a]Reviewed by Anderson et al. (1985)

ND, none detected

**Table 6. Methods for the analysis of NTA in water**

| Sample matrix | Sample preparation | Assay procedure[a] | Limit of detection | Reference |
|---|---|---|---|---|
| Water and sewage effluents | Add ion-exchange resin; stir; filter; add zinc-Zincon reagent | Colorimetric | 0.2 mg/l (as triNa salt) | Thompson & Duthie (1968) |
| Sewage effluents | Adjust pH to 2.0-2.5 with hydrochloric acid; add ferric nitrate solution; heat; add ammonium hydroxide/ammonium nitrate to raise pH to 3.9-4.1; cool; filter; add phenanthroline reagent | Colorimetric | 5 mg/l | Swisher et al. (1967) |
| Water | Deaerate with nitrogen gas; add indium (III) nitrate | DPP | 0.3 ppm | Haberman (1971) |
| Stream, sea- and sewage water | Add hydroxylamine sulfate solution; heat; cool; add acetate (chloride for saline solutions) electrolyte and bismuth nitrate solution; deaerate | DPP | 0.01 mg/l | Hoover (1973) |
| Water | Acidify with ascorbic and nitric acid; deaerate with nitrogen gas; add bismuth nitrate; determine before and after addition of bismuth | DPP | 0.05 mg/l | Haring & van Delft (1977) |
| Water | Convert to corresponding tri-$n$-butyl ester | GC/FID | Not reported | Warren & Malec (1972) |
| Tap water and sewage effluents | Isolate by anion-exchange chromatography; convert to tri-$n$-butyl ester | GC/FID | 1 ppb ($\mu$g/l) | Aue et al. (1972) |
| Tap water and sewage effluents | Convert to tri-$n$-butyl ester | GC/NPD, GC/MS/SIM | 1 $\mu$g/l | Games et al. (1981) |

[a]DPP, differential pulse polarography; GC/FID, gas chromatography/flame ionization detection; GC/NPD, gas chromatography/nitrogen phosphorus detection; GC/MS/SIM, gas chromatography/mass spectrometry/selective ion monitoring

# 3. Biological Data Relevant to the Evaluation of Carcinogenic Risk to Humans

## 3.1 Carcinogenicity studies in animals

**NTA and its salts**

*(a) Dietary administration*

**NTA**

*Mouse*: Groups of 50 male and 50 female B6C3F$_1$ mice, six weeks of age, were fed 7500 or 15 000 (maximum tolerated dose) ppm (mg/kg) commercial-grade NTA (purity, 99.5%) in the diet for 18 months and were killed at 21 months. Groups of 20 male and 20 female mice served as controls. More weight loss was observed in high- and low-dose females and in high-dose males than in controls; survival was comparable in treated and control animals of each sex. Hydronephrosis was detected in 8/44 high-dose males and 12/50 high-dose females, and animals of each sex had increased incidences of renal tumours, mostly adenocarcinomas: males—control, 0/20; low-dose, 5/49; high-dose, 24/44 ($p < 0.001$; $\chi^2$ for 2 × 3 contingency table); females—control, 0/20; low-dose, 0/39; high-dose, 4/50 ($p = 0.041$, test for linear trend) (National Cancer Institute, 1977).

*Rat*: Groups of 50 male and 50 female Fischer 344 rats, six weeks of age, were fed 7500 or 15 000 (maximum tolerated dose) ppm (mg/kg) commercial-grade NTA (99.5% pure) in the diet for 18 months and were killed at 24 months. Groups of 20 males and 20 females served as controls. A modest, dose-related decrease in body weight gain was observed; survival was comparable in treated and control animals of each sex. Renal interstitial fibrosis and tubular dilatation were found frequently. Increases were observed in the incidences of urinary-tract tumours, mainly tubular-cell adenomas and carcinomas, in males: control, 0/20; low-dose, 1/49; high-dose, 7/48 ($p = 0.006$, test for linear trend); and of transitional- and squamous-cell carcinomas of the urinary bladder in females: control, 0/18; low-dose, 2/45; high-dose, 12/48 ($p < 0.001$, test for linear trend). Increases were also seen in the incidences of phaeochromocytomas of the adrenal gland in females: control, 1/20; low-dose, 0/50; high-dose, 14/48 ($p < 0.001$; $\chi^2$ for 2 x 3 contingency table). The incidences of liver tumours, all considered to be neoplastic nodules [adenomas (Maronpot *et al.*, 1986)], were also increased in females: control, 2/15; low-dose, 8/49; high-dose, 22/49 ($p = 0.001$, test for linear trend) (National Cancer Institute, 1977).

**NTA, trisodium salt, monohydrate**

*Mouse*: Groups of 50 male and 50 female B6C3F$_1$ mice, six weeks of age, were fed 2500 or 5000 (maximum tolerated dose) ppm (mg/kg) commercial-grade NTA, trisodium salt, monohydrate (purity, 99.5%) in the diet for 18 months and were killed at 21 months. Groups of 20 male and 20 female mice served as controls. A dose-related decrease in body weight gain was observed in mice of each sex; survival was comparable in treated and control animals. No urinary-tract tumour was observed, but there was a dose-related increase in the incidence of haematopoietic tumours in male mice: control, 0/20; low-dose, 4/47; high-dose, 9/50 ($p = 0.015$, test for linear trend) (National Cancer Institute, 1977).

*Rat*: Groups of 50 male and 50 female Fischer 344 rats, six weeks of age, were fed diets containing 7500 or 15 000 (maximum tolerated dose) ppm (mg/kg) commercial-grade NTA, trisodium salt, monohydrate (purity, 99.5%) for 18 months and were killed at 24 months. Groups of 20 male and 20 female rats served as controls. A dose-related decrease in body weight was observed in rats of each sex; survival was comparable in treated and control animals. Evidence of renal inflammation was observed in low- and high-dose male and female rats, but no increase in the incidence of neoplasms was observed (National Cancer Institute, 1977).

In another feeding study, groups of 24 male and 24 female Fischer 344 rats, 51-55 days of age, were fed 0, 200, 2000 or 20 000 (maximum tolerated dose) ppm (mg/kg) commercial-grade NTA, trisodium salt, monohydrate (no impurity detected) in the diet for 104 weeks. Decreases in body weight and survival and hydronephrosis were observed in high-dose males. One papilloma of the urinary bladder was seen in a female given 2000 ppm; all other kidney and urinary-tract tumours were observed in males and females given the highest dose. Tubular-cell adenomas and adenocarcinomas of the kidney were observed in 4/24 males [$p = 0.004$, Cochran-Armitage test]; transitional-cell carcinomas developed in the renal pelvis in 4/24 males ($p = 0.003$, Cochran-Armitage test) and in the ureter in 8/24 males ($p < 0.001$, Cochran-Armitage test); and metastases were observed in 5/24 males. Tubular-cell adenomas and adenocarcinomas of the kidney developed in 4/24 females ($p = 0.003$, test for linear trend); transitional-cell carcinomas developed in the ureter in 6/24 females ($p < 0.001$, test for linear trend) and in the urinary bladder in 5/24 females ($p = 0.001$, test for linear trend); metastases were observed in 5/24 females (National Cancer Institute, 1977).

(b) *Administration in drinking-water*

**NTA, trisodium salt**

*Rat*: A total of 196 male, non-inbred Sprague-Dawley rats, weighing approximately 350 g, were given 0.1% NTA, trisodium salt [purity unspecified] in the drinking-water *ad libitum* for 704 days. A group of 192 untreated males served as controls. No difference in weight gain was observed between control and treated animals, but a higher proportion of treated rats died during the first 550 days of the study. An increase in the incidence of renal adenomas and adenocarcinomas was observed, with adenomas in 5/186 controls and 25 adenomas and four carcinomas in 29/183 treated animals ($p < 0.01$, Mantel-Haenszel test). In addition, renal tubular hyperplasia (grades III and IV) was observed 44/186 controls and 67/183 treated animals. There was no apparent difference in the frequency of severe nephritis between control and treated animals (Goyer *et al.*, 1981).

**NTA, disodium salt**

*Mouse*: Groups of 40 male and 40 female random-bred Swiss mice, eight weeks of age, were given 5 g/l NTA disodium salt, monohydrate [purity unspecified] in the drinking-water for 26 weeks and killed at 35-36 weeks. No increase in the incidence of tumours at any site was observed (Greenblatt & Lijinsky, 1974). [The Working Group noted the short duration of the experiment and the relatively low dose used.]

*Rat*: Groups of 15 male and 15 female MRC rats, eight to ten weeks of age, were given approximately 20 ml of drinking-water containing 0.5% NTA, disodium salt [purity unspecified] on five days a week for 84 weeks. All surviving animals were killed 104 weeks after the beginning of treatment. No significant difference in tumour incidence and no toxicity were observed (Lijinsky *et al.*, 1973). [The Working Group noted the small number of animals and the relatively low dose used.]

(c) *Administration with known carcinogens*[1]

*Rat*: In a two-stage carcinogenicity study of NTA, trisodium salt, monohydrate, four groups of 21 male Wistar rats, seven weeks old, received 0.05% *N*-nitroso(4-hydroxybutyl)butylamine (NHBBA) [purity unspecified] in the drinking-water for four weeks, after which they were fed 0 (NHBBA alone), 0.3%, 0.5% or 1.0% NTA, trisodium salt, monohydrate (purity, >95%) in the diet for 28 weeks, when all survivors were killed. An increased incidence of papillary or nodular [transitional-cell] hyperplasia of the urinary bladder was observed with all three doses of NTA, trisodium salt, monohydrate: NHBBA alone, 3/20; low-dose, 13/21; mid-dose, 18/18; high-dose, 17/17 [$p < 0.001$, Cochran-Armitage test]. An increase was also detected in the incidence of [transitional-cell] papillomas of the urinary bladder: NHBBA alone, 0/20; low-dose, 1/21; mid-dose, 8/18; high-dose, 12/17 [$p < 0.001$, Cochran-Armitage test]. There was also an increased incidence of transitional-cell carcinomas of the urinary bladder: NHBBA alone, 0/20; low-dose, 1/21; mid-dose, 2/18; high-dose, 7/17 [$p < 0.001$, Cochran-Armitage test]. In three additional groups that received 0.3, 0.5 or 1.0% NTA, trisodium salt, monohydrate without NHBBA, simple [transitional-cell] hyperplasia of the urinary bladder was observed frequently (Kitahori *et al.*, 1985).

In a similar study, five groups of 25-26 male Fischer 344 rats were given 0, 0.01% or 0.05% NHBBA [purity unspecified] in the drinking-water for four weeks and were then fed diets containing 0 or 2% NTA, trisodium salt, monohydrate (95.0% pure) for 32 weeks, at which time survivors were killed. In animals treated with 0.05% NHBBA plus NTA, trisodium salt, monohydrate, an increased incidence of papillary or nodular [transitional-cell] hyperplasia of the urinary bladder was observed: NHBBA, 13/26; NHBBA plus NTA, trisodium salt, monohydrate, 23/26 ($p < 0.01$). [Transitional-cell] papillomas of the urinary bladder were also observed in 8/26 rats gien NHBBA alone and in 18/26 also given the NTA compound ($p < 0.01$). In animals treated with the NTA compound alone, no hyperplastic or neoplastic lesion was observed (Fukushima *et al.*, 1985). [The Working Group noted the short duration of the experiment and the lack of specification of the statistical test used.]

---

[1]The Working Group noted that the four studies described were designed as two-stage carcinogenicity studies and could therefore not be evaluated as complete carcinogenicity studies.

In a further two-stage carcinogenicity study, eight groups of 24 male inbred Wistar rats, seven weeks of age, were fed a diet containing 0 or 1000 ppm (mg/kg) N-nitrosoethylhydroxyethylamine (NEHEA) (purity, 99.8%) for two weeks after which they were given 0, 3000, 10 000 or 30 000 ppm NTA, trisodium salt, monohydrate (95.0% pure) in the diet for 30 weeks, at which time survivors were killed. A significant increase in the incidence of renal tubular-cell tumours was observed in animals treated with NEHEA plus the mid and high doses of the NTA compound over that in animals treated with NEHEA alone: NEHEA alone, 4/24; low-dose, 5/22; mid-dose, 23/23 ($p < 0.01$); and high-dose, 23/23 ($p < 0.01$). In animals treated with the NTA compound alone, no renal tubular-cell tumour was observed (Hiasa et al., 1985). [The Working Group noted the short duration of the experiment.]

In a two-stage carcinogenicity study, groups of 15-20 male Wistar rats, weighing 130-150 g, were given drinking-water containing 0.2% N-nitrosobis(2-hydroxypropyl)amine (NDHPA; purity, 98%) for two weeks and were then fed 1% NTA (purity, 99%) or its trisodium salt, monohydrate (purity, 95%) in the diet for 30 weeks. The tumour incidences in the groups treated with NDHPA, with NDHPA plus NTA and with NDHPA plus NTA, trisodium salt, monohydrate were: urinary-bladder tumours (mainly papillomas)—1/20, 1/20 and 7/20 [$p = 0.004$, Cochran-Armitage test]; renal cell tumours—3/20, 15/20 and 10/20 [$p = 0.014$, Cochran-Armitage test]; and nephroblastomas—3/20, 4/20 and 11/20 [$p = 0.003$, Cochran-Armitage test] (Shimoyama, 1986).

### Solutions of NTA, disodium salt with metal salts

*Intraperitoneal injection*

*Mouse*: A group of 53 male and 21 female A/J mice, four weeks old, received daily intraperitoneal injections of solutions prepared from ferric nitrate and NTA, disodium salt (molar ratio of iron to NTA, 1:4; Fe-NTA), adjusted to pH 7.0 with $Na_2HCO_3$ at a level of 1.8-2.7 mg/kg bw iron, on six days per week for 12 weeks. The surviving animals were killed at 420 days. A further group of ten males and ten females was injected with equivalent amounts of NTA (reagent grade [purity unspecified]), and 20 males and 20 females were untreated. Fe-NTA was highly toxic to males: 28/53 died within 14 days, mainly from renal failure as a consequence of proximal tubular necrosis; no lethality was observed in females. Of the animals that survived to 420 days, 15/25 Fe-NTA-treated males ($p < 0.005$, $\chi^2$ test) and 1/21 Fe-NTA-treated females developed renal tubular-cell adenocarcinomas. The first tumours appeared at 50 days. Renal neoplasms did not occur in untreated controls or in mice treated only with NTA (Li et al., 1987). [The Working Group noted the short duration of the experiment.]

*Rat*: A group of 32 male Wistar rats [age unspecified] received six intraperitoneal injections per week of solutions of ferric nitrate and NTA, disodium salt, as described above, for two weeks (total dose, 100-150 mg iron per animal) and were kept for 240-260 days. Eight male rats served as untreated controls and eight as saline-treated controls. Eight animals in the treated group died during the study; serial sacrifices were made throughout the experiment. At termination of the study, 22/24 Fe-NTA-treated rats but no saline-treated or untreated control had developed renal adenocarcinomas (Okada & Midorikawa, 1982). [The Working Group noted the small number of animals used and the short duration of the study.]

Groups of 24 male Wistar rats, four weeks of age, received daily intraperitoneal injections of solutions prepared from ferric nitrate and NTA, disodium salt, as described above (5-7 mg iron/kg bw per day) or solutions prepared from aluminium chloride and NTA, disodium salt (Al-NTA; molar ratio of aluminium to NTA, 1:4; 1.5-2.0 mg aluminium/kg bw per day) on six days a week for up to three months and were killed at 52 weeks. Groups of ten males received injections of equivalent amounts of saline, solutions of NTA or solutions of aluminium chloride. Rats treated with Al-NTA or Fe-NTA had depressed weight gain and developed severe injury of the proximal convoluted tubules, polyuria and glucosuria. Fe-NTA-treated rats developed renal-cell carcinomas (14/18; $p < 0.05$); no such tumour was observed in the other groups (Ebina *et al.*, 1986). [The Working Group noted the small number of animals used and the short duration of the study.]

## 3.2 Other relevant biological data

(a) *Experimental systems*

(i) *Absorption, distribution, excretion and metabolism*

**NTA and its salts**

The absorption, distribution and excretion of NTA, trisodium salt have been reviewed (Anderson *et al.*, 1985). Absorption of NTA, disodium salt in rats and dogs ranged from 77% to 99% after single oral doses (Michael & Wakim, 1971). In a whole-body autoradiographic study, 0.93 mg [1-$^{14}$C-acetate]-NTA, trisodium salt was administered intravenously to NMRI albino mice and the same amount orally to C57Bl mice; heavy accumulation of radioactivity occurred in the skeleton, which persisted for 48 h, the longest interval studied (Tjälve, 1972).

The kidney attains concentrations of NTA greater than that in the plasma in rats with steady-state plasma NTA levels. The relatively high kidney concentrations of NTA can be attributed to high concentrations of NTA in small volumes of urine (Anderson, 1980).

In rats and dogs, the only route of excretion of absorbed NTA, disodium salt was *via* the urine, as shown by the absence of ingested NTA in the bile; in monkeys and rabbits, it was excreted in the faeces (Michael & Wakim, 1971).

NTA is not metabolized in mammals and is excreted rapidly by filtration in the kidney (Michael & Wakim, 1971; Budny, 1972; Chu *et al.*, 1978; Anderson *et al.*, 1985).

**Solutions of NTA, disodium salt with metal salts**

Repeated intraperitoneal injections of a solution of ferric nitrate and NTA, disodium salt (molar ratio, 2:1) resulted in deposition of iron in the parenchymal cells of the liver and in the pancreas and adrenal glands of rats and rabbits (Awai *et al.*, 1979). Iron uptake by rat liver was examined after a single intraperitoneal injection of $^{59}$Fe-NTA (Fe:NTA, 1:5 molar ratio) and of Fe-[$^{14}$C]-NTA (Fe:NTA, 1:1; prepared as above) to give 7.5 mg Fe/kg bw. Of the injected $^{59}$Fe, 30% was incorporated in the liver non-haem iron fraction by 3 h and was retained for 240 h; only 1% of the $^{14}$C injected as Fe-[$^{14}$C]-NTA was taken up by the liver by 3 h (Matsuura, 1983).

(ii) *Toxic effects*

**NTA and its salts**

The toxicology of NTA has been reviewed (Anderson *et al.*, 1985).

The oral $LD_{50}$ in rodents of NTA, trisodium salt, monohydrate was reported to be about 2 g/kg bw (Anderson *et al.*, 1985).

NTA is nephrotoxic. NTA and its trisodium salt have been shown to induce cytoplasmic vacuolation of renal proximal tubule cells, hydronephrosis, erosion and ulceration of the renal pelvic transitional epithelium and kidney hyperplasia in rats at dietary levels of 0.15% or more, in studies of 28 days or longer (Nixon, 1971; Mahaffey & Goyer, 1972; Nixon *et al.*, 1972; National Cancer Institute, 1977; Alden *et al.*, 1981; Merski, 1981; Alden & Kanerva, 1982a; Anderson *et al.*, 1982; Merski, 1982) and in mice at 0.5% or more (National Cancer Institute, 1977). In a comparison study in treated and untreated animals, all forms of renal toxicity, except hydronephrosis, basophilic hyperplasia of tubular cells and neoplasia, were reversed when treatment was discontinued (Alden & Kanerva, 1982b; Myers *et al.*, 1982). Ureters were swollen and showed alterations in epithelial morphology similar to those observed in the renal pelvis (Kanerva *et al.*, 1984).

The responses of Charles River and Fischer 344 rats to 1.5% NTA and 2% NTA, trisodium salt in the diet were evaluated in a four-week feeding study. In spite of different rates of ingestion, the two strains of animals had similar qualitative responses to NTA. Ingestion of NTA or its trisodium salt was associated with reduced growth, increased kidney:body weight ratio, increased urinary calcium, haematuria and the presence of crystalline NTA, calcium sodium salt in the urine (Anderson & Kanerva, 1979). Feeding a dose of 1.5% NTA (which induced bladder neoplasms) to rats was associated with a 50% decrease in the calcium concentration of bladder tissue, but with little change in magnesium, zinc, sodium or potassium levels (Anderson *et al.*, 1982).

No change in fat-free bone weight, total ash or percentage of ash was found in the tibias of rats fed NTA, trisodium salt for 91 days. When given for 30 days, the compound had no effect on serum alkaline phosphatase or on liver and kidney carbonic anhydrase (Michael & Wakim, 1973), but hepatic metallothionein levels were increased two fold following intraperitoneal administration of NTA (100 mg/kg bw) to male Swiss Webster mice (Goering *et al.*, 1985).

After NTA, trisodium salt was fed to male and female beagle dogs for 90 days at 0.03, 0.15 and 0.5% in the diet, urinary zinc excretion was significantly greater in dogs in the mid- and high-dose groups. NTA was deposited in bone (123-142 ppm at the 0.5% dose level), but this had no adverse effect (Budny *et al.*, 1973).

**Solutions of NTA with metal salts**

In the studies described below, animals were given solutions prepared from a ferric salt (usually ferric nitrate) and an NTA salt (usually NTA, disodium salt) in various molar ratios, as specified. In all cases, the solution contained an excess of either NTA or iron, which would be present in addition to the Fe-NTA complex in solution. The precise composition of the solutions was not further characterized by the authors.

Twenty-four hours after a single intraperitoneal injection of Fe-NTA (Fe:NTA, 1:4 molar ratio) to Wistar rats (Hamazaki *et al.*, 1985; Ebina *et al.*, 1986) or A/J mice (Li *et al.*, 1987), rats developed extensive necrosis of the renal proximal tubules, which progressed with multiple doses to partial renal degeneration, strictly confined to the proximal tubules. Sequalae were polyuria, glucosuria and aminoaciduria. In mice, the predominant autopsy finding among those (all males) that died within 14 days was renal tubular necrosis. Vitamin E protected Wistar rats against the nephrotoxic effects of Fe-NTA (Fe:NTA, 1:4—Okada *et al.*, 1987; Fe:NTA, unspecified—Hamazaki *et al.*, 1988). Mild diabetes has been reported after daily injection of Fe-NTA in rats and rabbits (Fe:NTA, 2:1—Awai *et al.*, 1979; Fe:NTA, 1:2-2.5—May *et al.*, 1980). Fe-NTA is a potent initiator of lipid peroxidation in the livers of rats (Fe:NTA, 1:1.5; Goddard *et al.*, 1986) and mice (Fe:NTA, 1:1.5; Goddard & Sweeney, 1983) injected intraperitoneally, in rat liver homogenates and hepatocyte suspensions (Fe:NTA, 1:1.5; Goddard *et al.*, 1986) and in Ehrlich ascites tumour cells (Fe:NTA, 1:5; Nakamoto *et al.*, 1986). It was reported in an abstract that oral administration of Fe-NTA [molar ratio unspecified] to male Fischer 344 rats increased the formation of 8-hydroxydeoxyguanosine in the kidney (Sai *et al.*, 1988).

Male Wistar rats given solutions prepared from aluminium chloride and NTA disodium salt (Al:NTA, 1:4; 1.5-2.0 mg Al/kg bw per day) by intraperitoneal injection for 14 days showed morphological damage in the liver and kidney, including diffuse mid-zonal coagulation necrosis of hepatocytes and acute proximal tubular necrosis of the kidney at day 4. Seven of ten rats given Al-NTA died within five days. When Al-NTA was given in a dose of 1.5-2.0 mg Al/kg bw per day for 54 days, metabolic acidosis was demonstrated and renal injury was severe, involving proximal tubular necrosis and granular casts in the distal tubules. From day 38 onwards, atrophy of the nerve cells of the cerebrum and demyelination of the brain stem were also observed (Ebina *et al.*, 1984, 1986).

(iii) *Effects on reproduction and prenatal toxicity*

Ten NMRI mice received 0.2% NTA in the drinking-water on days 6-18 of gestation; ten control mice received no treatment. A small difference in mean fetal weight was seen between the two groups on day 18, and the number of resorptions was slightly higher in the treated group. Skeletal and visceral examination did not reveal any teratogenic effect (Tjälve, 1972).

Groups of 20 mated female Charles River rats were given 0, 0.1 or 20 mg/kg bw NTA, trisodium salt, monohydrate (two groups for each dose) in the drinking-water on days 6-14 of gestation. Treatment did not affect the numbers of resorptions or fetuses, fetal body weight or development of the fetal skeleton. A significant increase in the incidence of hydronephrosis and bladder defects was observed in fetuses in some treated groups (Nolen *et al.*, 1972a).

NTA, trisodium salt did not induce reproductive toxicity in male or female Charles River CD rats in a two-generation study (0.1 or 0.5% in the diet) or in pregnant Charles River CD rats (0.1 or 0.5% in the diet on days 6-15 of pregnancy) or in rabbits (up to 250 mg/kg bw by gavage on days 7-16 of gestation; Nolen *et al.*, 1971).

The available studies provide no evidence that NTA or its salts enhance the reproductive toxicity of heavy metals in experimental animals (Nolen et al., 1972a,b; Scharpf et al., 1972, 1973; McClain & Siekierka, 1975).

(iv) *Genetic and related effects* (see Appendix 1)

**NTA and its salts**

NTA at concentrations up to 42.5 mM did not induce forward mutation or aneuploidy in *Aspergillus nidulans* (Crebelli et al., 1986). It did not induce respiration-defective mutants in *Saccharomyces cerevisiae* at a concentration of 4 g/l (Zetterberg, 1970), not did it induce sex-linked recessive lethal mutations in *Drosophila* in feeding and injection studies (Kramers, 1976—50 mM and 10 mM, respectively; Woodruff et al., 1985—4000 and 1000 ppm, respectively); however, it did induce aneuploidy (at $5 \times 10^{-2}$M; Costa et al., 1988a) and sex-chromosome loss (at 4000 ppm, Ramel & Magnusson, 1979) in *Drosophila*. NTA (0.5-5 µg/ml) did not induce sister chromatid exchange or chromosomal aberrations in the Chinese hamster CHO cell line in culture in the presence or absence of an exogenous metabolic system from Aroclor 1254-induced rat liver (Loveday et al., 1989). It was reported in an abstract to induce ploidy changes and endoreduplication in human lymphocytes *in vitro* (Bora, 1975). NTA did not cause dominant lethal mutation in mice *in vivo* at 125 mg/kg bw given intraperitoneally or 1000 mg/kg bw given orally (Epstein et al., 1972).

NTA, trisodium salt was not mutagenic to several strains of *Salmonella typhimurium* (Dunkel et al., 1985; Loprieno et al., 1985; Venier et al., 1987) or to *Escherichia coli* (Dunkel et al., 1985; Venier et al., 1987) in the presence or absence of an exogenous metabolic system from Aroclor 1254-induced rat liver (Dunkel et al., 1985; Loprieno et al., 1985; Venier et al., 1987), mouse liver or Syrian hamster liver or uninduced rat, mouse or Syrian hamster liver (Dunkel et al., 1985). It was not active in the SOS chromotest but gave positive results at a dose of 1 mg in differential toxicity tests in *E. coli* in the presence and absence of an exogenous metabolic system (Venier et al., 1987).

NTA, trisodium salt induced chromosomal aberrations at $2 \times 10^{-2}$M in *Vicia faba* (Kihlman & Sturelid, 1970); it induced micronuclei in *V. faba* at $2 \times 10^{-3}$M and in *Allium cepa* at $4 \times 10^{-3}$M (De Marco et al., 1986). NTA, trisodium salt was not mutagenic to *Saccharomyces pombe* or *Saccharomyces cerevisiae* (40 µg/ml) in the presence or absence of an exogenous metabolic system (Loprieno et al., 1985). The trisodium salt did not cause unscheduled DNA synthesis in primary cultures of rat hepatocytes at 0.5 or 1 mg/ml (Williams et al., 1982). It did not cause mutation at the *hprt* locus in Chinese hamster V79 cells *in vitro* at $10^{-2}$M (Celotti et al., 1987) and did not induce mutation at the TK locus in mouse lymphoma L5178Y cells *in vitro* in the presence or absence of an exogenous metabolic sytstem (630-2350 µg/ml or 524-1900 µg/ml, respectively; Mitchell et al., 1988). It did not induce sister chromatid exchange in the Chinese hamster CHO cell line ($10^{-3}$M, Ved Brat & Williams, 1984; 1.9 µg/ml, Loprieno et al., 1985; $2 \times 10^{-3}$M, Montaldi et al., 1985; 1 µg/ml, Venier et al., 1985) or in cultured peripheral lymphocytes from Balb/c and Balb/Mo mice ($10^{-3}$M; Montaldi et al., 1985). It induced chromosomal aberrations in rat kangaroo cells *in vitro* at $2 \times 10^{-2}$M (Kihlman & Sturelid, 1970), and it induced resistance to diphtheria toxin in a human epithelial-like cell line *in vitro* ($1.1 \times 10^{-5}$M; Grilli & Capucci, 1985). It did not induce sister chromatid exchange ($10^{-3}$M; Ved Brat & Williams, 1984) or chromosomal aberrations ($10^{-2}$M, Ved Brat & Williams, 1984; 7.5 × $10^{-3}$M, Montaldi et al., 1988) in cultured human peripheral lymphocytes. It did not induce micronuclei in mice *in vivo* (200-400 mg/kg bw; Montaldi et al., 1988).

As reported in an abstract, NTA, sodium calcium salt did not induce heritable translocations in mice *in vivo* after administration of 0.1% in drinking-water for seven weeks (Jorgenson et al., 1975).

**Solutions of NTA with metal salts**

Lead chromate ($PbCrO_4$) was mutagenic to *S. typhimurium* (Loprieno et al., 1985; Venier et al., 1987) and to *E. coli* (Venier et al., 1987) in the presence of NTA, trisodium salt, but not when tested alone. Similarly, lead chromate in a NTA, trisodium salt solution induced mutation in *Drosophila* (Costa et al., 1988) and mutations at the *hprt* locus in Chinese hamster V79 cells (Celotti et al., 1987). NTA, trisodium salt (2 × $10^{-3}$M-6 × $10^{-3}$M) enhanced the frequency of sister chromatid exchange in the Chinese hamster CHO cell line induced by the insoluble salts $CdCO_3$, $HgCl$, $PbSO_4$, $PbCrO_4$ and $NiCO_3$ (Loprieno et al., 1985; Montaldi et al., 1987), as well as that induced by insoluble chromates of Ba, Zn, Sr and Ca (Venier et al., 1985); no such enhancement was seen for soluble salts ($CdCl_2$, $K_2Cr_2O_7$, $HgCl_2$ and $NiCl_2$; Montaldi et al., 1987). Solutions of NTA:iron (2:1 molar ratio), with the iron as $FeSO_4$ and $FeCl_3$, caused chromosomal aberrations in the Chinese hamster CHO cell line only at millimolar concentrations (Whiting et al., 1981). NTA, trisodium salt (2 × $10^{-3}$M) enhanced the frequency of micronuclei and chromosomal aberrations induced in human lymphocytes by the insoluble salts $CdCO_3$, $HgCl$ and $PbSO_4$, and, to a lesser extent, that induced by $PbCrO_4$ and $NiCO_3$ (Montaldi et al., 1987). Transformation of Syrian hamster fibroblast BHK cells induced by Cr[VI] compounds was enhanced by the presence of NTA (Lanfranchi et al., 1988).

[The Working Group noted that when NTA or its salts and NTA in combination with metal salts caused a positive response, primarily in assays for chromosomal anomalies, the effects were seen only with very high concentrations of NTA.]

(b) *Humans*

(i) *Absorption, distribution, excretion and metabolism*

A capsule containing 10 mg [1-$^{14}$C]NTA in gelatin was given orally in fruit juice to each of eight male volunteers who had received no drugs for two weeks before entering the study. Twelve percent of the administered radioactivity was excreted in the urine and 77% in the faeces as unchanged NTA within 120 h of administration. A peak in the blood concentration (6.5 ng/g serum) occurred 1-2 h after dosing (Budny & Arnold, 1973).

(ii) *Toxic effects*

No data were available to the Working Group.

(iii) *Effects on reproduction and prenatal toxicity*

No data were available to the Working Group.

(iv) *Genetic and related effects*

No data were available to the Working Group.

## 3.3 Case reports and epidemiological studies of carcinogenicity to humans

No data were available to the Working Group.

# 4. Summary of Data Reported and Evaluation

## 4.1 Exposure data

Nitrilotriacetic acid and its sodium salts have been produced since the 1930s for use as metal chelating agents in household and industrial detergents, industrial water treatment, textile preparation and metal finishing. Occupational exposure to nitrilotriacetic acid and its salts may occur during its production and use, but data on levels are limited. Exposure to nitrilotriacetic acid, and presumably to its water-soluble metal complexes, occurs as a result of its presence in household detergents and in drinking-water.

## 4.2 Experimental carcinogenicity data

Nitrilotriacetic acid was tested for carcinogenicity by oral administration in the diet in mice and rats. It induced renal-cell adenocarcinomas in mice of each sex, renal-cell tumours in male rats and transitional- and squamous-cell carcinomas of the urinary bladder, hepatocellular adenomas and adrenal phaeochromocytomas in female rats.

Nitrilotriacetic acid, trisodium salt was tested for carcinogenicity in mice and rats by oral administration. When administered in the diet as the monohydrate, it induced haematopoietic tumours in male mice and benign and malignant tumours of the urinary system (kidney, ureter and bladder) in rats of each sex. When administered in drinking-water to male rats, it induced renal adenomas and adenocarcinomas.

In two-stage carcinogenicity studies in male rats by oral administration, nitrilotriacetic acid and its trisodium salt increased the incidence of urinary-tract tumours after pretreatment with different nitrosamines.

Solutions of nitrilotriacetic acid, disodium salt with ferric salts were tested in mice of each sex and in male rats by intraperitoneal administration. They induced renal adenocarcinomas in males of each species.

## 4.3 Human carcinogenicity data

No data were available to the Working Group.

## 4.4 Other relevant data

Nitrilotriacetic acid and its trisodium salt were nephrotoxic to rodents.

In a single study, nitrilotriacetic acid did not induce dominant lethal mutation in mice treated *in vivo*. Also in single studies, it did not induce chromosomal aberrations or sister chromatid exchange in Chinese hamster cells *in vitro*. In single studies, it induced aneuploidy and sex chromosome loss in *Drosophila* at high doses. In other studies, it did not induce sex-linked recessive lethal mutation in *Drosophila*. It was not mutagenic to fungi, and, in a single study, it did not cause aneuploidy in fungi.

In a single study, nitrilotriacetic acid, trisodium salt did not induce micronuclei in mice *in vivo*. It did not cause chromosomal aberrations or, in a single study, sister chromatid exchange in human peripheral lymphocytes *in vitro*, but, at a high dose in one study, it was mutagenic to a human epithelial-like cell line *in vitro*. It also caused chromosomal aberrations in rat kangaroo cells at a high dose in a single study, but it did not cause sister chromatid exchange or gene mutation or, in another study, unscheduled DNA synthesis in rodent cells *in vitro*. At high doses, it caused chromosomal aberrations in plants. It was not mutagenic to yeast or bacteria in the presence or absence of an exogenous metabolic system. It gave equivocal results for DNA damage in prokaryotes.

### 4.5 Evaluation[1]

There is *sufficient evidence* for the carcinogenicity of nitrilotriacetic acid and its sodium salts in experimental animals.

No data were available from studies in humans on the carcinogenicity of nitrilotriacetic acid and its salts.

In formulating the overall evaluation, the Working Group took note of the fact that nitrilotriacetic acid is liberated to some extent from nitrilotriacetate salts in solution.

**Overall evaluation**

Nitrilotriacetic acid and its salts are *possibly carcinogenic to humans (Group 2B)*.

# 5. References

Alden, C.L. & Kanerva, R.L. (1982a) The pathogenesis of renal cortical tumours in rats fed 2% trisodium nitrilotriacetate monohydrate. *Food chem. Toxicol.*, 20, 441-450

Alden, C.L. & Kanerva, R.L. (1982b) Reversibility of renal cortical lesions induced in rats by high doses of nitrilotriacetate in chronic feeding studies. *Food chem. Toxicol.*, 20, 935-937

Alden, C.L., Kanerva, R.L., Anderson, R.L. & Adkins, A.G. (1981) Short-term effects of dietary nitrilotriacetic acid in the male Charles River rat kidney. *Vet. Pathol.*, 18, 549-559

Aldrich Chemical Co. (1988) *1988-1989 Aldrich Catalog/Handbook of Fine Chemicals*, Milwaukee, WI, p. 1104

---

[1]For description of the italicized terms and criteria for making the evaluation, see Preamble, pp. 25-29.

## Summary table of genetic and related effects of nitrilotriacetic acid

| Nonmammalian systems | | | | | | | | | | | | | Mammalian systems | | | | | | | | | | | | | | | | | | | |
|---|---|---|---|---|---|---|---|---|---|---|---|---|---|---|---|---|---|---|---|---|---|---|---|---|---|---|---|---|---|---|---|---|
| Prokaryotes | | Lower eukaryotes | | | | Plants | | | Insects | | | | | In vitro | | | | | | | | | | | | | | In vivo | | | | |
| | | | | | | | | | | | | | Animal cells | | | | | | | Human cells | | | | | | | | Animals | | | | | | | Humans | | | | | |
| D | G | D | R | G | A | D | G | C | R | G | C | A | D | G | S | M | C | A | T | I | D | G | S | M | C | A | T | I | D | G | S | M | C | DL | A | D | S | M | C | A |
|   |   |   |   |   | -¹|   |   |   | - | +¹| +¹|   |   |   | -¹|   | -¹|   |   |   |   |   |   |   |   |   |   |   |   |   |   |   |   | -¹|   |   |   |   |   |   |

A, aneuploidy; C, chromosomal aberrations; D, DNA damage; DL, dominant lethal mutation; G, gene mutation; I, inhibition of intercellular communication; M, micronuclei; R, mitotic recombination and gene conversion; S, sister chromatid exchange; T, cell transformation

*In completing the tables, the following symbols indicate the consensus of the Working Group with regard to the results for each endpoint:*

–     considered to be negative
–¹    considered to be negative, but only one valid study was available to the Working Group
+¹    considered to be positive, but only one valid study was available to the Working Group

## Summary table of genetic and related effects of nitrilotriacetic acid, trisodium salt

| Nonmammalian systems | | | | | | | | | | | | Mammalian systems | | | | | | | | | | | | | | | | | |
|---|---|---|---|---|---|---|---|---|---|---|---|---|---|---|---|---|---|---|---|---|---|---|---|---|---|---|---|---|---|
| Prokaryotes | Lower eukaryotes | | | | Plants | | | | | Insects | | | In vitro | | | | | | | | | | | | | In vivo | | | |
| | | | | | | | | | | | | | Animal cells | | | | | | | Human cells | | | | | | Animals | | | | Humans |
| D | G | D | R | G | A | D | G | C | R | G | C | A | D | G | S | M | C | A | T | I | D | G | S | M | C | A | T | I | D | G | S | M | C | DL | A | D | S | M | C | A |
| ? | - | | - | | | | + | | | | + | | $-^1$ | $-^1$ | - | | | $+^1$ | | | | | | | | | + | $-^1$ | - | | | | | $-^1$ | | | | | | |

A, aneuploidy; C, chromosomal aberrations; D, DNA damage; DL, dominant lethal mutation; G, gene mutation; I, inhibition of intercellular communication; M, micronuclei; R, mitotic recombination and gene conversion; S, sister chromatid exchange; T, cell transformation

*In completing the tables, the following symbols indicate the consensus of the Working Group with regard to the results for each endpoint:*

? considered to be equivocal or inconclusive (e.g., there were contradictory results from different laboratories; there were confounding exposures; the results were equivocal)
− considered to be negative
+ considered to be positive for the specific endpoint and level of biological complexity
$-^1$ considered to be negative, but only one valid study was available to the Working Group
$+^1$ considered to be positive, but only one valid study was available to the Working Group

Anderson, R.L. (1980) The relationship of insoluble nitrilotriacetate (NTA) in the urine of female rats to the dietary level of NTA. *Food Cosmet. Toxicol.*, 18, 59-64

Anderson, R.L. & Kanerva, R.L. (1979) Comparisons of response of Fischer-344 and Charles River rats to 1.5% nitrilotriacetic acid and 2% trisodium nitrilotriacetate, monohydrate. *Food Cosmet. Toxicol.*, 17, 137-140

Anderson, R.L., Alden, C.L. & Merski, J.A. (1982) The effects of nitrilotriacetate on cation disposition and urinary tract toxicity. *Food chem. Toxicol.*, 20, 105-122

Anderson, R.L., Bishop, W.E. & Campbell, R.L. (1985) A review of the environmental and mammalian toxicology of nitrilotriacetic acid. *Crit. Rev. Toxicol.*, 15, 1-102

Aue, W.A., Hastings, C.R., Gerhardt, K.O., Pierce, J.O., II, Hill, H.H. & Moseman, R.F. (1972) The determination of part-per-billion levels of citric and nitrilotriacetic acids in tap water and sewage effluents. *J. Chromatogr.*, 72, 259-267

Awai, M., Narasaki, M., Yamanoi, Y. & Seno, S. (1979) Induction of diabetes in animals by parenteral administration of ferric nitrilotriacetate. A model of experimental hemochromatosis. *Am. J. Pathol.*, 95, 663-673

Bora, K.C. (1975) Effects of nitrolotriacetic acid (NTA) on chromosome replication and structure in human cells (Abstract No. 34). *Mutat. Res.*, 31, 325

Budny, J.A. (1972) Metabolism and blood pressure effects of disodium nitrilotriacetate ($Na_2NTA$) in dogs. *Toxicol. appl. Pharmacol.*, 22, 655-660

Budny, J.A. & Arnold, J.D. (1973) Nitrilotriacetate (NTA): human metabolism and its importance in the total safety evaluation program. *Toxicol. appl. Pharmacol.*, 25, 48-53

Budny, J.A., Niewenhuis, R.J., Buehler, E.V. & Goldenthal, E.I. (1973) Subacute oral toxicity of trisodium nitrilotriacetate ($Na_3NTA$) in dogs. *Toxicol. appl. Pharmacol.*, 26, 148-153

Celotti, L., Furlan, D., Seccati, L. & Levis, A.G. (1987) Interactions of nitroloacetic acid (NTA) with Cr(VI) compounds in the induction of gene mutations in cultured mammalian cells. *Mutat. Res.*, 190, 35-39

Chu, I., Becking, G.C., Villeneuve, D.C. & Viau, A. (1978) Metabolism of nitrilotriacetic acid (NTA) in the mouse. *Bull. environ. Contam. Toxicol.*, 19, 417-422

Costa, R., Russo, A., Zordan, M., Pacchierotti, A., Tavella, A. & Levis, A.G. (1988a) Nitrilotriacetic acid (NTA) induces aneuploidy in *Drosophila* and mouse germ-line cells. *Environ. mol. Mutagenesis*, 12, 397-407

Costa, R., Strolego, F. & Levis, A.G. (1988b) Mutagenicity of lead chromate in *Drosophila melanogaster* in the presence of nitrilotriacetic acid (NTA). *Mutat. Res.*, 204, 257-261

Crebelli, R., Bellincampi, D., Conti, G., Conti, L., Morpurgo, G. & Carere, A. (1986) A comparative study on selected chemical carcinogens for chromosome malsegregation, mitotic crossing-over and forward mutation induction in *Aspergillus nidulans*. *Mutat. Res.*, 172, 139-149

De Marco, A., Romanelli, M., Stazi, M.A. & Vitagliano, E. (1986) Induction of micronucleated cells in *Vicia faba* and *Allium cepa* root tips treated with nitrilotriacetic acid (NTA). *Mutat. Res.*, 171, 145-148

Dunkel, V.C., Zeiger, E., Brusick, D., McCoy, E., McGregor, D., Mortelmans, K., Rosenkranz, H.S. & Simmon, V.F. (1985) Reproducibility of microbial mutagenicity assays: II. Testing of carcinogens and noncarcinogens in *Salmonella typhimurium* and *Escherichia coli*. *Environ. Mutagenesis*, 7 (Suppl. 5), 1-248

Ebina, Y., Okada, S., Hamazaki, S. & Midorikawa, O. (1984) Liver, kidney, and central nervous system toxicity of aluminum given intraperitoneally to rats: a multiple-dose subchronic study using aluminum nitrilotriacetate. *Toxicol. appl. Pharmacol.*, 75, 211-218

Ebina, Y., Okada, S., Hamazaki, S., Ogino, F., Li, J.-L. & Midorikawa, O. (1986) Nephrotoxicity and renal cell carcinoma after use of iron- and aluminum-nitrilotriacetate complexes in rats. *J. natl Cancer Inst.*, 76, 107-113

Epstein, S.S., Arnold, E., Andrea, S., Bass, W. & Bishop, Y. (1972) Detection of chemical mutagens by the dominant lethal assay in the mouse. *Toxicol. appl. Pharmacol.*, 23, 288-325

Fukushima, S., Kurata, Y., Tamano, S., Inoue, K. & Ito, N. (1985) Promoting effect of trisodium nitrilotriacetate monohydrate on urinary bladder carcinogenesis in rats. *Jpn. J. Cancer Res.*, 76, 823-827

Games, L.M., Staubach, J.A. & Kappeler, T.U. (1981) Analysis of nitrilotriacetic acid in environmental waters. *Tenside Deterg.*, 18, 262-265

Gesellschaft Deutscher Chemiker (Society of German Chemistry) (1987) *Nitrilotriessigsaure* [Nitrilotriacetic Acid] (*Beratergremium fur umweltrelevante Altstoffe, Stoffbericht 5*) [Advisory Panel for Relevant Materials in the Environment, Substance Report 5], Weinheim, VCH Verlagsgesellschaft mbH, pp. 1-6

Goddard, J.G. & Sweeney, G.D. (1983) Ferric nitrilotriacetate: a potent stimulant of in vivo lipid peroxidation in mice. *Biochem. Pharmacol.*, 32, 3879-3882

Goddard, J.G., Basford, D. & Sweeney, G.D. (1986) Lipid peroxidation stimulated by iron nitrilotriacetate in rat liver. *Biochem. Pharmacol.*, 35, 2381-2387

Goering, P.L., Tandon, S.K. & Klaassen, C.D. (1985) Induction of hepatic metallothionein in mouse liver following administration of chelating agents. *Toxicol. appl. Pharmacol.*, 80, 467-472

Goyer, R.A., Falk, H.L., Hogan, M., Feldman, D.D. & Richter, W. (1981) Renal tumors in rats given trisodium nitrilotriacetic acid in drinking water for two years. *J. natl Cancer Inst.*, 66, 869-880

Greenblatt, M. & Lijinsky, W. (1974) Carcinogenesis and chronic toxicity of nitrilotriacetic acid in Swiss mice. *J. natl Cancer Inst.*, 52, 1123-1126

Grilli, M.P. & Capucci, A. (1985) Mutagenic effect of nitrilotriacetic acid on cultured human cells. *Toxicol. Lett.*, 25, 137-141

Haberman, J.P. (1971) Polarographic determination of traces of nitrilotriacetate in water samples. *Anal. Chem.*, 43, 63-67

Hamazaki, S., Okada, S., Ebina, Y. & Midorikawa, O. (1985) Acute renal failure and glucosuria induced by ferric nitrilotriacetate in rats. *Toxicol. appl. Pharmacol.*, 77, 267-274

Hamazaki, S., Okada, S., Ebina, Y., Fujioka, M. & Midorikawa, O. (1986) Nephrotoxicity of ferric nitrilotriacetate. An electron-microscopic and metabolic study. *Am. J. Pathol.*, 123, 343-350

Hamazaki, S., Okada, S., Ebina, Y., Li, J.-L. & Midorikawa, O. (1988) Effect of dietary vitamin E on ferric nitrilotriacetate-induced nephrotoxicity in rats. *Toxicol. appl. Pharmacol.*, 92, 500-506

Haring, B.J.A. & van Delft, W. (1977) Determination of nitrilotriacetic acid in water by derivative pulse polarography at a hanging mercury drop electrode. *Anal. chem. Acta*, 94, 201-203

Hiasa, Y., Kitahori, Y., Konishi, N. & Shimoyama, T. (1985) Dose-related effect of trisodium nitrilotriacetate monohydrate on renal tumorigenesis initiated with N-ethyl-N-hydroxyethylnitrosamine in rats. *Carcinogenesis*, 6, 907-910

Hoover, T.B. (1973) *Polarographic Determination of NTA (EPA-R2-73-254; US NTIS PB 222-940)*, Corvallis, OR, US Environmental Protection Agency, Office of Research and Monitoring

IARC (1987a) *IARC Monographs on the Evaluation of Carcinogenic Risks to Humans*, Suppl. 7, *Overall Evaluations of Carcinogenicity: An Udating of* IARC Monographs *Volumes 1 to 42*, Lyon, pp. 230-232

IARC (1987b) *IARC Monographs on the Evaluation of Carcinogenic Risks to Humans*, Suppl. 7, *Overall Evaluations of Carcinogenicity: An Udating of* IARC Monographs *Volumes 1 to 42*, Lyon, pp. 211-216

Jorgenson, T.A., Newell, G.W., Scharpf, L.G., Gribling, P., O'Brien, M. & Chu, D. (1975) Study of the mutagenic potential of nitrilotriacetic acid (NaCaNTA) in mice by the translocation test (Abstract No. 56). *Mutat. Res., 31*, 337-338

Kanerva, R.L., Francis, W.R., Lefever, F.R., Dorr, T., Alden, C.L. & Anderson, R.L. (1984) Renal pelvic and ureteral dilatation in male rats ingesting trisodium nitrilotriacetate. *Food chem. Toxicol., 22*, 749-753

Kihlman, B.A. & Sturelid, S. (1970) Nitrilotriacetic acid (NTA) and chromosome breakage. *Environ. Mutat. Soc. Newsl., 3*, 32-33

Kirk, P.W.W. & Lester, J.N. (1981) The determination of nitrilotriacetic acid in waters and waste waters. *Rev. anal. Chem., 5*, 207-224

Kirk, P.W.W., Perry, R. & Lester, J.N. (1982) Determination of nitrilotriacetic acid in waters and waste waters by gas-liquid chromatography, differential pulse polarography and a colorimetric method. *Int. J. environ. anal. Chem., 12*, 293-309

Kitahori, Y., Konishi, N., Shimoyama, T. & Hiasa, Y. (1985) Dose-dependent promoting effect of trisodium nitrilotriacetate monohydrate on urinary bladder carcinogenesis in Wistar rats pretreated with *N*-butyl-*N*-(4-hydroxybutyl)nitrosamine. *Jpn. J. Cancer Res. (Gann), 76*, 818-822

Kramers, P.G.N. (1976) Mutagenicity studies with nitrilotriacetic acid (NTA) and Citrex S-5 in *Drosophila*. *Mutat. Res., 40*, 277-280

Lanfranchi, G., Paglialunga, S. & Levis, A.G. (1988) Mammalian cell transformation induced by chromium(VI) compounds in the presence of nitrilotriacetic acid. *J. Toxicol. environ. Health, 24*, 251-260

Li, J.-L., Okada, S., Hamazaki, S., Ebina, Y. & Midorikawa, O. (1987) Subacute nephrotoxicity and induction of renal cell carcinoma in mice treated with ferric nitrilotriacetate. *Cancer Res., 47*, 1867-1869

Lijinsky, W., Greenblatt, M. & Kommineni, C. (1973) Feeding studies of nitrilotriacetic acid and derivatives in rats. *J. natl Cancer Inst., 50*, 1061-1063

Loprieno, N., Boncristiani, G., Venier, P., Montaldi, A., Majone, F., Bianchi, V., Paglialunga, S. & Levis, A.G. (1985) Increased mutagenicity of chromium compounds by nitrilotriacetic acid. *Environ. Mutagenesis, 7*, 185-200

Loveday, K.S., Lugo, M.H., Resnick, M.A., Anderson, B.E. & Zeiger, E. (1989) Chromosome aberration and sister chromatid exchange tests in Chinese hamster ovary cells *in vitro*. II. Results with 20 chemicals. *Environ. mol. Mutagenesis, 13*, 60-94

Mahaffey, K.R. & Goyer, R.A. (1972) Trisodium nitrilotriacetate in drinking water. Metabolic and renal effects in rats. *Arch. environ. Health, 25*, 271-275

Malaiyandi, M., Williams, D.T. & O'Grady, R. (1979) A national survey of nitrilotriacetic acid in Canadian drinking water. *Environ. Sci. Technol., 13*, 59-62

Maronpot, R.R., Montgomery, C.A., Jr, Boorman, G.A. & McConnell, E.E. (1986) National Toxicology Program nomenclature for hepatoproliferative lesions of rats. *Toxicol. Pathol., 14*, 263-273

Martell, A.E. & Smith, R.M. (1974) *Critical Stability Constants*, Vol. 1, *Amino Acids*, New York, Plenum, pp. 139-143

Matheson, D.H. (1977) *Nitrilotriacetic Acid (NTA) in the Canadian Environment* (Scientific Series No. 74), Ottawa, Inland Waters Directorate, Water Quality Branch

Matsuura, R. (1983) Uptake of iron and nitrilotriacetate (NTA) in rat liver and the toxic effect of Fe-NTA. *Acta med. Okayama, 37,* 393-400

May, M.E., Parmley, R.T., Spicer, S.S., Ravenel, D.P., May, E.E. & Buse, M.G. (1980) Iron nitrilotriacetate-induced experimental diabetes in rats. *J. Lab. clin. Med., 95,* 525-535

McClain, R.M. & Siekierka, J.J. (1975) The effects of various chelating agents on the teratogenicity of lead nitrate in rats. *Toxicol. appl. Pharmacol., 31,* 434-442

Merski, J.A. (1981) Acute structural changes in renal tubular epithelium following administration of nitrilotriacetate. *Food Cosmet. Toxicol., 19,* 463-470

Merski, J.A. (1982) Alterations of renal tissue structure during a 30-day gavage study with nitrilotriacetate. *Food chem. Toxicol., 20,* 433-440

Michael, W.R. & Wakim, J.M. (1971) Metabolism of nitrilotriacetic acid (NTA). *Toxicol. appl. Pharmacol., 18,* 407-416

Michael, W.R. & Wakim, J.M. (1973) Effect of trisodium nitrilotriacetate ($Na_3NTA$) on the metabolism of selected metal ions. *Toxicol. appl. Pharmacol., 24,* 519-529

Mitchell, A.D., Rudd, C.J. & Caspary, W.J. (1988) Evaluation of the L5178Y mouse lymphoma cell mutagenesis assay: intralaboratory results for sixty-three coded chemicals tested at SRI International. *Environ. mol. Mutagenesis, 12 (Suppl. 13),* 37-101

Monsanto Co. (1985) *Material Safety Data Sheet: NTA Powder and NTA 40% Solution*, St Louis, MO

Montaldi, A., Zentilin, L., Venier, P., Gola, I., Bianchi, V., Paglialunga, S. & Levis, A.G. (1985) Interaction of nitrolotriacetic acid with heavy metals in the induction of sister chromatid exchanges in cultured mammalian cells. *Environ. Mutagenesis, 7,* 381-390

Montaldi, A., Zentilin, L., Zordan, M., Bianchi, V., Levis, A.G., Clongero, E. & Paglialunga, S. (1987) Chromosomal effects of heavy metals (Cd, Cr, Hg, Ni and Pb) on cultured mammalian cells in the presence of nitrilotriacetic acid (NTA). *Toxicol. environ. Chem., 14,* 183-200

Montaldi, A., Mariot, R., Zordan, M., Paleologo, M. & Levis, A.G. (1988) Nitrilotriacetic acid (NTA) does not induce chromosomal damage in mammalian cells either *in vitro* or *in vivo*. *Mutat. Res., 208,* 95-100

Myers, M.C., Kanerva, R.L., Alden, C.L. & Anderson, R.L. (1982) Reversibility of nephrotoxicity induced in rats by nitrilotriacetate in subchronic feeding studies. *Food chem. Toxicol., 20,* 925-934

Nakamoto, S., Yamanoi, Y., Kawabata, T., Sadahira, Y., Mori, M. & Awai, M. (1986) Lipid peroxidation and cytotoxicity of Ehrlich ascites tumor cells by ferric nitrilotriacetate. *Biochim. biophys. Acta, 889,* 15-22

National Cancer Institute (1977) *Bioassays of Nitrilotriacetic Acid (NTA) and Nitrilotriacetic Acid, Trisodium Salt, Monohydrate ($Na_3NTA.H_2O$) for Possible Carcinogenicity (CAS No.139-13-9 (NTA); CAS No.18662-53-8 ($Na_3NTA.H_2O$))* (NCI-CG-TR-6; DHEW Publ. No. (NIH) 77-806), Bethesda, MD, US Department of Health, Education, and Welfare

Nixon, G.A. (1971) Toxicity evaluation of trisodium nitrilotriacetate. *Toxicol. appl. Pharmacol., 18,* 398-406

Nixon, G.A., Buehler, E.V. & Niewenhuis, R.J. (1972) Two-year rat feeding study with trisodium nitrilotriacetate and its calcium chelate. *Toxicol. appl. Pharmacol., 21,* 244-252

Nolen, G.A., Klusman, L.W., Back, D.L. & Buehler, E.V. (1971) Reproduction and teratology studies of trisodium nitrilotriacetate in rats and rabbits. *Food Cosmet. Toxicol.*, 9, 509-418

Nolen, G.A., Buehler, E.V., Geil, R.G. & Goldenthal, E.I. (1972a) Effects of trisodium nitrilotriacetate on cadmium and methyl mercury toxicity and teratogenicity in rats. *Toxicol. appl. Pharmacol.*, 23, 222-237

Nolen, G.A., Bohne, R.L. & Buehler, E.V. (1972b) Effects of trisodium nitrilotriacetate, trisodium citrate and a trisodium nitrilotriacetate-ferric chloride mixture on cadmium and methyl mercury toxicity and teratogenesis in rats. *Toxicol. appl. Pharmacol.*, 23, 238-250

Okada, S. & Midorikawa, O. (1982) Induction of the rat renal adenocarcinoma by Fe-nitrilotriacetate (Fe-NTA) (Jpn). *Naika Hokan*, 29, 485-491

Okada, S., Hamazaki, S., Ebina, Y., Li, J.-L. & Midorikawa, O. (1987) Nephrotoxicity and its prevention by vitamin E in ferric nitrilotriacetate-promoted lipid peroxidation. *Biochim. biophys. Acta*, 922, 28-33

Pouchert, C.J., ed. (1981) *The Aldrich Library of Infrared Spectra*, 3rd ed., Milwaukee, WI, Aldrich Chemical Co., p. 339

Pouchert, C.J., ed. (1983) *The Aldrich Library of NMR Spectra*, 2nd ed., Vol. 1, Milwaukee, WI, Aldrich Chemical Co., pp. 483-484

Pouchert, C.J., ed. (1985) *The Aldrich Library of FT-IR Spectra*, Vol. 1, Milwaukee, WI, Aldrich Chemical Co., p. 566

Procter & Gamble Co. (1981) *Submission to US Environmental Protection Agency, Summary of Indiana Monitoring Program for NTA*, Cincinnati, OH

Procter & Gamble Co. (1982) *Submission to US Environmental Protection Agency, Summary of Indiana Monitoring Program for NTA*, Cincinnati, OH

Procter & Gamble Co. (1983a) *New York Tap Water Monitoring for NTA, October 1981-June 1983, Submission to the New York State Department of Environmental Conservation*, Cincinnati, OH

Procter & Gamble Co. (1983b) *Summary of NTA Environmental Monitoring Program in Indiana, Submission to the New York State Department of Environmental Conservation*, Cincinnati, OH

Procter & Gamble Co. (1983c) *Canadian Tap Water Monitoring for NTA, Phase I—Ottawa—Carleton and Finch Ontario, and Phase II—Port Kells, British Columbia, Submission to the New York State Department of Environmental Conservation*, Cincinnati, OH

Ramel, C. & Magnusson, J. (1979) Chemical induction of non-disjunction in Drosophila. *Environ. Health Perspect.*, 31, 59-66

Riedel-de Haen (1984) *Laboratory Chemicals*, Hanover

Sadtler Research Laboratories (1980) *Standard Spectra Collection, 1980 Cumulative Index*, Philadelphia, PA

Sai, K., Takagi, A., Umermura, T., Kurokawa, Y. & Kasai, H. (1988) Studies on the formation of 8-hydroxydeoxyguanosine (8-OHdG) in the rat kidney by kidney carcinogens (Abstract No. P-36) (Jpn.). *Environ. Mutagenesis Res. Commun.*, 10, 74

Scharpf, L.G., Jr, Hill, I.D., Wright, P.L., Plank, J.B., Keplinger, M.L. & Calandra, J.C. (1972) Effect of sodium nitrilotriacetate on toxicity, teratogenicity, and tissue distribution of cadmium. *Nature*, 239, 231-233

Scharpf, L.G., Jr, Hill, I.D., Wright, P.L. & Keplinger, M.L. (1973) Teratology studies on methylmercury hydroxide and nitrilotriacetate sodium in rats. *Nature*, 241, 461-463

Shimoyama, T. (1986) Effects of trisodium nitrilotriacetate monohydrate, nitrilotriacetic acid and ammonium chloride on urinary bladder and renal tumorigenesis in rats treated with N-bis(2-hydroxypropyl)nitrosamine (Jpn.). *J. Nara med. Assoc.*, *37*, 610-632

Swisher, R.C., Crutchfield, M.M. & Caldwell, D.W. (1967) Biodegradation of nitrilotriacetate in activated sludge. *Environ. Sci. Technol.*, *1*, 820-827

Thompson, J.E. & Duthie, J.R. (1968) The biodegradability and treatability of NTA. *J. Water Pollut. Control Fed.*, *40*, 306-319

Tjälve, H. (1972) A study of the distribution and teratogenicity of nitrilotriacetic acid (NTA) in mice. *Toxicol. appl. Pharmacol.*, *23*, 216-221

Universities Associated for Research and Education in Pathology (1985) *Assessment of the Practical Risk to Human Health from the Use of Nitrilotriacetic Acid (NTA) in Household Laundry Products*, Bethesda, MD

US Environmental Protection Agency (1979) *Chemical Technology and Economics in Environmental Perspective. Task IV—Potential Worker and Consumer Exposures to Nitrilotriacetic Acid (NTA) in Detergents (EPA-560/11-79-008; NTIS PB-297-753)*, Washington DC

US Food and Drug Administration (1987) Boiler water additives. *US Code fed. Regul.*, *Title 21*, Part 173.310, pp. 117-120

Ved Brat, S. & Williams, G.M. (1984) Nitrilotriacetic acid does not induce sister-chromatid exchanges in hamster or human cells. *Food chem. Toxicol.*, *22*, 211-215

Venier, P., Montaldi, A., Gava, C., Zentilin, L., Tecchio, G., Bianchi, V., Paglialunga, S. & Levis, A.G. (1985) Effects of nitrilotriacetic acid on the induction of gene mutations and sister chromatid exchanges by insoluble chromium compounds. *Mutat. Res.*, *156*, 219-228

Venier, P., Gava, C., Zordan, M., Bianchi, V., Levis, A.G., De Flora, S., Bennicelli, C. & Camoinano, A. (1987) Interactions of chromium with nitrilotriacetic acid (NTA) in the induction of genetic effects in bacteria. *Toxicol. environ. Chem.*, *14*, 201-218

Warren, C.B. & Malec, E.J. (1972) Quantitative determination of nitrilotriacetic acid and related aminopolycarboxylic acids in inland waters. Analysis by gas chromatography. *J. Chromatogr.*, *64*, 219-237

Wendt, R.H., Payne, A.G. & Hopping, W.D. (1988) Nitrilotriacetic acid (NTA) environmental monitoring program in Indiana: 1979 to 1983. *Environ. Toxicol. Chem.*, *7*, 275-290

Whiting, R.F., Wei, L. & Stich, H.F. (1981) Chromosome-damaging activity of ferritin and its relation to chelation and reduction of iron. *Cancer Res.*, *41*, 1628-1636

Williams, G.M., Laspia, M.F. & Dunkel, V.C. (1982) Reliability of the hepatocyte primary culture/DNA repair test in testing of coded carcinogens and noncarcinogens. *Mutat. Res.*, *97*, 359-370

Woodiwiss, C.R., Walker, R.D. & Brownridge, F.A. (1979) Concentrations of nitrilotriacetate and certain metals in Canadian wastewaters and streams: 1971-1975. *Water Res.*, *13*, 599-612

Woodruff, R.C., Mason, J.M., Valencia, R. & Zimmering, S. (1985) Chemical mutagenesis testing in *Drosophila*. V. Results of 53 coded compounds tested for the National Toxicology Program. *Environ. Mutagenesis*, *7*, 677-702

W.R. Grace & Co. (1985) *Product Brochure: Hampshire Nitrilotriacetate (NTA)*, Lexington, MA, Organic Chemicals Division

Zetterberg, G. (1970) Negative results with nitrilotriacetic acid (NTA) as an inducer of gene mutation in some microorganisms. *Environ. Mutat. Soc. Newsl.*, *3*, 31-32

# INDUSTRY

# EXPOSURES IN THE TEXTILE MANUFACTURING INDUSTRY[1]

## 1. Historical Perspectives and Description of the Industry

### 1.1 Historical perspectives

Cloth and carpets have been made for thousands of years, and relics of ancient fabrics have been found throughout the world. Yarn was made as long ago as 8000 BC, and it is believed that grass and tree materials were the first substances used to make yarn-like strands of cloth (Marvin, 1973).

Mechanized production of textiles began in England at the end of the eighteenth century, as part of the industrial revolution. Since that time, the industrial production of textiles has spread rapidly to all parts of the world. During the last 20 years, much of the basic textile industry has shifted to developing countries.

Textile manufacture includes spinning, weaving, knitting, dyeing and finishing of all types of natural and synthetic fibres. Machines vary from primitive looms used in cottage industries to sophisticated machines in modern factories (Quinn, 1983). A glossary of some terms used commonly in the industry is given at the end of this volume (p. 279).

Textile workers are exposed to textile dusts (both natural and synthetic) throughout the textile manufacturing process. During spinning, weaving and knitting operations, the use of chemicals is limited. The most important chemicals used in these processes are sizing agents (e.g., starch) and yarn lubricants (spinning oil and polymers).

Workers in the cotton industry have been exposed to mineral lubricants used in the spindles during the operation called 'mule spinning' (twisting of yarn). This exposure has been evaluated previously (IARC, 1984). Mule spinning was discontinued in Italy in 1965 but may still be done elsewhere. Some countries have legislation prohibiting the use of oils for mule spinning other than those of animal or vegetable origin (Quinn, 1983).

The term 'dyestuff' refers to products used to impart colour to other materials and pertains to both dyes and pigments. Currently, the vast majority of textile dyes are synthetic

---

[1]Excluding the manufacture of asbestos textiles (IARC, 1977) and mule spinning with exposure to mineral oils (IARC, 1984)

products. The synthetic dyestuff industry has developed from the discovery of the first synthetic dye, mauve, in 1856 by Perkin (Travis, 1988). Soon after, in 1859, another important dye, magenta (see IARC, 1974), was prepared by Verguin. One of the most remarkable landmarks in the development of synthetic dyes was Griess' discovery of the diazo reaction in 1858 (Peters, 1975), which led to the development of the azo dyes. The most important dye structures (chromophores) include triphenylmethane compounds, indigoid and azo structures, azines, thiazines, anthraquinone derivatives and phthalocyanines (Munn & Smagghe, 1983). A profound technological advance was achieved in the 1950s when reactive dyes were discovered. These compounds react chemically with the fibre and provide properties of fastness not achieved with the earlier water-soluble dyes.

Dyestuff manufacturing has become one of the major sectors of the chemical industry. The Colour Index lists approximately 38 000 different commercial colourants involving 7000-8000 different chemical structures. World production of dyestuffs was estimated to be 600 000-700 000 tonnes (active substance) in 1978, of which 50-60% were used for textiles (Clarke & Anliker, 1980). In 1986, 107 000 tonnes of textile dyes were produced in the USA (Reisch, 1988).

Benzidine-based dyes (see IARC, 1987a) are an important group of synthetic colourants. In 1948, about 14 million kg were produced, representing about 21% of world dye production, by about 50 companies in 19 countries. The production of benzidine-based dyes decreased drastically in the USA during the 1970s and in 1980 (National Institute for Occupational Safety and Health, 1980), but they may still be used elsewhere.

Development in the field of textile finishing has also been rapid. Through the use of different finishing treatments, the properties of textiles can be enhanced in many respects. The most important chemical finishing processes for cotton fabrics include crease-resistant, flame-retardant, water-repellent, antisoiling and antimicrobial treatments.

Treatment for crease resistance is the most widely used process for cellulosic textiles (e.g., cotton, viscose) because all cellulose fibres are susceptible to wrinkling. For this purpose, formaldehyde (see IARC, 1987b)-based resins have been in common use since the 1950s, when 'permanent press' fabrics and garments became available on the market. The first type of resin used was urea-formaldehyde resin (see IARC, 1982). The first commercial product of this type was placed on the market in 1933. Melamine-formaldehyde resins (see IARC, 1982) have also been and still are used for crease resistance (Hurwitz, 1987).

A new class of crease-resistant finishing agent for textiles was introduced in the USA about 1949. The most important group of these chemicals was cyclic ethylene ureas, such as dimethylol ethylene urea (Hurwitz, 1987), which react with the cellulose fibre (Marsh, 1962). Application of the new finishing agents increased gradually as the popularity of so-called 'permanent press' garments increased in the 1950s. In 1959, dimethylol dihydroxy ethylene urea was described, and it has become the most commonly used crease-resistant finishing agent (Hurwitz, 1987). It is made from urea, formaldehyde and glyoxal and releases much less formaldehyde than the earlier urea and melamine resins. In the 1980s, the release of formaldehyde from dimethylol dihydroxy ethylene urea was further reduced by alkylation. Other low-formaldehyde processes have been developed (Vail, 1983).

The use of flame retardants in textiles has a long history. Sea water, clay and vinegar are examples of ancient flame retardants. Over the last three decades, much research has been conducted into the development of fire-retardant textiles for such uses as work clothes, upholstery, space research and military purposes (Nousiainen, 1988). The flame retardants that are currently used are either inorganic salts or reactive phosphorus and nitrogen compounds.

Inorganic salts are easier to apply and often less toxic than organic reactive flame retardants, but they dissolve during normal laundering processes. Organic flame retardants, such as tetrakis(hydroxymethyl)phosphonium chloride (THPC; see monograph, p. 95) and N-methylol dimethylphosphonyl propionamide (Pyrovatex CP), react with cellulosic fibres to form chemical bonds that are stable for 50 or more launderings. The first compound of this type (THPC) was introduced in 1953 by Reeves and Guthrie (Nousiainen, 1988) and has given rise to a number of variants involving phosphonium structures (Bogle, 1977). One of the most widely used, durable flame retardants, Pyrovatex CP, was patented in 1965 (Nousiainen, 1988). In the 1970s, tris(2,3-dibromopropyl)phosphate (see IARC, 1979a) was commonly used for textiles and plastics and in particular for children's sleepwear in the USA; however, the compound was found to have carcinogenic and mutagenic properties, and its production ceased by the end of the 1970s. Corresponding chemical structures, such as tris(2-chloroethyl)phosphate (see monograph, p. 195) and tris(dichloropropyl)phosphate, are still used. Decabromodiphenyl oxide (see monograph, p. 73), introduced in 1976, has been used as a flame retardant in textiles.

## 1.2 Description of the industry

A typical flow diagram for the transformation of raw cotton into finished fabric is presented in Figure 1. Raw cotton bales are opened, and the cotton may be blended with synthetic or other natural fibres at the opening line. The cotton is then delivered to the picking machines, which transfer the fibres to the cards. During these first stages, fibres may be transported by air currents (blowing). Cotton fibres are then processed at the card. From the card, the fibre strands are run on the drawing frame. The best quality cotton and cotton blend yarn undergoes combing before drawing. From the drawing frame, strands of parallel fibres are moved to the roving frame. The product, called 'roving', goes to the spinning frame, and part is spun into warp yarn and part into filling yarn. The remaining processes before weaving are to prepare the yarn for weaving. Spinning-frame warp yarn is transferred from a bobbin to a large spool. A large number of these packages are placed on a warping machine to make a beam of yarn (beaming). The two machines, called a spooler and a warper, are actually types of winding machines. Several beams are run together on the last machine before weaving, which is called a 'slasher'. In this process, a hot solution of starch is applied to the warp yarn to reduce breakage and damage in the weaving. Yarn may be dyed before it is woven; this is particularly true for wool. Weaving is accomplished on a machine called a loom. 'Finishing' in Figure 1 comprises preparation, dyeing, finishing and inspecting the fabric.

**Figure 1. Typical flow diagram for the transformation of fibre into fabric**[a]

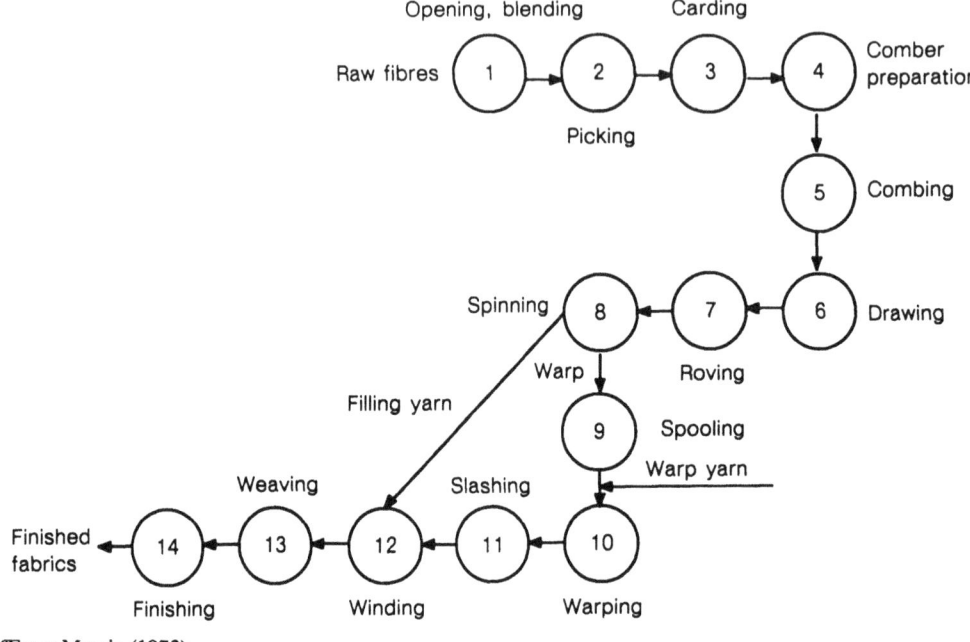

[a]From Marvin (1973)

Selected world production figures for woven cotton fabrics are given in Table 1, as an example of the recent production of basic textile products. In 1980, about 50% of world fibre production was accounted for by cotton, compared with about 70% in 1960 (Krol, 1985). Table 2 shows production figures for 1983 from the European Communities for some types of fabrics.

*(a) Fibre production*

Fabrics can be produced in two ways—by weaving and by knitting. Of these two processes, weaving is the older, being thousands of years old. The first knitting machine appeared in 1589 (Marvin, 1973).

The process of weaving involves the interlacing of two or more sets of yarn at right angles, the warp yarn running the length of the fabric and the filling yarn being inserted across the fabric. Each cross-wise insertion is called a pick. Knitting is the process of making a usable fabric from threads or yarns by arranging them into interlocking loops. The basic knit structure is called jersey fabric. In general, these same processes are followed for other fibres, both synthetic and natural.

Table 1. Selected production figures for woven cotton fabrics (in millions of square metres)[a]

| Area | 1976 | 1985 |
|---|---|---|
| Africa | 1 938 | 1 904 |
| America, North | 5 651 | 4 022 |
| America, South | 1 722 | 2 207 |
| Asia | 16 290 | 33 123 |
| Australia | 47 | 35 |
| Europe | 9 937 | 9 540 |
| Eastern Europe | 3 103 | 3 159 |
| European Communities | 4 726 | 4 714 |
| European Free Trade Association | 775 | 891 |
| China | NA | 15 202 |
| Egypt | 673 | 740 |
| France | 1 127 | 861 |
| Germany, Federal Republic of | 906 | 990 |
| India | 9 495 | 11 152 |
| Japan | 2 237 | 2 061 |
| Mexico | 523 | 510 |
| Nigeria | 367 | 285 |
| Poland | 979 | 887 |
| Portugal | 373 | 542 |
| Romania | 677 | 700 |
| South Africa | 126 | 139 |
| USA | 4 942 | 3 278 |
| USSR | 7 408 | 8 580 |

[a]From United Nations (1987)
NA, not available

Table 2. Production of fabrics in the European Communities, 1983[a]

| Type of fabric | Production (tonnes) |
|---|---|
| Cotton | 536 289 |
| Wool or animal hair | 162 803 |
| Synthetic | 436 081 |
| Total | 1 215 565 |

[a]From Commission of the European Communities (1988)

The yarn manufacturing process for synthetic fibres differs from that for cotton. The raw material is polymeric (plastic) material manufactured by the chemical industry. Synthetic fibre production involves melting of the polymer raw material and extrusion of the polymer melt through spinning heads or spinnerets. The production of the raw materials used to make yarn for synthetic textiles was not considered in this monograph. The description is included only for completeness.

*(b) Dyeing and finishing of fabrics*

The wet processing of textile fabrics is a combination of three separate operations: (i) preparing, (ii) dyeing and (iii) finishing. The combination is also sometimes referred to as finishing. A typical flow diagram for the dyeing and finishing of cotton fabric is presented in Figure 2. Most fabrics, except those prepared from wool, are dyed and finished after weaving. The end use of the textile determines whether it is dyed and/or finished.

**Figure 2. A typical flow diagram of the dyeing and finishing of cotton**[a]

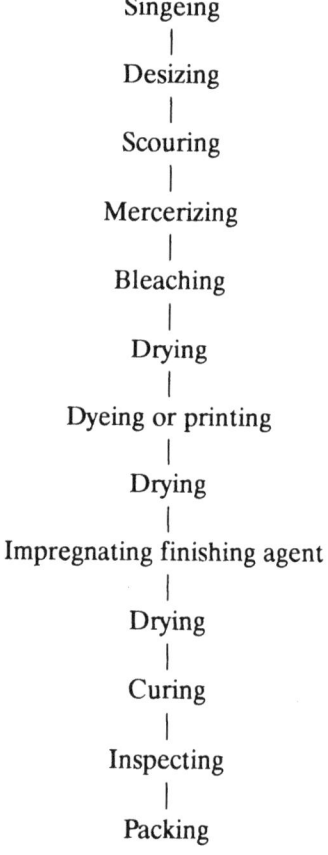

Singeing
|
Desizing
|
Scouring
|
Mercerizing
|
Bleaching
|
Drying
|
Dyeing or printing
|
Drying
|
Impregnating finishing agent
|
Drying
|
Curing
|
Inspecting
|
Packing

[a]From Marvin (1973)

(i) *Preparing*

Preparation involves the removal of undesirable materials from fabrics so that they can be dyed or finished in later processes. Different fabric materials are processed in different ways.

In *singeing*, unwanted surface hairs or filaments are removed with a flame. The aim of *desizing* is the elimination of sizing agents applied earlier to warp yarns. Sizing agents are normally starch or polyacrylates. In *scouring*, the fabric is boiled to remove the remaining sizing agents and impurities accompanying cellulose and other fibres. *Mercerization* is the short-term treatment of cotton fabrics with a sodium hydroxide solution, which changes the physical and chemical properties of fibres and increases their strength and capacity to absorb dye. Fabric *bleaching* is intended to eliminate natural substances that impart a grey shade to the fabric. Chlorine-releasing compounds (such as hypochlorites) and hydrogen peroxide (see IARC, 1985) are the most commonly used bleaching agents (Bukayev, 1984).

(ii) *Dyeing*

Solid colours are produced by either continuous or noncontinuous methods. Continuous processes are used for large-yardage cotton materials and for carpets, as well as for fabrics that contain 100% man-made fibres.

The aim of the dyeing process is to impart a certain colour to the fabric through application and fixing of dyes. Table 3 lists the major classes of dyes now used. In dyeing, the dye molecules penetrate the pores of the swollen fibres and are retained there by chemical or physical forces. Cotton is generally dyed after the yarn has been woven or knitted into fabric, while wool yarn is usually dyed before.

Dyes developed for cotton can be divided into three main groups: (i) water-soluble dyes, (ii) dyes soluble by alkaline reduction and (iii) dyes formed on the fibre. Water-soluble textile dyes are direct dyes that have an affinity for cellulose fibres and reactive dyes that interact chemically with cellulose fibre. All water-soluble dyes used in the textile industry are electrolytes. Dyes soluble by alkaline reduction include vat and sulfur dyes. Dyes formed on the fibre comprise azo and oxidation dyes obtained from the oxidation of certain amines (Bukayev, 1984).

Polyester is normally dyed with disperse dyes, which can contain different chromophores. Carrier compounds are used to improve the capacity of polyester to accept dyes and include biphenyl, chlorinated benzene, naphthalene and naphthalene derivatives and phthalimides. The use of carrier compounds can be partially avoided if the dyeing temperature is increased to 130°C or if the Thermosol method is used, in which disperse dye is fixed to polyester fibre by hot air. Wool/polyester blends, however, cannot be dyed at high temperatures, and carriers have to be used.

Wool and polyamides are normally dyed with acid dyes, metal complex dyes or chromium dyes. The preparation of polyamide for dyeing involves scouring, some form of setting treatment and, in some cases, bleaching. Raw wool is first scoured by the emulsification process, then bleached with hydrogen peroxide or sulfur dioxide and finally neutralized in a sodium carbonate bath (Niyogi, 1983).

Table 3. Important classes of textile dyes and related compounds[a]

| Class of compound | Major use | Major chemical structures |
|---|---|---|
| Acid dyes | Wool, polyamide | Azo (including premetallized dyes), anthraquinone, triphenylmethane, azine, xanthene, nitro and nitroso |
| Basic (cationic) dyes | Cotton | Triarylmethane, azo, azine, xanthene, thiazine, polymethine, oxazine and acridine |
| Direct dyes | Cotton, viscose | Diazo, triazo and polyazo, phthalocyanine, stilbene, oxazine and thiazole |
| Disperse dyes | Synthetic fibres (cellulose diacetate, cellulose triacetate, nylon, polyacrylic and polyester) | Simple azo, anthraquinone and nitroarylamine |
| Reactive dyes | Cotton, wool | Azo, anthraquinone, phthalocyanine and stilbene |
| Mordant dyes | Wool | Anthraquinone, azo, oxazine, triphenylmethane, nitroso and xanthene |
| Sulfur dyes | Cotton | Sulfur dyes |
| Vat dyes | Cotton, wool | Anthraquinone, polycyclic quinone and indigo |
| Optical brighteners | All fibres | Stilbene, dibenzothiophene, azole, coumarin and pyrazine |
| Dye carriers | Polyester, wool/polyester | Diphenyl, chlorinated aromatic hydrocarbon, benzoate and others |

[a]From Bateman (1978) and Reisch (1988)

Basic (cationic) dyes are used for dyeing acrylic fibres.

In printing, colour is applied to the fabric surface and is bound there by physical and chemical forces. The process is similar to that of dyeing. Sometimes, organic solvents (alcohols, ketones, esters, aliphatic and aromatic hydrocarbons) are used in printing dyes and for the cleaning of printing frames. Several printing techniques, i.e., direct, discharge and resist printing, are used. Printing is done by roller, flat and rotary machines.

(iii) *Finishing*

Finishing agents (Table 4) are used to make fabrics crease-resistant, shape-retaining, nonshrinking, flame-retardant, water-repellent, antisoiling and antistatic. Antimicrobial agents, such as antimildew agents, can also be added to fabrics. For cotton fabrics, crease-resistant treatment is the most important. This process involves impregnating the fabric with cyclic reactants such as dimethylol dihydroxy ethylene urea, and improves the crease resistance and dimensional stability of the fabric. Several agents can be applied simultaneously. Finishing involves steps of impregnation, drying and curing. Following the curing step, the textile may also be washed (Priha *et al.*, 1988).

Table 4. Typical finishing agents used in the textile industry[a]

| Type of agent | Typical chemicals | Use |
|---|---|---|
| Crease-resistant (durable press) | Urea-formaldehyde resin, melamine-formaldehyde resin, dimethylol ethylene urea, dimethylol dihydroxyethylene urea, carbamates, salt catalysts (e.g., magnesium chloride) | Cotton, viscose |
| Flame retardant | Tetrakis(hydroxymethyl)phosphonium salts, tris(2,3-dibromopropyl)phosphate, vinylphosphonate, decabromodiphenyl oxide, N-methyloldimethylphosphonyl propionamide (Pyrovatex CP) | Cotton, polyesters, polyamides, acrylics |
| Water repellent | Fluorocarbon compounds, silicones, zirconium-paraffin emulsions | Cotton |
| Antistatic | Tensides, polyethylene glycols, inorganic and organic salts, epoxy resins | Synthetic fibres |
| Antisoiling and soil-release | Aluminium, silicon and titanium oxides, starch, fluorocarbons, carboxymethyl cellulose, polymers (acrylates, epoxides) | Light-coloured textiles |
| Antimicrobial and related | | |
|    Antimildew | Pentachlorophenyl laurate, copper and zirconium compounds | Cotton (tent fabrics) |
|    Bactericide | Quaternary ammonium compounds, tributyltin oxide | Socks, foot-wear lining fabric |
|    Mothproofing | Dieldrin, pyrethroids, chlorinated aromatic sulfonamides, chlorinated urea derivatives | Wool, wool carpets |
| Softening agents | Tensides, polyethylene glycol, polysiloxanes | Synthetic fibres |

[a]From Priha et al. (1988)

## 2. Exposures in the Workplace

### 2.1 Introduction

The textile industry is one of the largest employers worldwide. Table 5 gives recent figures for the numbers of workers in textile manufacturing in many countries. Figure 3 illustrates some trends for the European Communities, Japan and the USA.

**Table 5. Numbers of workers (thousands) in the textile manufacturing industry (ILO code 321)**[a]

| Country or region | Workers (thousands) | Year |
|---|---|---|
| **AFRICA** | | |
| Botswana | 1 | 86 |
| Burundi | < 1 | 82 |
| Egypt | 291 | 79 |
| Ethiopia | 36 | 84 |
| Ghana | 16 | 79 |
| Kenya | 26 | 87 |
| Malawi | 7 | 85 |
| Mauritius | 4 | 87 |
| Nigeria | 66 | 80 |
| Sierra Leone[b] | < 1 | 81 |
| South Africa | 110 | 83 |
| Tanzania, United Republic of[c] | 38 | 80 |
| Zimbabwe | 21 | 85 |
| **AMERICA** | | |
| Argentina | 1 | 85 |
| Barbados[b] | 2 | 86 |
| Bolivia | 5 | 84 |
| Canada | 84 | 87 |
| Colombia | 51 | 86 |
| Cuba | 33 | 86 |
| Dominican Republic | 4 | 84 |
| Equador | 15 | 86 |
| ElSalvador | 18 | 83 |
| Guatemala | 7 | 86 |
| Haiti | 2 | 83 |
| Mexico | 48 | 87 |
| Antilles | < 1 | 82 |
| Nicaragua | 3 | 80 |
| Panama | < 1 | 85 |
| Puerto Rico | 3 | 87 |
| Uruguay | 18 | 86 |
| USA | 725 | 87 |
| Venezuela | 30 | 84 |
| Virgin Islands | 0 | 87 |

**Table 5 (contd)**

| Country or region | Workers (thousands) | Year |
|---|---|---|
| **ASIA** | | |
| Bangladesh | 280 | 84 |
| Brunei | <1 | 86 |
| China | 4745 | 87 |
| Hong Kong | 119 | 87 |
| India | 1708 | 85 |
| Israel | 88 | 84 |
| Japan | 673 | 84 |
| Jordan | 1 | 84 |
| Korea, Republic of | 402 | 86 |
| Malaysia | 39 | 81 |
| Philippines | 91 | 86 |
| Singapore | 3 | 86 |
| Sri Lanka | 41 | 86 |
| **EUROPE** | | |
| Austria | 42 | 87 |
| Belgium | 59 | 86 |
| Bulgaria | 121 | 86 |
| Cyprus | 2 | 87 |
| Czechoslovakia | 167 | 87 |
| Denmark | 15 | 86 |
| Finland | 15 | 87 |
| France[b] | 491 | 87 |
| Germany, Federal Republic of[b] | 582 | 86 |
| Greece | 61 | 83 |
| Hungary | 98 | 87 |
| Ireland | 10 | 87 |
| Luxembourg | <1 | 87 |
| Malta | 1 | 85 |
| Netherlands | 25 | 86 |
| Norway | 17 | 79 |
| Poland | 342 | 87 |
| Portugal | 134 | 85 |
| Romania | 412 | 85 |
| Spain | 170 | 87 |
| Sweden | 9 | 85 |
| Switzerland | 31 | 86 |
| Turkey | 180 | 84 |
| UK[b] | 559 | 87 |
| Yugoslavia | 281 | 87 |

**Table 5 (contd)**

| Country or region | Workers (thousands) | Year |
|---|---|---|
| **AUSTRALASIA** | | |
| Australia | 47 | 85 |
| New Zealand[b] | 38 | 87 |

[a]From International Labour Office (1988)
[b]ILO Category 32, which includes leather industry

**Figure 3. Employment trends in the textile industry[a]**

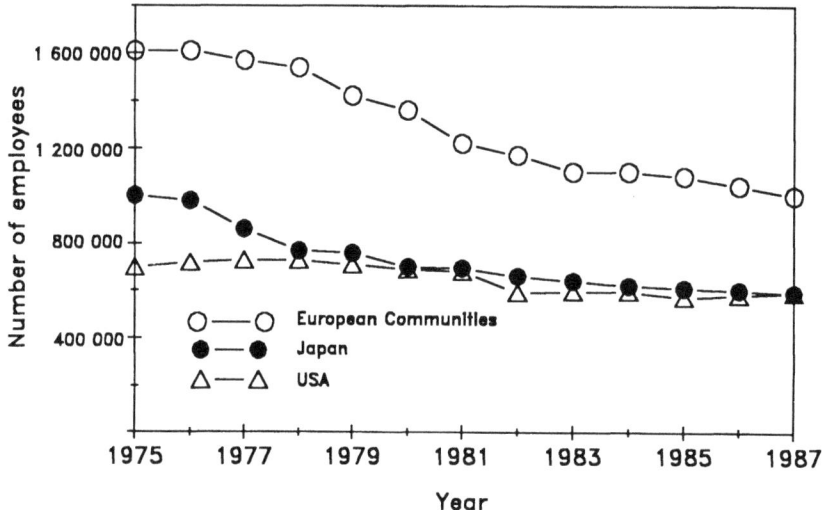

[a]From Commission of the European Communities (1988)

A wide variety of occupational health hazards are present in the textile manufacturing industry. The most ubiquitous exposure in textile mills is to organic dust, in particular to cotton dust. Chemical exposure in spinning and weaving is limited mainly to sizing agents and spinning oils. Raw cotton may be contaminated with bacteria, desiccants and defoliants; raw wool may be contaminated by pesticides from sheep dips. There are no data, however, to indicate the levels of desiccants, defoliants or pesticides in textile mills. During fabric preparation, workers can be exposed to a variety of bleaching, scouring, singeing and mercerizing agents. In dyeing, printing and finishing, chemicals are widely used and exposures may be highly complex.

In 1970, it was estimated that 60 000-75 000 persons in the USA were involved in dyeing and finishing processes (National Institute for Occupational Safety and Health, 1981). In dyeing and printing, workers are frequently exposed to dyes, a variety of acids such as formic, sulfuric and acetic acids, fluorescent brighteners, organic solvents and fixatives. Workers in the finishing operations are frequently exposed to crease-resistant agents, many of which release formaldehyde, and to flame retardants, such as organic phosphorus compounds, chlorinated hydrocarbons and carbamates. These exposures may occur simultaneously with physical hazards, including noise, vibration and heat.

The wide range of substances to which workers in textile manufacturing may be exposed is indicated in Table 6.

Table 6. Substances and classes of substances found in the textile manufacturing industry[a]

| Material | Principal use or source of emission |
| --- | --- |
| Acetic acid | Control of dye pH |
| Acid dyes | Dyeing |
| Ammonium sulfate | Control of dye pH |
| Basic dyes | Dyeing |
| Biphenyl | Dye carrier |
| Chlorendic acid | Flame retardant |
| Cotton dust | Opening, blending, carding, spinning, weaving, knitting |
| Cyclic ethylene ureas | Crease resistance |
| Decabromodiphenyl oxide | Flame retardant |
| Diammonium phosphate | Control of pH in wool dyeing |
| Dichloromethane | Fabric scouring |
| Dimethylformamide | Fabric finishing |
| 1,3-Diphenyl-2-pyrazoline | Fluorescent brightener |
| Direct dyes | Dyeing |
| Disperse dyes | Dyeing |
| Endotoxins | Organic fibre contaminant |
| Ethylene glycol monomethyl ether | Fabric printing |
| Formaldehyde resins | Crease resistance |
| Formic acid | Control of dye pH |
| Hydrogen peroxide | Fabric bleaching |
| Hypochlorites | Fabric bleaching, preparation, singeing |
| Inorganic salts (e.g., bromides, phosphates, chlorides) | Flame retardants and other uses |
| Monochlorobenzene | Fabric printing |
| Monosodium phosphate | Control of pH in jet-dye machines |
| Mordant dyes | Dyeing |
| Phenol | Printing |
| Pigment dyes | Dyeing and printing |
| Polyvinyl alcohol | Fabric preparation, mercerizing cotton |
| Reactive dyes | Cloth dyeing |

**Table 6 (contd)**

| Material | Principal use or source of emission |
|---|---|
| Sodium acetate | Dyeing of 100% polyester |
| Sodium bichromate | Chrome-dyeing process |
| Sodium carbonate | Fabric bleaching |
| Sodium hydroxide | Fabric bleaching, mercerizing, scouring |
| Sodium perborate | Antisoiling agent for polyester |
| Spinning oils | Lubricants |
| Starch | Sizing agent |
| Sulfur dyes | Dyeing |
| Sulfuric acid | Carbonizing process of wool dyeing, desizing |
| Tetrachloroethylene | Fabric scouring, dye carrier |
| Tetrakis(hydroxymethyl)phosphonium salts | Flame retardants |
| Tetrasodium pyrophosphate | Control of dye pH |
| Trichloroethylene | Dye carrier ingredient, scouring |
| Tris(2,3-dibromopropyl)phosphate | Flame retardant |
| Vat dyes | Dyeing |

[a]Adapted from Marvin (1973)

Very few data were available on the chemicals used, exposure levels and the numbers of workers involved in specific processes in developing countries. The exposure levels and chemicals used, in particular, dyes, could be quite different from those used elsewhere.

## 2.2 Organic dusts

### (a) Cotton

The largest single exposure in the textile manufacturing industry is to cotton dust. Airborne dust levels associated with various operations are presented in Table 7.

Methods for sampling cotton dust differ from country to country, and, therefore, different results may be obtained (De Rosa *et al.*, 1984). The best established apparatus for sampling cotton dust is the vertical elutriator (cut-off point, 15 μm respirable dust; Neefus *et al.*, 1977). This method is commonly used in the USA and was also recommended by a study group of the World Health Organization (1983). Occupational limits for exposure to cotton dust in various countries or regions are presented in Table 8.

Table 7. Concentrations of cotton dust in the work environment[a]

| Operation | No. of samples | Concentration (mg/m$^3$) Mean | Concentration (mg/m$^3$) Range | Sample type | Method[b] | Country | Reference |
|---|---|---|---|---|---|---|---|
| Opening, blending, cleaning | NA | 1.42 | 0.59–2.35 | R, area | VE | Egypt | Noweir (1975) |
| Spinning | NA | 0.2 | 0.14–0.26 | R, area | VE | Egypt | Noweir (1975) |
| Willowing | NA | 8.3 | max, 8.6 | T, NA | Filter[c] | India | Gupta (1969) |
| Winding room | NA | 0.9 | 0.9–1.0 | T, NA | Filter[c] | India | Gupta (1969) |
| Opening, blending | 9 | 1.8 | 0.28–6.36 | R, area | VE | USA | Jones et al. (1979) |
| Spooling, warping | 9 | 0.2 | 0.10–0.38 | R, area | VE | USA | Jones et al. (1979) |
| Opening | 9 | 0.89 | 0.28–2.43 | R, area | VE | USA | Hammad et al. (1981) |
| Cleaning | 7 | 15.8 | 9.98–19.4 | T, P | Filter[c] | USA | Hammad et al. (1981) |
| Blending | 6 | 6.4 | 1.6–11.1 | R, area | VE | USA | Hammad et al. (1981) |
| Blending | 6 | 8.8 | 3.2–14.5 | T, area | Filter[c] | USA | Hammad et al. (1981) |
| Twisting | 3 | 0.28 | 0.14–0.42 | R, area | VE | USA | Hammad et al. (1981) |
| Roving | 6 | 0.5 | 0.36–0.52 | R, area | VE | USA | Hammad et al. (1981) |
| Spinning | 112 | 1.5 | max, 30.0 | T, P | Filter[d] | UK | Hobson (1974) |
| Spinning | 84 | 1.1 | 0.59–1.59 | R, P | Filter[d] | UK | Cinkotai et al. (1984) |
| Carding | 24 | 4.63 | 1.45–7.81 | R, P | Filter[d] | UK | Cinkotai et al. (1984) |
| Opening | 26 | 1.6 | 0.42–2.90 | R, area | VE | China | Christiani et al. (1986) |
| Winding | 15 | 0.5 | 0.15–0.61 | R, area | VE | China | Christiani et al. (1986) |
| Carding, blowing | NA | NA | 0.06–5.28 | NA | NA | Hong Kong | Ong et al. (1985) |
| Other | NA | NA | 0.06–2.10 | NA | NA | Hong Kong | Ong et al. (1985) |
| Winding & twisting | 20 | 4.7 | 1.1–8.2 | T, area | Filter[c] | Cameroon | Takam & Nemery (1988) |
| Weaving | 20 | 6.0 | 5.1–6.8 | T, area | Filter[c] | Cameroon | Takam & Nemery (1988) |
| Winding & twisting | 6 | 2.0 | NA | T, P | Filter[c] | Cameroon | Takam & Nemery (1988) |
| Spinning | 6 | 8.9 | NA | T, P | Filter[c] | Cameroon | Takam & Nemery (1988) |
| Weaving | 6 | 4.5 | NA | T, P | Filter[c] | Cameroon | Takam & Nemery (1988) |

[a]R, respirable dust; VE, vertical elutriator (cut-off point, 15 μm); T, total dust; NA, not available; P, personal
[b]Filters analysed gravimetrically
[c]Open-faced cassette alone
[d]Open-faced cassette preceded by 12-in (30-cm) cube of 2-mm-mesh wire gauge to remove lint

Table 8. Occupational limits for exposure to cotton dust[a]

| Country or region | Year | Concentration (mg/m³) | Interpretation[b] |
|---|---|---|---|
| Czechoslovakia | 1987 | 2 | TWA |
| Denmark | 1987 | 0.5 | TWA |
| Finland | 1987 | 1 | TWA |
| German Democratic Republic | 1987 | 5 | TWA (8.75 h) |
| Germany, Federal Republic of | 1988 | 1.5 | TWA |
| India | 1987 | 0.2 | TWA |
| | | 0.6 | STL |
| Indonesia | 1987 | 1 | TWA |
| Mexico | 1987 | 0.2 | TWA |
| Netherlands | 1987 | 0.2 | TWA |
| Norway | 1987 | 0.5 | TWA |
| Sweden | 1987 | 0.5 | TWA (VE) |
| Switzerland | 1987 | 1.5 | MAC |
| Taiwan | 1987 | 1 | TWA |
| UK | 1987 | 0.5 | TWA (spinning to winding and weaving) |
| | | 5 | TWA (all other processes) |
| USA[c] | | | |
| OSHA | 1988 | 0.2 | TWA (yarn industry, VE) |
| | | 0.75 | TWA (slashing and weaving, lint-free VE) |
| | | 0.5 | TWA (all other textile operations, lint-free VE) |
| ACGIH | 1988 | 0.2 | TWA (VE) |
| NIOSH | 1983 | 0.2 | TWA (lint-free, VE) |
| USSR | 1987 | 2 | MAC |
| Yugoslavia | 1987 | 5 | TWA |

[a]From Cook (1987); Deutsche Forschungsgemeinschaft (1988); National Institute for Occupational Safety and Health (1988); American Conference of Governmental Industrial Hygienists (1989)
[b]TWA, time-weighted average (8-h); STL, short-term level (30 min); VE, occupational level as determined by vertical elutriation (cut-off point, 15 μm respirable dust); MAC, maximum allowable concentration (8-h). All occupational exposure limits are for total dust unless noted; the values are not comparable, as different sampling methods were used.
[c]OSHA, Occupational Safety and Health Administration; ACGIH, American Conference of Governmental Industrial Hygienist; NIOSH, National Institute of Occupational Safety and Health.

(b) *Wool*

Wool dust concentrations were quantified in a wool carpet weaving facility in Turkey using a filter method [not further specified]; levels varied within the plant, the highest being found in the opening area (3.4 mg/m³) and the lowest in the spinning area (1.7 mg/m³; Özesmi *et al.*, 1987).

(c) *Flax*

Respirable airborne flax dust was collected with a vertical elutriator in a flax mill in Alexandria, Egypt. The mean levels in mechanical textile operations ranged from 0.60 mg/m$^3$ in winding to 4.03 mg/m$^3$ in carding; those in the manual processing area varied from 1.54 mg/m$^3$ in spinning to 9.8 mg/m$^3$ in hackling (Noweir, 1975). [The Working Group noted that the number of samples collected was not reported.]

(d) *Hemp*

In an evaluation of mean respirable airborne levels of hemp dust collected with a horizontal laminar elutriator/filter in a Yugoslav textile mill, spinners had the highest levels of exposure (2.7 mg/m$^3$) and carders the lowest (0.9 mg/m$^3$; Valic & Žuškin, 1971).

## 2.3 Dyes and their components

(a) *Textile dyes*

Over 5000 workers were estimated to be potentially exposed to benzidine-derived dyes (see IARC, 1987a) in the USA textile dyeing and finishing industry in 1972-74 (National Institute for Occupational Safety and Health, 1977). In a study in a textile dyeing plant in the USA, four of ten dyers potentially exposed to benzidine-derived dyes had benzidine (see IARC, 1987c) or monoacetylbenzidine, a metabolite of benzidine, in their urine (National Institute for Occupational Safety and Health, 1978). Five of 20 workers involved in weighing benzidine-derived dyes in three UK textile mills had benzidine in their urine; all five worked in the same factory (Meal *et al.*, 1981).

About 16 000 workers are potentially exposed to textile dyes in the Finnish textile industries. Dyers' mean exposure to total dust in three dyehouses varied from 0.4 to 4.1 mg/m$^3$, depending on the dye type and other parameters; the corresponding mean dye concentrations were 0.02-0.12 mg/m$^3$. The proportion of dyes (mainly indigo) in this dust varied from 1.6 to 12% (Schimberg & Vuorinen, 1986).

(b) *Trichloroethylene* (see IARC, 1979b, 1987d)

About 22 000 workers were estimated to be potentially exposed to trichloroethylene in the US textile manufacturing industry in 1972-74 (National Institute for Occupational Safety and Health, 1977). Samples collected in the breathing zone of workers at two US textile mills during the weighing of dyes indicated a mean exposure to trichloroethylene of 0.38 ppm (2.04 mg/m$^3$), with a range of 0.11-0.56 ppm (0.59-3.01 mg/m$^3$; Bateman, 1978).

(c) *Acetic acid*

Samples collected in the breathing zone of workers at two US textile mills during the weighing of dyes indicated a mean exposure to acetic acid of 13 ppm (32 mg/m$^3$), with a range of 1-40 ppm (2.45-98 mg/m$^3$; Bateman, 1978).

(d) *Biphenyl*

Potential exposure to biphenyl in the USA is considerable because of its high production volume and widespread use as a dye carrier (National Cancer Institute, 1985a). High airborne concentrations were measured in a dyehouse in a Finnish textile factory in the early 1970s, due to the use of open-type dyeing machines. In this workplace survey, short-term (15-30 min) biphenyl concentrations were 7.5-44 mg/m³. In two later surveys in Finnish textile factories when closed-pressure dyeing machines were used, biphenyl concentrations were under 0.05 mg/m³ (Priha *et al.*, 1988).

### 2.4 Finishing agents and their components

Exposure to formaldehyde (see IARC, 1982, 1987b) is common in the finishing process. About 20 000 employees were estimated to be exposed to formaldehyde in US textile finishing plants in 1979 (Goodson, 1984). As indicated in Table 5, large numbers of workers are employed in the textile manufacturing industry in developing countries; however, no data were available on the numbers employed in the finishing process or on levels of exposure to formaldehyde. Measurements in a US textile printing and finishing plant indicated that during treatment of printed fabrics before finishing, operators had an 8-h time-weighted average (TWA) exposure to formaldehyde of 1.2 ppm (1.5 mg/m³), while chemical finishers had an 8-h TWA of 0.7 ppm (0.85 mg/m³; Keenlyside & Elliott, 1981). Levels of formaldehyde in US textile mills treating nylon fabric were reported to have ranged from 1 ppm to 11 ppm (1.2-13.4 mg/m³) in 1955; by 1979, however, these levels had fallen to 0.1-1.4 ppm (0.12-1.7 mg/m³; Ward, 1984). [The Working Group noted that duration of sampling was not reported.]

Formaldehyde levels in Finnish textile factories in 1975-78 and in the Swedish textile industry are given in Table 9.

**Table 9. Airborne formaldehyde concentrations in Finnish and Swedish textile factories during selected finishing processes**

| Process/work | No. of samples | Formaldehyde concentration (mg/m³)[a] | |
|---|---|---|---|
| | | Mean | Median |
| Finland[b] | | | |
| Crease-resistance treatment | 52 | 0.5 | 0.4 |
| Flame-retardant treatment | 67 | 2.5 | 1.2 |
| Other treatments | 17 | 0.4 | 0.4 |
| Mixing of finishing resin | 8 | 1.1 | 0.3 |
| Fabric warehouse | 6 | 1.1 | 1.1 |
| Sweden[c] | | | |
| Crease-resistance treatment | 29 | 0.2 | 0.2 |
| Flame-retardant treatment | 2 | 1.5 | NA |

[a]Area sampling time ranged from 30-60 min
[b]From Nousiainen & Sundquist (1979)
[c]From Rosén *et al.* (1984)
NA, not available

Formaldehyde is also present in textile dust derived from finished cellulosic fibres for crease-resistant and flame-resistant textiles (Rosén et al., 1984). Unstable N-methylol and other unstable bonds are easily hydrolysed and metabolized to formaldehyde (Vail, 1983; Priha et al., 1988), and exposure via the skin may take place during contact with finished textiles. Formaldehyde is a common skin sensitizer in textile and clothing industries (Hatch & Maibach, 1986). Due to such problems, regulations limiting formaldehyde levels in fabric have been drawn up in some countries, including Japan and Finland. Formaldehyde concentrations ranging from 32 to 855 mg/kg were measured in textiles marketed in Finland (Priha et al., 1988).

Exposure to other chemicals occurs in the textile manufacturing industry (see Table 6), but quantitative data were not available to the Working Group.

## 2.5 Other agents

### (a) Bacteria and endotoxins

Endotoxin levels of 0.02-2.5 µg/m$^3$ have been observed in cardrooms of the US cotton, flax and jute industries, on filters containing dust collected on vertical elutriators (Rylander & Morey, 1982). The mean endotoxin content in airborne, unwashed cotton dust in a model US cardroom was found to range from 40.3 ± 4.1 to 390.2 ± 22.6 ng/mg. Washing the cotton reduced the endotoxin concentrations to a range of 7.4 ± 1.0 to 21.6 ± 4.0 ng/mg. These samples were collected with a cascade impactor preceded by a vertical elutriator (Olenchock et al., 1983).

Evaluation of area airborne levels of endotoxins in two cotton mills in Shanghai, China, collected with a vertical elutriator, revealed mean (range) levels of 0.002 (0.001-0.02)-0.53 (0.32-0.71) µg/m$^3$ (Kennedy et al., 1987). Evaluation of the levels of airborne endotoxins present in the work environment of a wool carpet-weaving plant in Turkey showed that the weaving process was the dustiest and contained the highest levels (maximal level, 31.2 µg/g wool dust) compared to the washing process (mean level, 0.7 µg/g wool dust). The range of endotoxin levels at the various processes was 0.1-31.2 µg/g wool dust (Özesmi et al., 1987).

Samples of airborne bacteria were collected with an Anderson viable sampler in 21 English cotton spinning mills. The mean concentrations of endo agar bacteria were 270 ± 140 − 6150 ± 3380 organisms/m$^3$, and those of the nutrient agar bacteria between 1200 ± 540 and 89 300 ± 21 300 organisms/m$^3$ (Cinkotai & Whitaker, 1978).

### (b) Ethylene glycol monomethyl ether

During use of a printing press in a textile printing plant in Massachusetts, USA, the average level of ethylene glycol monomethyl ether originating from cleaning agents was 8.0 ppm (30 mg/m$^3$; Ohi & Wegman, 1978). [The Working Group noted that the range of levels and the number of samples collected were not reported.]

### (c) Tetrachloroethylene (perchloroethylene) (see IARC, 1979c; 1987e)

About 6600 employees were estimated to be potentially exposed to tetrachloroethylene in the US textile manufacturing industry in 1972-74 (National Institute for Occupational Safety and Health, 1977). Tetrachloroethylene is used for scouring (mainly of double knits), sizing, desizing and as a dye carrier (National Cancer Institute, 1985b).

*(d) Monochlorobenzene*

During use of a printing press in a textile printing plant in Massachusetts, USA, the average airborne level of monochlorobenzene originating from cleaning agents was 15.0 ppm (69 mg/m$^3$; Ohi & Wegman, 1978). [The Working Group noted that the range of levels and the number of samples collected were not reported.]

*(e) Other solvents*

Results of a survey conducted in several Finnish textile manufacturing facilities in 1975-78 are given in Table 10.

Table 10. Exposure to common solvents used in the Finnish textile printing industry, 1975-78[a]

| Solvent | No. of samples | Concentration (ppm) [mg/m$^3$] | |
|---|---|---|---|
| | | Mean | Median |
| Acetone | 57 | 40 [95] | 1.0 [2.4] |
| n-Butanol | 28 | 7.7 [23] | 3.8 [11] |
| n-Butyl acetate | 60 | 3.8 [16] | <0.1 [<0.4] |
| Dichloromethane | 18 | 66 [230] | 30 [104] |
| Ethyl acetate | 35 | 31 [96] | 4.8 [15] |
| Hydrocarbon solvent (white spirit) | 52 | [230] | [167] |
| 1-Propanol | 15 | 16 [39] | <0.1 [2.5] |

[a]From Nousiainen & Sundquist (1979); study covered preparation of printing plates and rolls and cleaning of presses

*(f) Oil mist*

In Finland, workers have been exposed to average levels of 1.4 mg/m$^3$ (51 samples) oil mist, which results from the use of yarn lubricants in the weaving, knitting and fixing of cotton-polyamide yarn (Nousiainen & Sundquist, 1979).

*(g) Sodium hydroxide*

In a survey conducted in Finnish textile factories in 1975-78, mean airborne concentrations of sodium hydroxide were 1.7-6.8 mg/m$^3$ during mercerizing, bleaching, scouring and mixing operations (Nousiainen & Sundquist, 1979).

## 3. Biological Data Relevant to the Evaluation of Carcinogenic Risk to Humans

### 3.1 Carcinogenicity studies in animals

No data were available on the carcinogenicity of textile dusts to experimental animals.

### 3.2 Other relevant data

(a) *Experimental systems*

(i) *Absorption, distribution, excretion and metabolism*

No data were available to the Working Group.

(ii) *Toxic effects*

Studies on the toxic effects of exposures to dusts in the textile industry in experimental animals and in in-vitro systems have concentrated on three main areas: (i) identification of animal models that imitate human responses to inhaled dusts and that develop airway diseases similar to those of humans (Walker *et al.*, 1975; Kutz *et al.*, 1980; Ellakkani *et al.*, 1984, 1985, 1987; Witek *et al.*, 1988); (ii) identification of active components of dusts responsible for immediate and delayed airway responses, such as bronchoconstriction and recruitment of cells involved in the release of leukotrienes, histamine and other mediators of airway tone (Antweiler, 1960; Rylander & Snella, 1976; Buck *et al.*, 1986); and (iii) use of in-vitro cell systems or organ explants to evaluate the cytotoxicity and other effects of dusts and dust extracts (Johnson *et al.*, 1986; Thomson *et al.*, 1986). The findings from these lines of research do not appear to have immediate relevance to an evaluation of the potential carcinogenicity of exposures in the textile industry.

(iii) *Effects on reproduction and prenatal toxicity*

No data were available to the Working Group.

(iv) *Genetic and related effects*

No data were available to the Working Group.

(b) *Humans*

(i) *Absorption, distribution, excretion and metabolism*

No data were available to the Working Group.

(ii) *Toxic effects*

Effects on human health in the textile industry, apart from those arising from exposures to chemicals associated with textile manufacturing, are limited almost entirely to respiratory disease arising from inhalation of organic dust and to microbial contamination arising from vegetable and animal fibres. Other health effects reported include some dermatitis and possible increases in mortality rates from cardiovascular disease.

Respiratory disease, including byssinosis, bronchitis, acute and chronic changes in lung function and heightened airway reactivity, have been the subject of intensive study in the primary textile industries utilizing cotton, soft hemp, flax, wool and some other vegetable textile fibres (sisal, jute, manila, St Helena hemp). The worldwide prevalence of byssinosis, clinical manifestations, epidemiological studies, environmental and health assessments, and the relationship between exposure to cotton, flax and soft hemp dust and byssinosis, together with recommended permissible exposure limits, have been reviewed (World Health Organization, 1983).

There is further epidemiological evidence of the importance of endotoxins arising from gram-negative organisms as etiological agents in provoking acute airway constriction and symptoms of byssinosis among cotton textile workers (Castellan et al., 1984; Malmberg, 1985; Rylander et al., 1985; Castellan et al., 1987; Rylander, 1987). Textile workers exposed to unscoured wool also develop lung function abnormalities consistent with byssinosis (Zuskin et al., 1976). Respiratory symptoms consisting of bronchitic wheeze, breathlessness and persistent rhinitis, conjunctivitis and chills, which are related to concentrations of dust (contaminated with endotoxin), have been reported in Yorkshire wool textile workers (Love et al., 1988) and as byssinosis among carpet weavers exposed to wool contaminated with endotoxins (Özesmi et al., 1987).

Health effects following acute and chronic exposure to cotton dust, including mill fever, pulmonary function, chest tightness (byssinosis), hyperreactive airways and chronic bronchitis, have been summarized as the 'Manchester criteria' (Rylander et al., 1987).

Case reports of both primary irritant and contact dermatitis, often occurring together, have been published. Nearly all of these reports refer not to occupational dermatitis related to exposure to textile dyes and other chemical irritants and sensitizers found in the textile industry, but rather to dermatological reactions to wearing garments made of irritating fibres and/or containing chemical residues (Hatch & Maibach, 1985, 1986). Occupational dermatoses, including contact and irritant dermatitis, have been attributed to mechanical irritation, dyes, synthetic detergents, oil products and microbes (Reinhard & Tronnier, 1970; Sokolova, 1972; Kieć-Świerczyńska, 1982; Makushkina, 1983; Mathur et al., 1985).

Reviews of UK Registrar General death rates from 1891 to 1932 revealed high rates of respiratory and cardiovascular disease among cotton textile workers (Registrar General, 1897, 1908, 1923, 1927, 1938). These data were reanalysed in the light of subsequent studies of respiratory disease among Lancashire cotton textile operatives: after correcting for respiratory causes of death, excesses in cardiovascular morality were still noted, particularly among carding machine stripper and grinders, who traditionally have the dustiest jobs in textile mills (Schilling & Goodman, 1951). A subsequent mortality study of cotton textile workers revealed low rates for all causes of death, including respiratory disease, heart disease and cancer (Henderson & Enterline, 1973). A cohort employed in two North Carolina cotton mills also had no overall increase in mortality from nonmalignant respiratory disease; however, the rate doubled between persons with low duration of exposure and those with high duration. Significantly increased mortality from cardiovascular disease was also observed among men and women in yarn processing areas (Merchant & Ortmeyer, 1981).

(iii) *Effects on reproduction and prenatal toxicity*

Data from the Finnish National Board of Health hospital discharge register and the national census were used to analyse spontaneous abortions by occupational exposure of mothers and husbands for 1973-76. Using logistic regression models in which adjustment was made for several potential risk factors (age, place of residence, parity), relative risks (RRs) for spontaneous abortion were found to be increased among women employed as spinners (odds ratio, 1.3; 95% confidence interval (CI), 0.96-1.9), fabric inspectors (1.5; 0.96-2.4) and weavers (1.4; 1.1-1.9) over those in women employed in manufacturing (Lindbohm *et al.*, 1984).

In a study of prematurity and low birth weight in the region of Montréal, Canada, no increased risk was observed among women employed in the textile industry: 16 pre-term and 18 low birthweight babies were observed among 186 pregnancies (McDonald *et al.*, 1988).

An analysis of birth records in the state of Washington, USA (1980-81) revealed an increased risk for fetal death among offspring of women employed in the textile industry (RR, 1.5; 95% CI, 1.2-1.9; 71 cases) (Vaughan *et al.*, 1984).

(iv) *Genetic and related effects*

No data were available to the Working Group.

## 3.3 Epidemiological studies of carcinogenicity to humans[1]

A lack of data on occupational exposure was a major obstacle to an evaluation of specific risks in the textile manufacturing industry. 'Textile industry' and 'textile work' were frequently used as general terms, with no further specification, to include a wide range of exposures and occupations. In the text below, the terminology of the authors was used, and only the distinctions that appeared in the papers are made. Textile workers were also sometimes grouped jointly with garment workers and those in other occupations, so that estimates of the risks for workers in textile manufacturing may be biased.

Studies of occupational groups in which the Working Group considered there was probably a high proportion of garment workers or which included workers who manufactured dyes were not considered; however, in a number of studies, particularly those based on mortality statistics, the proportion of nontextile workers in joint occupational groups was unknown. In those cases, the study was included but it was considered to be of only limited importance for an evaluation of carcinogenic risk in the textile manufacturing industry.

Considerable differences may have existed in levels or patterns of exposure or in the presence of modifying or confounding factors in the occupational groups that have been studied, which may have produced apparently contradictory findings. A further difficulty in

---

[1]Calculations of statistical significance that were done by the Working Group are given in square brackets in the text.

evaluating carcinogenic risk in the textile industry is that many of the major studies—of different types—addressed risks for cancers at many sites. Some studies reported only statistically significant results, while others also reported negative findings. In order to make an unbiased evaluation, all the reported data, irrespective of statistical significance, were taken into account.

In the following, the design of studies that addressed cancer at several sites is summarized first. Then, the results of these and other studies are presented, by site, in the order given in the International Classification of Diseases. In general, duration of exposure appeared to have no effect on risk for workers in the textile industry; this aspect is therefore mentioned only when an effect was seen. Few of the studies were specifically designed to study the risk for cancer associated with working in the textile industry. The reported associations are therefore often incidental findings in studies in which many risk factors were considered.

(a) *Descriptions of studies of cancers at multiple sites*

(i) *Mortality/morbidity statistics*

Versluys (1949) analysed the registrations of 49 245 (23 318 men and 25 927 women) deaths from carcinoma in the Netherlands in the period 1931-35. For men in certain occupations, the distribution of deaths by site was compared to the distribution in all men.

Occupational mortality in England and Wales has been examined in a series of studies for the periods 1949-53 (Office of Population Censuses and Surveys, 1958), 1959-63 (Office of Population Censuses and Surveys, 1971; Logan, 1982) and 1970-72 (Office of Population Censuses and Surveys, 1978; Logan, 1982), and for Great Britain in 1979-80 and 1982-83 (Office of Population Censuses and Surveys, 1986). These compilations are referred to as the 1951, 1961, 1971 and 1981 decennial supplements, respectively. All analyses involved the calculation of age-adjusted standardized mortality ratios (SMRs), based on national mortality rates. For the 1951 supplement, only statistically significant results are given, and the study did not report overall cancer mortality in male textile workers. Before the 1981 supplement, married women were classified according to the occupation of their husband, whereas single women were classified according to their own occupation; this yielded overall cancer SMRs among textile workers of 106 in 1961 and 105 in 1971 for married women and 115 in 1961 and 148 in 1971 for single women (Logan, 1982). In 1981, the proportionate mortality ratio (PMR) for cancers at all sites in female textile workers aged 20-59 years was 91.

Guralnick (1963) published a report on mortality and occupation based on the entries of occupation and industry on the death certificates of men between the ages of 20-64 years who had died in the USA in 1950. The population at risk in each occupation and age class was estimated from the 1950 census figures. Expected deaths were calculated from the cause-, age- and ethnic-specific mortality rates for the entire US population. SMRs were reported only for sites for which >20 cases were observed.

Delzell and Grufferman (1983) investigated the distribution of causes of death among white female textile workers who had died in North Carolina (USA) during 1976-78. A total of 4462 deaths had occurred among women whose usual occupation, as recorded on the death certificate, had been in the textile industry and who were at least 15 years of age at death. It was estimated that 86% of the classifiable industries manufactured textile mill products and 14% manufactured clothing and other fabricated textile products. Expected deaths were calculated from the distribution of causes of death among other white female residents of North Carolina. Results were presented for selected cancer sites only.

In several studies, the Swedish Cancer Environment Register was used to study cancer incidence in 1961-79. Occupation was classified according to 1960 census records, and all analyses were standardized for sex, birth cohort and geographical region (Malker *et al.*, 1986a,b, 1987; McLaughlin *et al.*, 1987).

Olsen and Jensen (1987) analysed 93 810 cases of cancer registered in Denmark in 1970-79. These were linked to the Supplementary Pension Fund employment records, and age-standardized proportional incidence ratios (SPIRs) were estimated for various branches of industry. The observed number of cancer cases was allocated to the industry in which the cancer patient had been employed for the longest time.

A proportionate mortality study of 6113 male textile workers 16 years of age or more who had resided and had died in the State of Rhode Island (USA) during the period 1968-78 was carried out by Dubrow and Gute (1988). Information on occupation was retrieved from death certificate files, and all those coded as textile industry were double-checked against the original statements on the death certificates. The cause-specific mortality pattern of textile workers was compared with that of other Rhode Island decedents.

Another proportionate mortality study was conducted among carpet and textile workers in five counties in north-west Georgia, USA, a region with a very high percentage of textile industry employment (O'Brien & Decouflé, 1988). The study was based on mortality records, 1970-84, of white men aged 20-74 years at death. Statements about occupation and industry were abstracted from 1356 retrievable death certificates. For 28.5% of the decedents, the usual industry had been textile or carpet/textile. The final study group comprised 240 decedents who were classified as likely or possibly to have been production workers; for 91, no specific occupation in the textile industry was given. The number of expected deaths was calculated on the basis of the cancer mortality of other residents in the study area and that of all Georgia residents.

(ii) *Cohort studies*

Henderson and Enterline (1973) examined the mortality at ages 15-64 years of two cohorts of white male cotton textile workers at three mills in Georgia, USA, engaged in the processing of raw cotton into woven fabric. The first cohort consisted of 5822 men who had worked at some time in the mills between 1938 and 1941, and the second of 6316 men who were working in the same mills during 1948-51. A total of 1772 men were members of both cohorts and had probably worked at least eight to ten years in the cotton textile mills. The mortality experience of these textile workers was examined through 30 June 1963. The number of expected deaths was calculated from the age-specific death rates for white males in Georgia for 1940, 1950 and 1960; rates for 1945 and 1955 were obtained by interpolation. A total of 1134 deaths (SMR, 81) were reported during the study period; death certificates were available for 87% of these. The observed:expected ratio was consistently lower than 1.00 for deaths from cancers at all sites and for those from digestive, respiratory and urinary cancers. Exposure was specified only as 'work in cotton textile mills'; however, the authors stated that 'some' of the workers had been engaged in dyeing cotton yarn. Smoking was excluded as a possible explanation of the findings on the basis of previous investigations which had shown similar smoking habits in cotton industry workers and the rest of the population. [The Working Group noted that no data were provided on the completeness of follow up.]

A proportionate mortality study was based on 1429 death certificates preserved by a section of the National Union of Dyers, Bleachers and Textile Workers in Bradford (UK) for persons exposed before 1936 and followed for 1957-68 (Newhouse, 1978). Only data on cancers of the digestive system, lung and bladder were given. The authors noted that with this study design they would not have detected cancer cases with a latency shorter than 20 years.

A cohort of 2844 persons (2119 men, 725 women) employed for 'some time' at two cotton mills in North Carolina (USA) during 1937-40 was studied by Merchant and Ortmeyer (1981). Complete job history and vital status were available for 1444 persons (1062 men, 382 women), and mortality over 1940-75 was analysed. The number of expected deaths was calculated on the basis of race-, sex- and age-specific death rates for the US population in the same calendar period. Exposure to cotton dust was classified into four categories: 1, high exposure, including 'preparation activities' such as opening, blending, carding and work in the waste house; 2, moderate exposure corresponding to 'yarn processing', including spinning, warping, winding, spooling and beaming; 3, moderate to low exposure, including slashing, weaving and cloth handling; and 4, variable but generally low exposure, comprising 'other' jobs, such as finishing, packing, maintenance and administrative-clerical. A total of 513 deaths (SMR, 98) was seen. Overall SMRs for all malignant neoplasms tended to decrease with increased presumed exposure to cotton dust. Site-specific data were given only for cancer of the trachea, bronchus and lung; risks at other sites were reported not to be elevated.

(iii) *Case-control studies*

Detailed personal interviews were sought with a random 10% sample of all persons with invasive tumours newly diagnosed during a three-year period in eight areas of the USA surveyed in the Third National Cancer Surveys (Williams *et al.*, 1977). Interviews were obtained with 3539 men and 3937 women (57% of the original sample). The proportions of specific, main lifetime industries and occupations among patients with cancer at one site were compared with those of patients with cancers at other sites combined as a control group, while controlling for other variables such as age, sex, smoking and drinking habits, and educational level. 'Textile mill products' was classified as main lifetime industry for 11 male (0.3%) and 24 female (0.6%) patients. As a second analytical approach, the recent industries of patients who were interviewed were compared to those of people in industries at the same locations as those of the patients in the Third National Cancer Surveys, using the US 1970 census tabulations. Only sites and work categories 'showing an association' were reported. No association of any type of cancer with working in the textile industry was found.

During 1956-65, all persons referred to the Roswell Park Memorial Institute, Buffalo, NY, USA, were asked prior to diagnosis of disease to report their lifetime occupational history (Decouflé *et al.*, 1978). In total, 6434 white males and 7515 white females were selected for the study. The ratio of persons in a given occupation to those whose lifetime employment had consisted almost entirely of clerical jobs among cases of cancer at specific sites was compared with the ratio in controls without neoplastic disease, taking age into account. The categories considered included 'operatives in textile mills', 'spinners' and 'weavers'; only statistically significant findings were generally reported.

A subset of the data presented by Decouflé et al. (1978) was analysed in order to examine the possible cancer risk pertaining to occupations in which exposure to dust was suspected (Bross et al., 1978). The study was limited to men. RRs adjusted for age, smoking and ethnicity were calculated as in the previous study. Only sites for which the RR was >2 were reported.

In a case-control study of cancer registrations in men aged 18-54 in three English counties during the period 1975-80, occupational histories were obtained by postal questionnaire from 1533 patients (52.1% of the 2942 cases identified) or next-of-kin (Coggon et al., 1986a,b). Eighteen cancer sites were examined, and each was compared with all other cancers combined. All analyses were adjusted for age, county of residence, source of the history (patient or relative) and smoking history.

A case-control study of cases of cancer at different sites and occupational exposure to nine organic dusts was conducted in the area of Montréal, Canada (Siemiatycki et al., 1986). Histologically confirmed cases of cancer at 19 sites newly diagnosed between September 1979 and June 1983 among male residents aged 37-70 were ascertained in 19 major hospitals. The number of eligible subjects was 2610, but completed interviews were obtained for only 2180 (83.5%); 19% of these were obtained from next-of-kin. The questionnaire was designed to obtain a detailed description of each job the subject had had in his working lifetime, as well as information on important potential confounders. A team of chemists and hygienists translated each job reported in the questionnaires into a list of potential exposures in accordance with all available information about each situation. This analysis covered nine cancer sites for which at least 100 subjects had been interviewed. Each series of subjects with a common tumour was compared with one or more controls drawn from among cases of cancer at the other sites included in the study. Exposure information was used to set up three exposure levels for each organic dust: 'unexposed', 'doubtful' and 'substantial'. The types of dust relevant to textile manufacturing were cotton, wool and synthetic fibres.

The case-control approach was used to examine mortality from five cancers—oesophagus, pancreas, cutaneous melanoma, kidney and brain—among men aged 18-54 in three English counties during the periods 1959-63 and 1965-79 (Magnani et al., 1987). For each case, four controls were selected from deaths from other causes during the same year, matched for age, sex and residence. Occupations of cases and controls were identified from death certificates, and a matched analysis was performed.

*(b) Oral and pharyngeal cancer*

In his study of death registrations in the Netherlands, Versluys (1949; see p. 238) observed four deaths from these cancers among male weavers and workers in woollens, whereas 7.1 were expected.

A study of death registrations for oral and pharyngeal cancers in men aged 15-64 in England and Wales in 1959-63 (Moss & Lee, 1974) showed 31 deaths among male textile workers as compared with 17.5 expected on the basis of national age-specific rates (RR, 1.8; $p = 0.001$). The site-specific RRs were 2.0 for cancer of the tongue (nine deaths; $p < 0.05$), 2.3 for cancer of the mouth (eight deaths; $p < 0.05$) and 1.5 for pharyngeal cancer (14 deaths; not significant). The overall RRs for oral and pharyngeal cancer were 4.3 in fibre preparers (11 deaths; $p < 0.0001$), 1.3 in spinners, winders and warpers (five deaths), 0.68 in weavers and knitters (three deaths), 1.9 in bleachers, dyers and finishers (six deaths) and 1.7 in miscellaneous textile workers (six deaths). Data on the type of fibre worked with were not directly available; however, in an expanded series of 19 deaths in fibre preparers, 18 were in wool workers and only one in a cotton worker, whereas a ratio of less than 2:1 would have been expected on the basis of census data. [The Working Group noted that this study was a further analysis of a previously reported incidental finding and that information on tobacco and alcohol consumption was not available.]

Delzell and Grufferman (1983; see p. 238) found a PMR of 100 (95% CI, 60-150; 18 deaths) among white female textile workers in North Carolina (USA) for cancers of the oral cavity and pharynx; Dubrow and Gute (1988; see p. 239) reported a PMR of 86 (95% CI, 65-115; 39 deaths) for men in the textile industry in Rhode Island (USA), and O'Brien and Decouflé (1988; see p. 239) gave a PMR of 80 (95% CI, 40-150; eight deaths) for male carpet and textile workers in Georgia (USA).

Olsen and Jensen (1987; see p. 239) found four cases of cancer of the buccal cavity and pharynx (SPIR, 35; 95% CI, 13-93) among Danish men manufacturing textiles, and two (36; 9-144) among those in spinning, weaving and finishing. The data for women were seven cases (122; 58-255) and two cases (93; 23-371), respectively.

In the case-control study of Decouflé et al. (1978; see p. 240) at the Roswell Park Memorial Institute in upstate New York, men and women employed as operatives in textile mills had elevated risks for cancer of the buccal cavity and pharynx after controlling for smoking. Eleven deaths were observed among both men (RR, 2.2; not significant) and women (RR, 1.9; $p = 0.04$). The findings for other male textile workers were not reported. No case was found in female spinners or weavers, but the findings for other female textile workers were not reported.

In a case-control study in the north-west region of England (Moss, 1976), 32 of 57 women with squamous-cell carcinomas at oral and pharyngeal sites reported having worked with textiles for at least two years at some time in their lives, as compared with 19 of 57 age-matched female breast cancer controls from the same hospital [crude odds ratio [OR], 2.6; $p = 0.02$]. The ORs were highest for women who had worked in spinning and related jobs ([crude OR, 3.7] seven cases) for at least ten years.

A case-control study of oral and pharyngeal squamous-cell cancer in the two main textile regions of England involved interviews with 280 cases and 280 age- and sex-matched controls with cancers other than those of the bladder, skin, nasal cavity and sinuses, and larynx (Whitaker et al., 1979). Overall, 86 cases and 77 controls had had at least two years' experience in textile work. [The matched OR was 1.2 (95% CI, 0.8-1.9).]

Coggon et al. (1986b, see p. 241) found no case of oral cancer among male textile workers in three English counties.

In a case-control study of oral and pharyngeal cancer among women in the southern USA, subsequent to a correlation study (Blot & Fraumeni, 1977), occupational histories were taken into consideration (Winn et al., 1981). Cases and controls were identified from hospitals and from death certificate diagnoses in North Carolina. A total of 255 cases were identified (156 from hospital records and 99 from death certificates), and two female controls were sought for each case, matched for age, race, source of ascertainment and county of residence. Completed interviews were obtained for 232 cases (91%) and 410 controls (82%); next-of-kin were interviewed for 51% of the cases and for 21% of the controls. After controlling for oral use of snuff, no increased risk (RR, 1.0) was found to be associated with employment in the textile industry—a major employer of women in North Carolina.

A further analysis (Winn et al., 1982) allowed categorization of each job a study subject had held in the textile, hosiery and apparel industries according to probable exposure to each of four agents: dusts, dyes, finishing chemicals and oil mists. Overall, neither the crude nor the tobacco-adjusted RR for oral cancer in relation to employment in the production of textiles was significantly raised. Too few women had worked in job titles involving exposure to dyes, finishing chemicals or oil mists to permit meaningful analyses, but 65 female textile workers had held potentially dusty jobs; spinners and spoolers predominated in this category. [The crude overall OR for workers in presumably dusty jobs was 1.4 (0.83-2.4). Adjustment for tobacco use was not reported for workers in this category, but made little change in different subcategories.] Risk did not increase with duration of exposure.

(c) *Cancers of the oesophagus and stomach*

In the death registration study of Verluys (1949; see p. 238) in the Netherlands, 116 deaths from stomach cancer (PMR, 121) and nine deaths from oesophageal cancer (PMR, 64) occurred in men in weaving and working in woollens.

In the decennial supplements of the UK Registrar General (see p. 238), one of the most consistent findings for male textile workers was an elevated risk for stomach cancer. In the 1951 supplement, an excess of stomach cancer was noted in bleaching, dyeing and finishing workers (SMR, 127; 65 deaths) and in dyehouse workers (SMR, 144; 36 deaths) in the textile industry; the SMRs were 139 in 1961, 149 in 1971 and 111 in 1981. Increased mortality from cancer of the oesophagus was noted in none of the supplements. For women, the most consistent site-specific finding was also an excess of stomach cancer: SMR, 147 in 1961 and 107 in 1971 in married women, and 164 and 157, respectively, in single women (Logan, 1982). In the 1981 supplement, there was little evidence of an increased risk for cancer of the stomach among female textile workers, but there was a suggestive increase in rates for oesophageal cancer (PMR, 191; not significant). [The Working Group noted that socioeconomic status was not taken into consideration in these studies.]

In the occupational mortality study of Guralnick (1963; see p. 238) of US men, a slight increase in the number of deaths from stomach cancer was seen (42 observed; SMR, 156) among operatives and allied workers in yarn, thread and fabric mills. [The Working Group assumed that, since cancer of the oesophagus was not mentioned, fewer than 20 cases were seen.]

Delzell and Grufferman (1983; see p. 238) found PMRs of 80 (95% CI; 40-170; eight deaths) for oesophageal cancer and 100 (95% CI, 90-120; 28 deaths) for stomach cancer from the death certificates of female textile workers in North Carolina, USA.

Olsen and Jensen (1987; see p. 239) found no case of oesophageal cancer; but for stomach cancer, 16 cases (87; 95% CI, 53-142) were seen in men in the manufacture of textiles, and eight cases (SPIR, 83; 41-166) in those in spinning, weaving and finishing. Among women in textile manufacture, the SPIRs were 56 (8-400; one case) for oesophageal cancer and 131 (80-214; 16 cases) for stomach cancer; among women in spinning, weaving and finishing, seven cases of stomach cancer (142; 68-297) were observed.

In the proportionate mortality study of Dubrow and Gute (1988; see p. 239) in Rhode Island (USA), textile workers classified as 'operatives' engaged in dyeing and finishing showed significantly increased mortality from cancer of the oesophagus (12 observed; PMR, 215; 95% CI, 125-371). The PMR for stomach cancer for all male textile workers was 98 (80-120; 78 deaths).

In the proportionate mortality study of O'Brien and Decouflé (1988; see p. 239) in Georgia (USA) among carpet and textile workers, a suggestive increase was noted for cancer of the oesophagus (PMR, 150; 70-270; ten deaths). The PMR for stomach cancer was 110 (50-210; nine deaths).

In the study of Henderson and Enterline (1973; see p. 239) among men in Georgia (USA), a nonsignificant increase in mortality from cancer of the digestive system was noted, only among cotton textile workers in the second of the two cohorts studied (20 observed; SMR, 151.5 [95% CI, 92.5-234]).

Newhouse (1978; see p. 240) observed an age- and period-adjusted PMR of 115 for cancer of the digestive system (122 deaths) among members of the National Union of Male Dyers, Bleachers and Textile Workers in Bradford (UK).

In the case-control study of Bross *et al.* (1978; see p. 241), a statistically significant elevated risk, larger than 2.0, was seen for cancer of the stomach and a nonsignificant elevated risk of the same magnitude for cancer of the oesophagus among men with occupational exposures to dust admitted to the Roswell Park Memorial Institute in New York State (USA).

In the case-control study of Siematycki *et al.* (1986; see p. 241) among men in Montréal, Québec (Canada), the OR for stomach cancer was 0.4 (95% CI, 0.2-1.0; five cases) for working with cotton, 0.9 (0.4-1.9; seven cases) for working with wool and 0.8 (0.3-2.0; six cases) for working with synthetic fibres.

Coggon *et al.* (1986b, see p. 241) found RRs of 1.0 (one case) for oesophageal cancer and 1.4 (six cases) for stomach cancer among men in the UK textile industry; and Magnani *et al.* (1987; see p. 241) found an OR of 2.7 (0.4-16.0) for oesophageal cancer for men working in the textile industry in three English counties.

*(d) Colorectal cancer*

In the death registration study of Versluys (1949; see p. 238) in the Netherlands, there were 11 deaths from cancer of the small intestine (PMR, 69) and 12 from rectal cancer (PMR, 86).

In the study of Guralnik (1963; see p. 238) of occupational mortality among US men, increased numbers of deaths from cancer of the intestine and rectum (ICD 152-154) were seen among spinners and weavers in the textile industry (SMR, 162; 21 deaths) and among operatives and allied workers in yarn, thread and fabric mills (SMR, 130; 39 deaths).

In the study of Delzell and Grufferman (1983; see p. 238) of white female textile workers in North Carolina (USA), the PMR was 100 for cancers of both the colon (95% CI, 80-120; 115 deaths) and rectum (90-120; 21 deaths).

Olsen and Jensen (1987; see p. 239) found that 48 cases of cancer of the small intestine, colon and rectum (SPIR, 107; 95% CI, 81-142) had been registered among Danish men in the manufacture of textiles and 25 (SPIR, 107; 72-158) in those employed in spinning, weaving and finishing. For women, the SPIRs were 120 (94-153; 64 cases) and 153 (23-371; 32 cases), respectively.

Dubrow and Gute (1988; see p. 239) noted a statistically significant increase in mortality from cancer of the rectum (72 observed; PMR, 128; 95% CI, 104-158) among male textile workers in Rhode Island (USA). The elevated mortality from rectal cancer turned out to be statistically significant in the occupational category 'operatives, except transport', which included 63.2% of the decedents; 47 deaths were observed, yielding a PMR of 134 (95% CI, 102-175). Within the textile manufacturing categories, decedents engaged in 'dyeing and finishing' showed a significantly increased PMR for rectal cancer (174; 115-264; 21 observed). The PMR for cancer of the colon for all male textile workers was 90 (140 deaths).

In the proportionate mortality study of O'Brien and Decouflé (1988; see p. 239) among male textile workers in Georgia (USA), the PMRs were 80 (50-130; 16 deaths) for cancer of the colon and 48 (two deaths) for rectal cancer.

In the case-control study of Williams *et al.* (1977; see p. 240), the RR for rectal cancer for working in textile mills was 6.8 (three cases) among men and 3.2 (two cases) among women in the Third National Cancer Surveys in the USA.

In the case-control study of Decouflé *et al.* (1978; see p. 240) on admissions to the Roswell Park Memorial Institute in New York State (USA), the RR for colorectal cancer in male operatives in textile mills was 1.7 (eight cases); that for women was 0.6 (11 cases).

Vobecky *et al.* (1983) designed a case-control study to investigate further a previously suggested association between large-bowel cancer and working in a carpet factory also manufacturing synthetic fibres (from acetate and polypropylene (Vobecky *et al.*, 1984)) in Québec (Canada) on the basis of five cases observed in young men (Vobecky *et al.*, 1978). Cases occurring between 1 January 1965 and 31 December 1976 in 24 communities from which the carpet factory was likely to draw its manpower were identified, using medical records from local hospitals. Controls were chosen at random from all people living in the same communities and matched for sex, age and residence. There were 224 cases of large-bowel cancer and 224 controls available for study. Telephone interviews were attempted for all subjects or their next-of-kin, resulting in 207 pairs of cancer patients and matched controls (103 male and 104 female pairs). Thirty-five cancer patients had a history of employment [length unspecified] in a carpet factory *versus* 28 controls—a statistically nonsignificant difference. Among males, the number of patients who had worked in the factory was 29 *versus* 17 controls ($p < 0.05$). No association was found among women.

Vobecky *et al.* (1984) tried to address the question of whether the increased risk noted in the previous study was confined to any particular section of the plant. Analysis was limited to 34 male cases and 101 controls for whom an employment history was available. A significantly elevated risk was found for working in 'textile' (RR, 3.0; $p < 0.03$). An elevated risk (RR, 2.1; $p < 0.025$) was also observed for working in two extrusion departments of the plant; the risk was higher among those who had worked in these departments after 1974 (RR, 6.3; $p < 0.002$) and for longer than ten years ([RR, 4.7]; $p < 0.002$).

In order to investigate possible relationships between employment in the textile industry and cancers of the colon and prostate, suggested by a correlation study (Blair & Fraumeni, 1978), a case-control study was conducted using death certificates (Hoar & Blair, 1984). South Carolina (USA) was selected because a large proportion of the state's population is employed in the textile industry. Cases were residents of selected counties who had died during 1970-78. One control for each cancer death was selected from state mortality data, matched for year of death, race, sex, county and age at death. The 1975 and 1976 Industrial Directories were used to identify the manufacturing activity in all companies named on death certificates. For the study of colon cancer, 820 pairs of cases and controls were available; no significant result was obtained in relation to textile work.

Coggon *et al.* (1986b, see p. 241) reported RRs of 5.9 (three cases) for colon cancer and 0.8 (one case) for cancer of the rectum among male textile workers in three English counties.

In the case-control study of Siemiatycki *et al.* (1986, see p. 241) in Montréal, Québec (Canada), when the risk of 'substantial' exposure to synthetic fibres was compared with 'unexposed', the risk for colorectal cancer was elevated (22 exposed cases; OR, 1.5; 95% CI, 0.8-2.9). Also of borderline significance was the increased risk for rectal cancer from exposure to wool dust [number not reported]. When data were further analysed by logistic regression techniques to take into account all potential confounders, both occupational and nonoccupational, the association of exposure to wool dust with rectal cancer fell towards the null value. Results for the association between exposure to synthetic fibres and colorectal cancer were: 'doubtful exposure', 12 exposed cases (OR, 3.3; 95% CI, 1.3-8.2); 'substantial exposure', 22 cases (OR, 1.5; 0.9-2.7); 'substantial exposure' >15 years, 16 exposed cases (OR, 3.0; 1.4-6.6).

(e) *Nasal cavity cancer* (see Table 11)

In a study in England and Wales (excluding the Oxford region), Acheson *et al.* (1972) compared the occupations of 80 male cases of adenocarcinoma of the nasal cavity with those of 85 male cases of other nasal cancers matched for age, region and year of registration. The occupations of cases were also compared with the occupational distribution of working and retired men in the 1961 census. Two cases of adenocarcinoma occurred in male textile workers compared with 0.8 expected on the basis of the census data [SMR, 250; 95% CI, 30-903].

Two controls with other nasal cancers were also textile workers. Seven cases of adenocarcinoma or other nasal cancers occurred in female textile workers. No exposure to wood dust was reported. [The Working Group noted that expected numbers could not be calculated for women.]

Table 11. Studies of nasal cavity cancer among workers in the textile industry

| Type of study and reference (country) | Sex | No. of cases in textile workers | Relative risk[a] | 95% confidence interval | Comments |
|---|---|---|---|---|---|
| *Mortality and morbidity statistics* | | | | | |
| Acheson et al. (1972) (England and Wales) | M | 2 | 2.5 | 0.30-9.0 | |
| Acheson et al. (1981) (England and Wales) | M | 10 | 0.95 | 0.46-1.8 | |
|  | F | 5 | 2.2 | 0.70-5.1 | |
| Malker et al. (1986a) (Sweden) | M | 8 | 2.4* | NA | |
|  | F | 3 | 3.0 | NA | |
| Dubrow & Gute (1988) (USA) | M | 4 | 1.4 | NA | |
| Olsen (1988) (Denmark) | M | 1 | 1.6 | NA | Spinners and weavers |
|  | F | 2 | 5.6 | NA | |
| *Case-control studies* | | | | | |
| Bross et al. (1978) (USA) | M | NA | >2.0* | NA | No numbers given |
| Brinton et al. (1985) (USA) | M | 12 | 0.8 | 0.4-1.7 | Textile and clothing industry |
|  | F | 22 | 2.1 | 1.1-4.3 | |
| Ng (1986) (Hong Kong) | M,F | 14 | 2.9 | 1.1-7.9 | Nasal cavity and sinus; mainly weavers |
| Roush et al. (1987) (USA) | M | 17 | 0.7 | 0.4-1.3 | Sinonasal and nasopharyngeal; formaldehyde-associated textile work |

[a]Standardardized mortality ratios were converted to relative risks for comparison
*$p < 0.05$
NA, not available

In a survey of nasal cancer in England and Wales in 1963-67, information on occupation at the time of diagnosis was obtained from interviews, hospital notes and death certificates (Acheson et al., 1981). Of the 925 male cases, ten were in textile workers, as compared with 10.5 expected on the basis of age-specific national census data (SMR, 95; [95% CI, 46-175]). In women, five of 677 nasal cancers were in textile workers, as compared to 2.3 expected [SMR, 217; 70-507].

The Swedish Cancer-Environment Register (see p. 239) was used to study nasal cancer incidence (Malker et al., 1986a). Elevated risks for work in the textile industry were observed for both men (SIR, 180; 12 cases) and women (SIR, 260; four cases). The occupational category of textile worker was also associated with elevated risks for both men (SIR, 240; eight cases; $p < 0.05$) and women (SIR, 300; three cases). Only one of the eight cases among men was an adenocarcinoma; two were squamous-cell carcinomas and the others of other histological types. The authors noted that the smoking habits of this cohort were comparable to those of the general Swedish population.

Dubrow and Gute (1988; see p. 239) found a PMR of 141 (four deaths) for nasal cancer among male textile workers in Rhode Island (USA).

Olsen (1988) analysed all 382 cases of cancers of the sinonasal cavities diagnosed in 1970-84 in Denmark, many of which were the same as those described by Olsen and Jensen (1987). One male case (SPIR, 158) and two female cases (SPIR, 559) were recorded for the occupational category of spinning and weaving of textiles.

In the case-control study of Bross et al. (1978; see p. 241), male operatives in US textile mills had a statistically significant elevated risk, larger than 2.0, for cancer of the 'nose'.

Brinton et al. (1985) explored in detail the association they had noted previously between the occurrence of nasal cancer and working in the textile and clothing industry (Brinton et al., 1977, 1984). The case series included patients 18 years or older diagnosed with primary malignancies of the nasal cavities and sinuses at four hospitals in North Carolina and Virginia (USA) between 1 January 1970 and 31 December 1980. For cases alive at the time the study was conducted, two hospital controls were selected, matched for hospital, year of admission, age, sex, race and residence. Patients with diagnoses of neoplasms of the buccal cavity and pharynx, oesophagus, nasal cavity and sinuses, larynx, benign tumours of the respiratory system, other diseases of the upper respiratory tract and mental disorders were excluded from the control group. For deceased cases, two matched control series were selected—one from hospitals and one from among deceased individuals identified through state vital statistics offices. Telephone interviews with study subjects or with their next-of-kin were completed for 160 of 193 cases and 290 controls (178 of 232 hospital controls and 112 of 140 death certificate controls). Twelve male cases and 28 male controls reported employment in the textile or clothing industry (RR, 0.82; 95% CI, 0.4-1.7), whereas 22 female cases and 20 female controls reported such employment (RR, 2.1; 95% CI, 1.1-4.3). Women who had worked for fewer than ten years were at higher risk (12 exposed cases; RR, 3.9; 95% CI, 1.4-11.0) than those who had worked for ten years or more (seven exposed cases; RR, 1.4; 95% CI, 0.5-3.8). Women first employed fewer than 20 years before diagnosis had a much higher risk (nine exposed cases; RR, 5.8; $p < 0.05$) than those first employed earlier (12 exposed cases [RR, 1.4]). Among women, an increased risk of borderline significance was found to be associated with exposure to dust (RR, 2.3; 95% CI, 0.9-5.5). The textile industries listed in the employment histories included primarily textile and cotton mills, clothing manufacture and hosiery; no occupation predominated. The primary origin of dust was cotton. The association of work in the textile industry with specific histological types of tumour was also investigated. An increased risk for adenocarcinoma was found in both women (RR,

2.5; 95% CI, 0.7-9.0) and men (RR, 2.5; 95% CI, 0.7-8.3), and the risk for adenocarcinomas associated with working in dusty conditions was elevated among both men (RR, 4.7; 95% CI, 1.2-17.8) and women (RR, 3.4; 95% CI, 0.8-14.1). The increases in risk were not affected by tobacco use or by employment in other high-risk industries.

A case-control study in Hong Kong (Ng, 1986) of 225 cases of nasal cavity and sinus cancer in persons 18 years old or more diagnosed in 1974-81, and of 226 controls with other cancers matched for treatment centre, year, age, sex, race and resident status gave an OR for textile work of 2.9 (95% CI, 1.1-7.9; 14 cases). The OR was 7.4 (1.2-45.1; seven cases) for persons who had been employed for at least 15 years in textile work. The ORs for weavers and other textile workers, adjusted for employment years, were 4.7 (1.2-19.2; nine cases) and 1.8 (0.4-7.3; five cases), respectively. The study included an additional control group of 224 persons with nasopharyngeal cancer, among whom there was a similar proportion of textile workers as in the case group, suggesting that textile workers also have elevated risks for this cancer type. Only two of the 225 cases in the study had worked with furniture or wood dust; it was not known whether they had worked with textiles.

A case-control study designed to examine potential associations between nasopharyngeal and sinonasal cancer and formaldehyde-related occupations failed to reveal any increased risk for persons in the textile industry (Roush *et al.*, 1987). Newly diagnosed cases were identified through the Connecticut Tumor Registry from among males who had died of any cause between 1935 and 1975, and controls were drawn randomly from men who had died in Connecticut in the same period. Information on occupation was obtained from death certificates and city directories. Among the 198 sinonasal and 173 nasopharyngeal cancer cases, there were, respectively, ten and seven cases whose formaldehyde-related occupation had been in 'textiles' *versus* 43 controls with such occupations out of a total of 605. The resulting OR was 0.7 (95% CI, 0.4-1.3).

*(f) Laryngeal cancer*

Kennaway and Kennaway (1936) examined death certificates for cases of cancer of the lung and larynx in men from England and Wales in 1921-32, and calculated age-adjusted mortality ratios based on the 1921 and 1931 censuses. For the occupational category 'cotton spinners and piecers (mule, ring, cap or flyer)', the RR was 1.5 (31 deaths) for laryngeal cancer. For the category of 'cotton strippers and grinders and card-room jobbers', the RR was 0.6 (two deaths), and, for the category of cotton weavers, the RR was 0.8 (22 deaths).

Versluys (1949; see p. 238) observed four deaths from cancer of the larynx (PMR, 103) among death registrations for male weavers and workers in woollens in the Netherlands.

In the 1981 decennial supplement of the UK Registrar General (see p. 238), there was little evidence of an increased risk for cancer of the larynx among female textile workers.

In their study of death certificates, Delzell and Grufferman (1983; see p. 238) found a PMR for laryngeal cancer of 280 (95% CI, 100-730; five deaths) among white female textile workers in North Carolina (USA); Dubrow and Gute (1988; see p. 239) reported a PMR of 108 (24 deaths) among male textile workers in Rhode Island, and O'Brien and Decouflé

(1988; see p. 239) found five deaths (PMR, 110) among male carpet and textile workers in Georgia.

Olsen and Jensen (1987; see p. 239) found three cases (41; 95% CI, 13-127) among male workers manufacturing textiles and one case (28; 4-199) among male spinners, weavers and finishers. Among women, there were five cases (SPIR, 235; 98-566) and one case (117; 16-831) in the two categories, respectively.

Decouflé et al. (1978; see p. 240) in their case-control study at the Roswell Park Memorial Institute, New York (USA), reported an increased, statistically nonsignificant RR of 2.0 for cancer of the larynx (five cases; adjusted for smoking) among male operatives in the textile industry, while in a subset of the same cohort, Bross et al. (1978; see p. 241) found increases of the same magnitude among male operatives in textile mills.

A case-control study was conducted in southern Ontario (Canada) between 1977 and 1979 on the role of tobacco, alcohol, asbestos and nickel in the etiology of cancer of the larynx (Burch et al., 1981). Cases were ascertained through hospitals which served the study area for radiotherapy, and for each case an individually matched neighbourhood control was selected, matched on age and sex. Of 258 cases ascertained, 204 (79%) were interviewed; the same number of controls were interviewed out of a total of 315 eligible controls. Questions were asked on demographic data, smoking, alcohol use and detailed occupational history, including information on exposures, which allowed the investigation of occupational exposures other than asbestos and nickel. Estimates of RR were obtained by an individually matched case-control analysis; only numbers for discordant pairs were presented. Elevated risk was observed for individuals who reported exposure to textile dusts; in five of the pairs, the case had been exposed and the control not, but in none of the pairs had the control been exposed and the case not.

A further case-control study was conducted in the Greater Augusta area, Georgia, USA (Flanders et al., 1984) involving all persons with newly diagnosed, histologically confirmed squamous-cell laryngeal cancer, who were resident in one of seven counties of Georgia and who were treated at one of the ten hospitals in the area between 1 September 1974 and 30 September 1979. By reviewing hospital medical records, potential controls matched by age, area of residence, history of tobacco smoking and alcohol drinking were identified for each case. Final matching was carried out for age, sex, alcohol and tobacco history, area of residence and source of medical care, and was successful for 85 of 353 potential controls and for 42 of 64 potential cases. For each occupational category in which at least 15 subjects had worked, laryngeal cancer rate ratios were estimated by comparing the incidence rate among those who had worked at least six months in that occupational category with the rate among those who had not. Only numbers for discordant pairs were presented. The rate ratio for all textile processors was 1.5 (at least seven cases; 90% CI, 0.6-3.9). For workers who separated, filtered or dried textile fibres, a statistically significantly increased risk for laryngeal cancer was found (at least nine cases; RR, 3.2; 90% CI, 1.3-8.0). In a further analysis, subjects were categorized as exposed only if they had worked for at least five years in a given occupation; in addition, only work experience during the time frame from the age of 14 until five years before diagnosis was considered to be relevant exposure. In this subset, the estimated rate ratio for the occupation 'all textile processors' was 4.2 (at least four cases; 90% CI, 1.0-22.4) and that for separating, filtering and drying was 5.6 (at least five cases; 90% CI, 1.4-29.1) in comparison with those who had never worked in the trade.

A case-control study in Denmark in the period 1980-82 involved interviews with all 326 incident cases of laryngeal cancer under 75 years of age and 1134 community controls matched for age and sex (Olsen & Sabroe, 1984). Cases and controls were asked about their present, latest and longest-held occupation and to describe their work place and type of work. The RRs, adjusted for age, sex, tobacco and alcohol consumption, were 1.0 (95% CI, 0.4-2.9; six cases) for any exposure to textile dyes, 1.4 (0.8-2.7; 16 cases) for exposure to wool dust and 1.5 (0.8-2.6; 20 cases) for exposure to cotton dust.

Coggon et al. (1986a; see p. 241) found a RR of 2.4 (one case) for laryngeal cancer among male textile workers in three English counties.

*(g) Lung cancer*

Kennaway and Kennaway (1936) examined death certificates of cases of cancer of the lung and larynx in men in England and Wales in 1921-32 and calculated age-adjusted mortality ratios based on the 1921 and 1932 censuses. For the occupational category 'cotton spinners and piecers (mule, ring, cap or flyer)', the RR was 0.3 (seven deaths) for lung cancer. For the category of 'cotton strippers and grinders and card-room jobbers', the RR was 0.3 (one death); and for the category of cotton weavers, the RR was 0.5 (13 deaths).

Versluys (1949; see p. 238) observed five deaths from lung cancer (PMR, 43) among death registrations of men in the Netherlands working as weavers and workers in woollens.

In the 1951 decennial supplement of the UK Registrar General (see p. 238), a decreased risk for lung cancer was noted among male bleaching, dyeing and finishing workers (SMR, 73; 77 deaths), and one of the most consistent findings in male textile workers in 1961, 1971 and 1981 was a decreased risk for this cancer (SMR, 85 (Logan, 1982), 88 and 94, respectively). Roman et al. (1985) analysed the 1971 data according to married women's own occupation and noted a decreased risk for lung cancer in textile workers, particularly in weavers (SMR, 71; 34 deaths). In the 1981 supplement, the PMR for lung cancer in female textile workers was 141 (39 deaths).

Guralnik (1963; see p. 238) reported that US male labourers in textile mill products had elevated mortality due to cancer of the lung (23 observed; SMR, 192).

In Los Angeles County, USA, all death certificates mentioning lung cancer for the period 1968-70 and all newly diagnosed cases of lung cancer reported in 1972-73 were examined in relation to statements on occupation and industry abstracted from death certificates and hospital admission sheets, respectively (Menck & Henderson, 1976). The study was limited to white males in the age group 20-64 years, and the total number of white males at risk for each occupation/industry was estimated from census figures. Expected deaths/incident cases were calculated for each specific occupation/industry from the age-specific rates of cancer for all occupations/industries. The ratios of observed deaths plus incident cases to expected deaths plus incident cases were then calculated. There were 27 deaths and 20 incident cases of lung cancer in the industry category 'textile, apparel', yielding a SMR of 119, which was statistically nonsignificant. Smoking was not controlled for.

In their death certificate analysis, Delzell and Grufferman (1983; see p. 238) reported a PMR of 90 (106 deaths) for white female textile workers in North Carolina (USA).

In the cancer registry study of Olsen and Jensen (1987; see p. 239) in Denmark, there was a moderately decreased risk for cancer of the lung and trachea in men (SPIR, 88; 95% CI, 70-111; 73 cases) and women (82; 56-120; 26 cases) employed in textile manufacture and in men (91; 66-125; 39 cases) and women (75; 39-143; nine cases) employed in spinning, weaving and finishing.

In the proportionate mortality study of Dubrow and Gute (1988; see p. 239) in male textile workers in Rhode Island (USA), lung cancer mortality was lower than expected, except among 'service workers' (24 cases) and workers manufacturing 'synthetic and silk only' (eight cases) for each of whom a 30% statistically nonsignificant elevation was noted. O'Brien and Decouflé (1988; see p. 239) found a PMR of 100 (90-110; 138 deaths) in male carpet and textile workers in Georgia (USA).

Henderson and Enterline (1973; see p. 239) reported a low observed:expected ratio for respiratory cancer (0.55) in their cohort study of mortality among male textile workers in Georgia. Newhouse (1978; see p. 240) observed 103 cases of lung cancer with 109.3 expected among male dyers, bleachers and textile workers in Bradford (UK).

Merchant and Ortmeyer (1981; see p. 241) found that overall SMRs for lung cancer tended to decrease with increased presumed exposure to cotton dust. Only in the 'other' job category was a small increase in SMR observed; workers in this category also had potential exposure to asbestos, cutting oils, solvents and dyes. The principal dye used was indigo. On the basis of cross-sectional data on North Carolina textile workers, the smoking habits of cotton textile workers were considered to be similar to those of other workers and the rest of the population. [The Working Group noted the small proportion of the cohort included in the analysis.]

In the case-control study of Williams et al. (1977; see p. 240), as part of the US Third National Cancer Survey, a suggestive increase in cancer of the lung was noted among male patients who had worked with textile mill products (RR, 2.6; three cases).

Decouflé et al. (1978; see p. 240) found that men admitted to the Roswell Park Memorial Institute (New York, USA) who had been employed as operatives in the textile mill industry had an elevated but statistically nonsignificant risk for lung cancer (RR, 1.5; nine cases; adjusted for smoking).

A comparison was made of death certificate statements on usual occupation and kind of industry for 858 white males who had lived in coastal counties of Georgia (USA) and who had died of primary lung cancer during 1961-74 with those for 858 controls (Harrington et al., 1978). Each death certificate of a case was matched by age at death within one year, year of death within six years, sex, race and county of usual residence to a death certificate of a person who had succumbed to conditions other than lung cancer, chronic respiratory disease or bladder cancer. There were seven cases and eight controls in the industrial category 'textiles'; the matched pair analysis yielded an estimated RR of 0.88.

Milne *et al.* (1983) conducted a case-control study comparing lung cancer deaths *versus* deaths from all other cancers occurring in a county of California (USA) between 1958 and 1962. Usual occupation and industry of employment were extracted from death certificates. The 925 deaths from lung cancer were compared with 6420 deaths from all other cancers. The age-adjusted RR associated with textile manufacturing among males was 1.9, based on five exposed cases and 13 exposed controls; the result was statistically nonsignificant. [The crude RR was 2.7 (98% CI, 1.0-7.1)]. No data regarding textile industry were reported for female workers, and information on tobacco use was not available.

Coggon *et al.* (1986a, see p. 241) found a RR of 0.3 (one case) for cancer of the bronchus in their case-control study of male textile workers in three English counties.

In the case-control study of Siemiatycki *et al.* (1986; see p. 241), in Canada, the ORs for lung cancer were 0.8 (95% CI, 0.4-1.3; 25 cases) for people working with cotton, 0.5 (0.3-1.0; 15 cases) for those working with wool and 0.5 (0.2-1.1; 11 cases) for those working with synthetic fibres.

A case-control study of lung cancer mortality in persons aged 14-60 was conducted in Prato, Italy (Buiatti *et al.*, 1979). Information on occupation from death certificates was verified by interviews with next-of-kin. The RR for lung cancer mortality in textile workers compared with that of other residents was 2.0 in men ([95% CI, 1.4-2.7]; 42 deaths) and 4.8 in women ([95% CI, 0.9-14.0]; three deaths). Workers who had been employed only in the reprocessing of textiles to serve as raw material (nine deaths) or in dyeing (six deaths) had lung cancer mortality rates six to nine times higher than expected, whereas mortality was not markedly elevated in persons who had been involved only in spinning or weaving. [The Working Group noted that no adjustment was made for age or smoking habits.]

In a case-control study in Florence and Prato, Italy (Paci *et al.*, 1987), 65 of 441 cases ot male lung cancer admitted during 1980-83 had been nonasbestos textile workers, as compared with 127 of 1075 hospital controls matched for age, sex and smoking habits (OR, 1.5; 95% CI, 0.98-2.3). The analysis was adjusted for area of residence, age and smoking habits. The elevated risk was greatest (OR, 2.4; 95% CI, 1.2-4.8; 16 cases) for the period 15-24 years from first employment in the industry. The authors concluded, however, that the elevated lung cancer risk may have been due to asbestos exposure in rag-sorting, weaving and refining.

A population-based case-control study in urban Shanghai (China) involved interviews with 1405 newly diagnosed lung cancer patients and 1495 general population controls (Levin *et al.*, 1987). Women were interviewed in 1984-86 and men in 1984-85. The analysis included adjustment for smoking and 'if necessary' for age, sex, education, place of birth, dietary vitamin A and previous history of chest diseases. The RR for cotton textile employment was 0.7 (95% CI, 0.6-0.9; 169 cases). This decrease in risk was observed for both men and women and for smokers and nonsmokers. The reductions in risk tended to be greater for lung cancer cell types other than adenocarcinoma. Low risks were observed in virtually all occupations in the cotton textile industry, and there was little difference in risk according to self-reported exposure to textile dust. In a subset of 733 newly diagnosed male lung cancer cases and 760 controls, the OR for employment in the textile industry was 0.7 (0.5-1.0; Levin *et al.*, 1988).

Possible explanations have been sought for the low rates of lung cancer observed in most studies. Ashley (1967) calculated SMRs for lung cancer in each of the county boroughs of England and Wales for the years 1958-63. The overall lung cancer SMR was 89 in the eight towns in which cotton textiles were an important industry, and 87 in the four county boroughs in which the wool industry assumed major importance. He found that the lung cancer deficit was associated with an excess of chronic bronchitis, and the findings were not related to the degree of air pollution or population density. He suggested that chronic lung disease associated with textile work may confer protection against carcinogenic substances. In a further analysis using multiple regression, Ashley (1969) found lower SMRs for lung cancer in both men and women in coal and textile towns, controlling for population density, social class, smoke pollution and sulfur dioxide pollution.

Enterline et al. (1985) proposed several possible explanations for the lower than expected mortality from respiratory cancer found among cotton textile workers. The first was based on the hypothesis that cotton textile workers in dusty operations smoke, on average, less than other workers and the rest of the population. The second possible explanation was that exposure to cotton dust may stimulate mucus production, which might protect against carcinogens such as cigarette smoke. The third explanation, which the authors considered most likely, was based on the evidence that endotoxins, which are found in airborne cotton dust, are potent anticancer agents.

[The Working Group noted that data on smoking habits were not available in most of the studies of lung cancer in textile workers, but, when data were available, adjustment for cigarette smoking made little difference to the findings.]

*(h)   Bladder cancer* (see Table 12)

Versluys (1949; see p. 238) reported five deaths from bladder cancer (PMR, 93) among death registrations of male weavers and workers in woollens in the Netherlands.

**Table 12. Studies of bladder cancer among workers in the textile industry**

| Type of study and reference (country) | Sex | No. of cases in textile workers | Relative risk[a] | 95% confidence interval | Comments |
|---|---|---|---|---|---|
| *Mortality and morbidity statistics* | | | | | |
| Versluys (1949) (Netherlands) | M | 5 | 0.93 | NA | |
| Office of Population Censuses and Surveys (1961-1981); Logan (1982) (UK) | M | 1 | 1.1<br>1.2<br>0.73 | NA<br>NA<br>NA | 1961<br>1971<br>1981 |
| Delzell & Grufferman (1983) (USA) | F | 13 | 1.00 | 0.7-1.5 | Textile workers |

Table 12 (contd)

| Type of study and reference (country) | Sex | No. of cases in textile workers | Relative risk[a] | 95% confidence interval | Comments |
|---|---|---|---|---|---|
| Olsen & Jensen (1987) (Denmark) | M | 28 | 0.86 | 0.59-1.3 | Textile manufacture |
| | F | 13 | 1.1 | 0.62-1.8 | |
| | M | 13 | 0.77 | 0.45-1.3 | Spinning, weaving, finishing |
| | F | 6 | 1.3 | 0.57-2.8 | |
| Malker et al. (1987) (Sweden) | M | 147 | 1.1 | NA | Textile industry |
| | M | 49 | 1.1 | NA | Cotton industry |
| Dubrow & Gute (1988) (USA) | M | 58 | 0.85 | 0.68-1.07 | Textile workers |
| O'Brien & Decouflé (1988) (USA) | M | 8 | 1.2 | 0.6-2.5 | Carpet and textile workers |

*Cohort studies*

| | | | | | |
|---|---|---|---|---|---|
| Henderson & Enterline (1973) (USA) | M | 9 | 1.6 | 0.75-3.1 (cohort 1) | Urinary system including bladder |
| | M | 5 | 1.4 | 0.44-3.2 (cohort 2) | |
| Newhouse (1978) (UK) | M | 14 | 1.1 | NA | Dyers, Bleachers and Textile Workers' Union members |

*Case-control studies*

| | | | | | |
|---|---|---|---|---|---|
| Wynder et al. (1963) (USA) | M | 8 | 2.7 | 0.75-9.8 | Textile workers |
| | F | 10 | 2.2 | 0.71-6.6 | Garment workers |
| Anthony & Thomas (1970) (UK) | M | 50 | 2.2 | NA | Textile workers |
| | F | 24 | <1 | NA | |
| | M+F | 9 | 7.7 | NA | Weaver } Employment |
| | M+F | 11 | 2.9 | NA | Finisher } for ≥20 yrs |
| | M+F | 8 | 3.4 | NA | Dyer } |
| Decouflé et al. (1978) (USA) | F | 6 | 2.6 | NA | Operatives in textile mills; adjusted for smoking |
| Tola et al. (1980) (Finland) | M | 1 | 0.50 | 0.05-5.3 | Textile workers |
| | F | 1 | 0.32 | 0.04-2.9 | |
| Cartwright (1982) (UK) | M+F | 24 | 1.3 | 0.8-2.4 | Dye users |
| Najem et al. (1982) (USA) | M+F | 5 | 0.9 | 0.3-2.7 | Textile industry |
| Silverman et al. (1983) (USA) | M | 7 | 0.7 | 0.3-1.8 | Textile industry |
| | M | 2 | 0.5 | 0.1-2.7 | Textile workers; lower urinary tract |
| Schoenberg et al. (1984) (USA) | M | 12 | 0.61 | 0.30-1.2 | Textile mill workers |

Table 12 (contd)

| Type of study and reference (country) | Sex | No. of cases in textile workers | Relative risk[a] | 95% confidence interval | Comments | |
|---|---|---|---|---|---|---|
| Morrison et al. (1985) (USA, UK, Japan) | M<br>M<br>M | 30<br>79<br>16 | 0.9<br>0.9<br>1.0 | 0.6-1.4<br>0.7-1.2<br>0.6-1.6 | Boston<br>Manchester<br>Nagoya | Textile workers; lower urinary tract |
| Vineis & Magnani (1985) (Italy) | M | 21 | 1.8 | 0.9-3.6 | Textile industry | |
| Maffi & Vineis (1986) (Italy) | F | 11<br>2<br>2<br>3<br>4<br>5 | 1.9<br>∞<br>4.0<br>2.6<br>5.6<br>2.6 | 0.85-4.2<br><br>0.6-26.9<br>0.4-15.5<br>1.1-29.2<br>0.8-8.1 | Textile industry<br>Carders<br>Twisting machine operator<br>Winding machine operator<br>Other winders and twisters<br>Weavers (power loom) | |
| Coggon et al. (1986b) (UK) | M | 5 | 1.3 | NA | Textile workers; bladder and renal pelvis | |
| Siemiatycki et al. (1986) (Canada) | <br>M | <br>17<br>15<br>21 | <br>1.6<br>1.3<br>1.2 | <br>0.9-3.0<br>0.7-2.4<br>0.7-2.1 | 'Substantial' exposure to:<br>Synthetic fibres<br>Wool fibres<br>Cotton fibres | |
| Corisco et al. (1987) (Spain) | M | 5 | 4.9 | 0.7-34.9 | Textile industry | |
| Jensen et al. (1987) (Denmark) | M+F | 56 | 1.7 | 1.1-2.4 | Textile and leather industry | |
| Claude et al. (1988) (FRG) | M<br>M | 35<br>8 | 1.7<br>0.73 | 0.98-2.9<br>0.29-1.8 | Textile industry<br>Textile workers | |
| Gonzáles et al. (1988) (Spain) | M+F | 19<br>8<br>10<br>2 | 2.1<br>4.4<br>1.9<br>0.33 | 0.82-5.1<br>1.2-16.8<br>0.71-5.0<br>0.06-1.9 | Textile industry<br>Dyeing and printing<br>Weaving<br>Spinning | |
| Gonzáles et al. (1989) (Spain) | M<br>F<br>M<br>F<br>M<br>F | 41<br>11<br>10<br>9<br>11<br>1 | 1.9<br>6.4<br>3.5[b]<br>21.2[b]<br>1.3[b]<br>0.34[b] | 1.1-3.1<br>1.3-30.0<br>1.3-9.3<br>1.5-298<br>0.5-3.1<br>0.1-7.7 | Textile industry<br><br>Weavers<br><br>Dyers<br> | |

**Table 12 (contd)**

| Type of study and reference (country) | Sex | No. of case in textile workers | Relative risk[a] | 95% confidence interval | Comments |
|---|---|---|---|---|---|
| Risch et al. (1988) (Canada) | M | 21[c] | 1.5 | 0.61-4.0 | Dyeing |
| | M | | 4.6 | 1.1-31.6 | Dyers employed 8-28 yrs before diagnosis |
| | M | 61[c] | 1.1 | 0.65-2.0 | All fabric dust |
| | F | 39[c] | 1.1 | 0.50-2.2 | |
| | M | 18[c] | 0.76 | 0.28-2.0 | Cotton dust |
| | F | 12[c] | 1.4 | 0.44-4.9 | |
| | M | 10[c] | 1.3 | 0.35-5.0 | Synthetic fabrics dust |
| | M | 13[c] | 0.91 | 0.30-2.9 | Wool dust |
| | F | 12[c] | 1.1 | 0.32-3.6 | |

[a]Standardized mortality ratios, standardized incidence ratios, standardized proportional incidence ratios and proportional mortality ratios were converted to relative risks for comparison
[b]Conditional logistic regression analysis
[c]Total number of subjects exposed (cases and controls)

In the UK Registrar General's decennial supplements for 1961, 1971 and 1981 (see p. 238), the SMRs for cancer of the bladder were 109, 123 (Logan, 1982) and 73, in men, respectively. In the 1981 supplement, there was little evidence of an increased risk for bladder cancer among female textile workers.

Delzell and Grufferman (1983; see p. 238) reported a PMR of 100 (13 deaths) among white female textile workers in North Carolina (USA).

In the cancer registry study of Olsen and Jensen (1987; see p. 239), the SPIRs for bladder cancer were 86 for men in textile manufacturing (95% CI, 59-125; 28 cases) and 107 for women (62-184; 13 cases) and 77 for men in spinning, weaving and finishing (45-133; 13 cases) and 127 for women (57-283; six cases).

The Swedish Cancer-Environment Register (see p. 239) was used to study male bladder cancer incidence in 1961-79 (Malker et al., 1987). Of the 11 702 cases of bladder cancer, 147 were in workers in the textile industry (SIR, 108), 49 of whom had worked in the cotton industry (SIR, 108). There were 62 cases in the occupational category of textile worker (SIR, 91) and 32 cases in carpet makers (SIR, 129).

Dubrow and Gute (1988; see p. 239) found a PMR of 85 (95% CI, 68-107; 58 deaths) for bladder cancer among male textile workers in Rhode Island (USA), and, in their proportionate mortality study, O'Brien and Decouflé (1988; see p. 239) noted a suggestive increase for cancer the bladder (PMR, 120; 60-250; eight cases) among male carpet and textile workers in Georgia (USA).

In the cohort study of Henderson and Enterline (1973; see p. 239) in the USA, an exception to the generally low observed:expected ratios for cancer deaths was cancer of the urinary system. In the first cohort, nine cases were observed between 1938 and 1963 versus 5.5 expected (SMR, 164 [95% CI, 74.8-310.6]); in the second cohort, five cases were observed between 1948 and 1963, whereas 3.7 were expected (SMR, 135 [43.9-315.4]). Among workers belonging to both cohorts, two cases were observed, while 1.6 were expected (SMR, 125). [The Working Group noted that the proportion of cases of cancer of the urinary system that were bladder cancer was not specified.]

Newhouse (1978; see p. 240) found 14 cases of bladder cancer with 13.1 expected (PMR, 110) among male bleachers, dyers and textile workers in Bradford (UK).

Histologically confirmed bladder cancer cases and controls were interviewed at seven main hospitals in the New York metropolitan area from January 1957 to December 1960 (Wynder *et al.*, 1963). In total, 300 male cases and 70 female cases were matched individually by age and sex to controls who were patients from the same hospitals, excluding those with cancer of the respiratory system or upper alimentary tract as well as those with myocardial infarction. The interview included data on occupation, age, race, smoking habits and residence. Eight male cases and three controls were classified as textile workers [crude RR, 2.7; 95% CI, 0.75-9.8]. Seven of the cases and one control had been employed in the textile industry for five or more years. Among female study subjects, ten cases and five controls had been engaged in the textile or garment industry [crude RR, 2.2; 0.71-6.6]. The possible role of exposure to dyes in certain textile operations was suggested. [The Working Group noted that exclusion from the control group of patients with tobacco-related diseases might introduce a bias with regard to bladder cancer.]

In a case-control study in Leeds, UK, 1422 bladder cancer cases were identified in 1959-67, and the occupational histories of 812 male cases and 218 female cases were compared with those of 390 surgical controls and 341 controls with other cancers (Anthony & Thomas, 1970). Controls were matched on age, sex and residence and (for 340 male and 50 female cases) for smoking history. Comparisons with the two control groups yielded similar findings. For textile workers, the crude OR for bladder cancer in men was 2.2 ($p < 0.01$), whereas the RR in women was less than 1.0. The RRs were particularly elevated in persons who had worked for 20 years or more as weavers (RR, 7.7; nine cases), finishers (RR, 2.9; 11 cases) and dyers (RR, 3.4; eight cases).

Decouflé *et al.* (1978; see p. 240), in their case-control study of admissions to a hospital in New York State (USA), found that female operatives in textile mills were at high, but statistically nonsignificant, risk for cancer of the bladder (RR, 2.6; six cases; adjusted for smoking).

The occupational histories of 180 of the 274 cases of bladder cancer that occurred in the industrial part of Finland in 1975-76 were compared with those of 180 hospital controls matched for age and sex (Tola *et al.*, 1980). Two cases and five controls gave textile worker as their predominant occupation [crude OR, 0.39; 95% CI, 0.1-1.9].

Cartwright (1982) conducted a case-control study of 991 cases of bladder cancer in West Yorkshire (UK) in the period 1978-80. All prevalent cases were matched with one hospital control and all newly diagnosed cases were matched with two, by health district, age and sex. Cases and controls were interviewed regarding their occupational history. The RR associated with the dyeing of woollens was 1.3 (95% CI, 0.8-2.4; 24 cases). [The Working Group noted that no data were given concerning other jobs in the textile industry.]

Najem et al. (1982) conducted a case-control study of bladder cancer in two northern counties of New Jersey (USA). The study was based on 75 prevalent cases admitted to four private clinics and two community hospitals in 1978. Two controls for each case were derived from the consecutive admission lists of the same clinic or hospital, matched on age, place of birth, sex, race and residence, excluding patients with a history of any neoplasm or with 'tobacco-related' heart disease. Interviewers were aware of the subjects' status as a case or control. Lifetime occupational history was determined beginning at age 16; study subjects were classified as having been employed in a particular industry if they had worked in that industry for at least one year. Five cases and ten controls had worked in the textile industry, yielding an estimated RR of 0.9 (95% CI, 0.3-2.7).

A population-based case-control study was conducted in Detroit, MI (USA) with the purpose of identifying industries and occupations in which workers might have an increased risk for cancer of the lower urinary tract (Silverman et al., 1983). The case series consisted of all 420 histologically confirmed, newly diagnosed cases of carcinoma of the lower urinary tract (bladder (95%), renal pelvis, ureter and urethra) in 60/61 hospitals of the tricounty area, occurring between December 1977 and November 1978 among male residents between the ages of 21 and 84 years. The controls were selected from the general male population of the study area and matched to the cases for age. Analysis was restricted to white males. Interviews were completed for 303 cases and 296 controls. Seven cases and ten controls had ever been employed in the 'textiles' industry (RR, 0.7; 95% CI, 0.3-1.8). Analysis by occupational category revealed two cases and four controls who had ever been employed as a 'textile worker' (RR, 0.5; 95% CI, 0.1-2.7).

As part of the National Cancer Institute study of the geographic distribution of bladder cancer mortality in the USA, the association between occupational exposure and bladder cancer risk was examined in a case-control study in New Jersey (Schoenberg et al., 1984), similar in design to the study described above. Analysis was restricted to 658 white male cases 21-84 years old, diagnosed during 1978-79, and 1258 white male controls. For working in a textile mill the OR was 0.61 (95% CI, 0.30-1.2; 12 cases).

A collaborative study of environmental risk factors for bladder cancer was carried out in Boston, USA (1976-77), Manchester, UK (1976-78), and Nagoya, Japan (1976-78; Morrison et al., 1985). Cases were male patients 21-89 years old with an initial diagnosis of a primary neoplasm of the lower urinary tract (bladder, ureter, renal pelvis, urethra). A pathology review indicated that virtually every case had a transitional- or squamous-cell tumour; 95% of the tumours occurred in the bladder. Controls were selected from electoral registers in such a way as to ensure an age and sex distribution similar to that of the cases. Subjects or their proxies were interviewed according to a standardized schedule; employment histories were obtained by interview. The 'textiles' group included both the textile industry and manufacture of cloth and cloth garments. Analysis was restricted to persons for whom smoking history was known; there were 430 such cases and 397 such controls in Boston, 399 cases and 493 controls in Manchester, and 226 cases and 443 controls in Nagoya, which were about 60% of the original numbers. In none of the study areas was the RR for bladder cancer elevated among 'textile' workers. In Boston, the estimated RR was 0.9 (90% CI, 0.6-1.4); in Manchester, the RR was 0.9 (0.7-1.2), and that in Nagoya 1.0 (0.6-1.6).

A case-control study in the province of Turin, Italy, involving interviews with 512 male cases of bladder cancer between 1978-83 and 596 age-matched male hospital controls (Vineis & Magnani, 1985) gave an OR of 1.8 (95% CI, 0.9-3.6) for employment in the textile industry. Adjustment for smoking did not affect the OR, but it fell to 0.9 when only cases and controls living in the city of Turin were considered. The authors suggested that this indicated the possibility of a selection bias. [The Working Group considered that this may have been due to different referral patterns of cases and of controls.]

In a hospital-based case-control study among female residents of the province of Turin, Italy between 1981-83 (Maffi & Vineis, 1986), 11 of 55 patients with bladder cancer had been employed in the textile industry for at least six months, as compared with 17 of 202 general surgical controls (cardiac and thoracic surgery excluded). The age-adjusted OR was 1.9 (95% CI, 0.85-4.2). The following jobs in the textile industry showed elevated risks: carder (two cases, no control), twisting machine operator (OR, 4.0; 95% CI, 0.6-26.9; two cases), winding machine operator (2.6; 0.4-15.5; three cases), other winders and twisters (5.6; 1.1-29.2; four cases) and weavers (2.6; 0.8-8.1; five cases).

Coggon *et al.* (1986b; see p. 241) reported a RR of 1.3 (five cases) for cancer of the bladder and renal pelvis among male textile workers in three English counties.

In the case-control study of Siematycki *et al.* (1986; see p. 241) in Montréal (Québec, Canada), the association of 'substantial' exposure with synthetic fibres and bladder cancer was statistically significant (OR, 1.8; 95% CI, 1.0-3.2, on the basis of logistic regression analysis; 17 cases). For exposure to wool, the OR was 1.3 (0.7-2.4; 15 cases), and for exposure to cotton, the OR was 1.2 (0.7-2.1; 21 cases), on the basis of analogous analysis.

Corisco *et al.* (1987) studied 180 male patients 41-87-years old with histologically proven bladder urothelioma and 180 age-matched healthy volunteer controls in Madrid, Spain. Five cases and one control were textile workers (OR, 4.9; 95% CI, 0.7-34.9). [The Working Group noted the potential for bias from using volunteer controls.]

A case-control study in Copenhagen (Denmark) involved interviews with 371 patients with bladder cancer diagnosed in 1979-81 and 771 general population controls matched for age and sex (Jensen *et al.*, 1987). All analyses were adjusted for age and sex. A RR of 1.7 was observed for ever having worked in the textile and leather industry (95% CI, 1.1-2.4; 56 exposed cases); however, there was only a weak association with duration of employment.

Claude *et al.* (1988) conducted a case-control study in northern Federal Republic of Germany which involved interviews with 531 male cases of cancer of the lower urinary tract occurring during the period 1977-85 and 531 age-matched, male hospital controls chosen primarily from urological wards. The matched RR for textile workers was 0.73 (95% CI, 0.29-1.8; eight exposed cases) and that for the textile industry, 1.7 (95% CI, 0.98-2.9; 35 exposed cases).

In a case-control study of bladder cancer in the county of Mataro, Spain, in 1978-81 (Gonzáles *et al.*, 1988), 19/57 cases and 21/107 controls reported past employment in the textile industry (OR, 2.2; 95% CI, 1.0-4.7). The case group included newly diagnosed and prevalent cases identified through a hospital registry and deceased cases identified through a death registry. Controls were selected from the same registries as the cases, matched on sex, age, residence and date of hospitalization or death. For each case, one control was chosen with cancer other than of the bladder or lung, and one with a non-neoplastic disease. The OR decreased slightly to 2.1 (95% CI, 0.82-5.1) when the analysis was adjusted for tobacco smoking. The risk was particularly elevated for textile workers who worked in dyeing or printing (OR, 4.4; 95% CI, 1.2-16.8). The risk for weaving was 1.9 (0.71-5.0) and that for spinning, 0.33 (0.06-1.9).

Gonzáles *et al.* (1989) performed a further study involving interviews with 497 prevalent and newly diagnosed cases of bladder cancer in five provinces of Spain in 1985-86, 583 hospital controls and 530 population controls matched by age, sex and residence. A matched analysis adjusted for smoking and other high-risk occupations gave ORs for textile work of 1.9 in men (95% CI, 1.1-3.1; 41 cases) and 6.4 in women (1.3-30.0; 11 cases). The mean latent period since time of first employment to diagnosis of the cancer was 41 years. When analysed by conditional logistic regression, the highest risk was for the subgroup of weavers in both men (OR, 3.5; 1.3-9.3; ten cases) and women (OR, 21.2; 1.5-298; nine cases); the RR for textile dyers was 1.3 in men (0.5-3.1; 11 cases) and 0.34 in women (0.1-7.7; one case). [The Working Group noted that the numbers of cases on which the final analysis was based were not presented, and also noted the discrepancy between the crude (3.6, as computed by the Working Group) and logistic OR (21.2) for female weavers.]

The occupational factors possibly linked to the incidence of cancer of the bladder in the provinces of Alberta and southern Ontario (Canada) were investigated in a case-control study based on all urothelial and other primary malignant tumours of the bladder newly diagnosed in 1979-82 among male and female residents aged 35-79 years (Risch *et al.*, 1988). Controls were identified randomly from population listings and individually matched to cases by sex, age and residence; of the eligible cases and controls, 67% and 53% were interviewed, respectively, and, for the analysis, 781 matched case-control sets were available. For male cases who had been employed in 'dyeing of cloth' for at least six months eight to 28 years before diagnosis, a significant association was found (OR, 4.6; 95% CI, 1.1-31.6; adjusted for smoking). A significant trend with duration of employment was also noted. No increased risk was associated with exposure to cotton dust, wool dust or dye.

[The Working Group noted that data on smoking habits were not available in most of the studies of bladder cancer in textile workers, but, when data were available, adjustment for cigarette smoking made little difference to the findings.]

*(i)   Haematopoietic malignancies*

In the study of death certificates of white women in the USA by Delzell and Grufferman (1983; see p. 238), the ratio of observed:expected deaths was significantly increased for non-Hodgkin's lymphoma (1.7; 95% CI, 1.2-2.3; 51 deaths). A suggestive increase (1.2; 0.8-1.6; 45 deaths) in the number of leukaemia deaths was also noted. Information on type of textile manufacturing or on specific jobs and duration of employment was not available.

Dubrow and Gute (1988; see p. 239) found PMRs of 104 (95% CI, 57-191; nine deaths) for Hodgkin's disease; 92 (65-129; 28 deaths) for non-Hodgkin's lymphoma; and 73 (53-100; 31 deaths) for leukaemia among male textile workers in Rhode Island (USA).

In the proportionate mortality study of O'Brien and Decouflé (1988; see p. 239) among male carpet and textile workers in Georgia (USA), ten deaths from lymphocytic leukaemia were observed, where 3.4 would have been expected (PMR, 290; 95% CI, 140-540). For non-Hodgkin's lymphoma, six deaths were seen (PMR, 70; 30-160); for Hodgkin's disease and multiple myeloma, three deaths each (expected, 2.9 and 4.1, respectively); and for all leukaemia, 19 deaths (PMR, 150; 90-240).

In the cancer registration study of Olsen and Jensen (1987; see p. 239) in Denmark, the risk for Hodgkin's disease was elevated in men in both textile manufacturing (214; 95% CI, 96-476; six cases) and spinning, weaving and finishing (312; 117-831; four cases); there were only two cases (39; 10-155) among women in textile manufacture and none among those in spinning, weaving and finishing. Other figures for men in the two occupational categories were: for non-Hodgkin's lymphoma, six cases (87; 40-198) and four cases (124; 47-330); for acute leukaemia, four cases (129; 48-344) and two cases (134; 34-536); for other leukaemia, three cases (51; 16-158) and three cases (99; 32-307); and for other haematopoietic cancers, 14 cases (126; 75-213) and four cases (72; 27-192).

Coggon *et al.* (1986b), in their case-control study of men in three English counties (see p. 241), found RRs of 0.8 (three cases) and 1.2 (one case) for Hodgkin's disease and 1.4 (five cases) and 3.0 (two cases) for non-Hodgkin's lymphoma for working in the textile industry and among textile workers, respectively.

Schumacher and Delzell (1988) performed a death certificate-based case-control study to investigate associations between occupation and non-Hodgkin's lymphoma in men aged 35-75 in North Carolina (USA), focusing mainly on farming and the textile manufacturing industry. The 501 cases were in men who had been residents of the state and whose death certificates mentioned non-Hodgkin's lymphoma. Controls were selected from all non-neoplastic deaths among male residents of North Carolina in the same periods, and were frequency matched to cases on year of death, age and race. A total of 569 controls were selected. The usual occupation and industry, as listed on the death certificate, was coded by a person who was unaware of the subjects' status as a case or a control. The RR for non-Hodgkin's lymphoma among white males employed in the textile industry (59 cases and 68 controls) was 0.81 (90% CI, 0.59-1.1) and that for black textile workers (six cases and five controls) was 2.4 (90% CI, 0.88-6.6). The specific occupation of 'dye workers' within the textile industry was listed for only one case and no control.

In the case-control study of Siemiatycki *et al.* (1986; see p. 241), the OR by logistic regression analysis for the association between 'substantial' exposure to cotton dust and non-Hodgkin's lymphoma was 1.9 (95% CI, 1.0-3.7; 11 cases) and that for 'substantial' exposure for more than years was 3.0 (1.3-7.2; seven exposed cases). When only textile processing workers with 'substantial' exposure to cotton dust were considered, the OR was 12.6 (4.7-33.3). Other workers exposed to cotton dust had no excess risk.

A case-control study in Yorkshire, UK, in 1979-84 involved interviews with 248 patients with Hodgkin's disease and 489 other hospital patients without current malignant disease, matched by health district, sex and age (Bernard et al., 1987). Thirty cases and 51 controls were textile workers [crude OR, 1.2; 95% CI, 0.73-1.9].

*(j) Other cancers*

Delzell and Grufferman (1983, see p. 238) observed eight deaths (PMR, 220; 95% CI, 100-500) from cancer of the *thyroid* among white female textile workers in North Carolina (USA). In the proportionate mortality study of O'Brien and Decouflé (1988, see p. 239) among male carpet and textile workers in Georgia (USA), a suggestive increase for cancer of the thyroid (two observed, 0.5 expected) was seen.

Versluys (1949; see p. 238) reported a PMR of 184 (21 cases) for cancer of the *liver* among male weavers and workers in woollens in the Netherlands. In a study of *biliary tract* cancer in Sweden, using the Swedish Cancer-Environment Registry (see p. 239), 23 of 1304 male cases of *gall-bladder cancer* (SIR, 150) and seven of 764 other biliary tract cancers (SIR, 60) had worked in the textile industry in 1960 (Malker et al., 1986b). There were 11 cases of gall-bladder cancer (SIR, 150) and four cases of other biliary tract cancers (SIR, 70) in spinners, weavers and knitters.

In the cancer registry study of Olsen and Jensen (1987; see p. 239), elevated risks were observed for cancer of the *pancreas* in men (SPIR, 168; 95% CI, 110-258; 21 cases) and women (123; 74-204; 15 cases) employed in textile manufacture and in men (170; 94–307; 11 cases) and women (145; 69-305; seven cases) in the industrial subcategory of spinning, weaving and finishing textiles. Bross et al. (1978; see p. 241), in their case-control study of admissions to the Roswell Park Memorial Institute (New York State, USA), reported a statistically significant elevated risk, larger than 2.0, for cancer of the pancreas among male operatives in textile mills; and, in the case-control study of Magnani et al. (1987; see p. 241) in three English counties, occupation in the textile industry resulted in an OR for men of 1.6 (95% CI, 0.3-8.2) for pancreatic cancer.

Delzell and Grufferman (1983; see p. 238) found significantly increased PMRs for cancer of the *cervix* (210; 95% CI, 160-280; 59 observed) and for unspecified genital cancer (270; 150-470; 16 observed) in white female textile workers in North Carolina (USA). In the cancer registry study of Olsen and Jensen (1987; see p. 239), the SPIRs for cancer of the cervix uteri were 132 (95% CI, 107-163; 86 cases) for textile manufacture and 136 (96-193; 31 cases) for spinning, weaving and finishing. However, in the UK Registrar General's 1981 decennial supplement (see p. 238), there was little evidence of an increased risk for cancer of the cervix.

O'Brien and Decouflé (1988; see p. 239) observed five deaths from *testicular* cancer among carpet and textile workers in Georgia (USA), whereas 1.8 were expected (PMR, 270; 95% CI, 90-630); all occurred in young men, who had probably spent relatively little time in the industry.

Bross et al. (1978; see p. 241) reported a nonsignificantly elevated risk (larger than 2.0) for cancer of the *prostate* among operatives in textile mills. In the study of Hoar and Blair (1984; see p. 246), 1037 pairs of cases and matched controls were available for the study on prostatic cancer. An increased risk for prostatic cancer of borderline statistical significance was found for black workers under 65 years of age at death (OR, 2.5; 95% CI, 1.0-6.4; 15 cases). Among white males, increased risks for prostatic cancer were found in two subcategories of the textile industry: broad-woven fabric mills (OR, 4.0; 0.5-35.8) and dyeing and finishing occupations (OR, 2.0; 0.5-8.0). Siemiatycki et al. (1986; see p. 241) reported ORs for prostatic cancer of 1.0 (95% CI, 0.6-1.8; 16 cases) for working with cotton, 0.9 (0.4-1.8; nine cases) for working with wool and 0.7 (0.3-1.7; seven cases) for working with synthetic fibres, among male textile workers in Montréal, Québec, Canada.

Olsen and Jensen (1987; see p. 239) observed an increased risk for *melanoma* of the skin among cases of cancer registered for men involved in textile manufacture (SPIR, 189; 95% CI, 107-333; 12 cases) and spinning, weaving and finishing (224; 101-499; six cases), but not in women (98; 62-156; 18 cases; and 101; 45-225; six cases, respectively). In the 1981 decennial supplement of the UK Registrar General (see p. 238), there was little evidence of an increased risk for either melanoma or cancer of the *connective tissue*. Delzell and Grufferman (1983, see p. 238) found a significantly increased PMR for cancer of connective tissue (260; 95% CI, 130-520; ten observed cases) among white female textile workers in North Carolina (USA).

A case-control study in Copenhagen and Sjaelland island (Denmark) involved interviews in 1979-82 with 96 male and female patients less than 80 years old with cancer of the *renal pelvis and ureter* and with 288 controls selected from admissions to the same hospital for diseases other than of the urinary tract or other smoking-related diseases (Jensen et al., 1988). Controls were matched for age and sex, and analyses were adjusted for age, sex and lifetime tobacco consumption. The case group included eight textile workers (OR, 0.9; 95% CI, 0.4-2.4).

Siemiatycki et al. (1986; see p. 241) reported ORs for cancer of the *kidney* of 1.1 (95% CI, 0.5-2.7; seven cases) for working with cotton, 1.0 (0.3-3.0; five cases) for working with wool and 0.8 (0.2-2.8; four cases) for working with synthetic fibres among male textile workers in Montréal, PQ (Canada).

The Swedish Cancer-Environment Registry (see p. 239) was used to estimate age-standardized incidence ratios for *intracranial gliomas* (McLaughlin et al., 1987). Of the 3394 intracranial gliomas in men, 35 were in textile workers (SIR, 90; adjusted for age and region). A total of 1035 intracranial gliomas were seen in women, but the findings for textile workers were not reported; a SIR of 230 (15 cases) was found for female wool workers.

Van Steensel-Moll et al. (1985) conducted a case-control study in the Netherlands of 519 *children* under the age of 15 years with acute lymphocytic leukaemia diagnosed in 1973-80 and 507 controls matched for age, sex and municipality. Questionnaires were mailed to the children's parents. All analyses were adjusted for age and sex. Birth order and social class were not found to be confounders. Eight case mothers and two control mothers had worked in the textile industry during pregnancy (OR, 4.2; 95% CI, 1.0-17.7).

## 4. Summary of Data Reported and Evaluation

### 4.1 Exposure data

The textile manufacturing industry employs over ten million workers throughout the world. The industry includes the spinning, weaving, knitting, dyeing and finishing of numerous types of natural and synthetic fibres. The products include fabrics, yarns and carpets.

Textile workers are exposed to textile-related dusts throughout the manufacturing process. During spinning, weaving and knitting operations, exposure to chemicals is generally limited.

In dyeing and printing operations, workers are frequently exposed to dyes (including those based on benzidine as well as a variety of acids and bases), optical brighteners, organic solvents and fixatives. Workers in finishing operations are frequently exposed to crease-resistance agents (many of which release formaldehyde), flame retardants (including organophosphorus and organobromine compounds) and antimicrobial agents. In the dyeing, printing and finishing processes, workers typically have multiple exposures, which can vary with time and process.

### 4.2 Experimental carcinogenicity data

No data were available to the Working Group.

### 4.3 Human carcinogenicity data

*Oral and pharyngeal cancers*

Five studies of mortality and morbidity statistics did not indicate an increased risk for cancers at these sites. In the USA, a hospital-based case–control study showed an association between cancer of the buccal cavity and pharynx and textile work for both men and women working in textile mills. Of four case–control studies conducted in the UK, one had no case of oral cancer in textile workers, another showed an elevated risk for oral and pharyngeal cancers particularly among male fibre preparers, the third demonstrated an increased risk among female textile workers employed in spinning and weaving, and the fourth showed a small increase in risk in textile workers. A case–control study in the USA showed no increase, but a further study suggested a slightly increased risk for women potentially exposed to dust in the textile industry.

*Cancers of the oesophagus and stomach*

Ten studies based on mortality or incidence statistics in four countries were available to the Working Group. Seven of them showed an increased risk for stomach cancer among textile workers, and another showed an increase only among women in textile manufacturing. Oesophageal cancer risk was found to be elevated in three of these studies, and, in one of these, the increase was significant among a group of workers engaged as operatives in dyeing and finishing. In none of these studies was socioeconomic status taken into consideration. Two cohort studies, one in the USA and one in the UK, found moderate increases in mortality from cancer of the 'digestive system', without further specification. A case–control study in the USA showed an increased risk for stomach and oesophageal cancer. A Canadian case–control study did not show an increased risk for stomach cancer associated with exposure to cotton, wool or synthetic fibre dusts. Two case–control studies were conducted in the UK; one showed an increased risk for cancer of the stomach but not of the oesophagus, and the other showed an increase for oesophageal cancer.

*Colorectal cancer*

Of six large studies based on routinely collected cancer incidence or mortality data, two showed an elevated risk for colorectal cancer among textile workers; one showed an elevated risk for rectal cancer and a decreased risk for cancer of the colon. The incidence of cancers of the large bowel was reported to be increased in sequential case–control studies on workers in the synthetic fibres unit of a carpet factory in Canada. In another case–control study in Canada, the incidence of colorectal cancer was found to be significantly associated with exposure to synthetic fibre dust; the study took possible confounders into consideration. In two case–control studies, one in the UK and one in the USA, increased risks for cancers of the colon and rectum were observed, respectively, but there were few cases. A further case–control study in the USA showed an increased risk for colorectal cancer in men and a decreased risk in women; however, a large case–control study in the USA showed no evidence of an association between cancer of the colon and work in the textile industry.

*Nasal cancer*

Five studies based on mortality and morbidity statistics consistently showed increased risks for nasal cancer in textile workers, one in women only. In the USA, a hospital-based case–control study showed a significantly elevated risk in men employed as operatives in textile mills. In another study in the USA, an increased risk was noted among female textile and garment workers, predominantly in those first employed fewer than 20 years before diagnosis; an elevated risk for adenocarcinoma of the nasal cavity was noted among men and women in dusty operations. A significantly elevated risk related to duration of employment was found for textile workers in Hong Kong, particularly among weavers. Another study in the USA did not show an increased risk among men employed in formaldehyde-associated textile work.

*Laryngeal cancer*

Three mortality studies and one study of national mortality statistics in the UK revealed no association between textile work and laryngeal cancer. One US and one UK mortality study suggested a borderline positive association between textile work and laryngeal cancer; one Danish record-linkage study suggested a positive association only for women. Four case–control studies reported positive associations; and two further case–control studies showed positive associations between textile processing and exposures to textile dust and laryngeal cancer when controlling for alcohol and tobacco use.

*Lung cancer*

Four studies based on national mortality statistics in the UK found decreased risks for lung cancer among male textile workers; one of the studies showed a decreased risk among women and one showed an increased risk. Of seven further studies based on routinely collected cancer mortality or incidence statistics, five showed a decreased risk for lung cancer in textile workers and one an increased risk. Two cohort studies in the USA revealed a decreased risk for lung cancer among textile workers; in one, the decreased risk was associated with increased presumed exposure to cotton dust. One cohort study in the UK showed no increased risk. Of four case–control studies in the USA, two showed relative risks greater than 2.0, one showed a smaller increase in risk and one showed a decreased risk for lung cancer in textile workers. A case–control study in Canada showed a moderately decreased risk for lung cancer in textile workers, particularly among those working with wool or synthetic fibres. Two case–control studies in Italy showed an elevated risk for lung cancer in textile workers. A case–control study in China also showed a decreased risk for lung cancer in cotton textile workers.

*Bladder cancer*

Of three studies based on national mortality statistics in the UK, two showed an increased risk for bladder cancer among textile workers. Of six other studies based on routinely collected mortality or incidence statistics, two reported increased risks among textile workers and one showed an increased risk only for women. Two cohort studies, one in the USA and one in the UK, showed moderately increased risks.

Of a total of 19 case–control studies in which bladder cancer in textile workers was investigated, 14 showed elevated risks. These include five studies in which the risk for dyers was examined (two in the UK, one in Canada and two in Spain), all of which reported elevated risks. In the Canadian study, there was a nearly five-fold increase in risk in workers who had been employed for at least six months during the period eight to 28 years before diagnosis, and there was a trend with duration of exposure.

Four studies also addressed risks in weavers (the two Spanish studies, a study in the UK and a study in Italy), and all reported an elevation of risk of approximately two fold or more.

The findings of the 13 case–control studies that did not specifically address risks in dyers or weavers (five in the USA, one each in the UK, Canada, Denmark, Finland, the Federal Republic of Germany, Italy and Spain, and a collaborative study in the USA, UK and Japan) are less consistent: eight reported elevated risks and five reported decreased risks among textile workers.

Data on smoking habits were not available in most of the studies on textile workers. When they were available, adjustment for cigarette smoking made little difference to the findings.

### Haematopoietic malignancies

One mortality study of white female textile workers in the USA showed a positive association between work in manufacturing textile mill products and non-Hodgkin's lymphoma. Two further US mortality studies of textile and of textile and carpet manufacturers reported no increase in risk. A Danish record-linkage morbidity study gave no evidence of an increased risk for this cancer among men or women in textile manufacturing. A case-control study in the UK showed a moderately increased risk, on the basis of a few cases, and a case-control study in the USA showed no significant association between non-Hodgkin's lymphoma and employment in the textile industry. A Canadian case-control study showed a positive association between non-Hodgkin's lymphoma and 'substantial' exposure to cotton dust, which became stronger when analysis was limited to textile processing workers exposed to cotton dust.

A Danish record-linkage morbidity study based on a small number of cases reported a borderline positive association for Hodgkin's disease among men engaged in spinning, weaving and finishing. Two US mortality studies and two UK case-control studies found a nonsignificant association between textile work and Hodgkin's disease. One mortality study reported a significant positive association between leukaemia and textile work.

### Other cancers

Two mortality studies reported a borderline positive association between *thyroid* cancer and work in the textile industry.

One mortality study reported an elevated but nonsignificant association between cancer of the *liver* and working with textiles. A similar association was reported for cancer of the *gall-bladder* in another mortality study.

In one record-linkage morbidity study and in one case-control study, the risk for cancer of the *pancreas* was elevated in men working in the textile industry; in a further case-control study, the risk was increased, but not significantly so.

A mortality study and a record-linkage morbidity study reported a significant association between *cervical cancer* and textile work, while examination of mortality statistics gave little evidence of such an association. These studies were not controlled for social class.

A single mortality study found an increase in the number of deaths from *testicular cancer* among carpet and textile workers.

One case-control study showed a borderline increase in risk for *prostatic cancer* among black but not white textile workers; for white workers, increased risk was seen in two subcategories of the industry. One further case-control study showed no significant association between prostatic cancer and work in the textile industry; another showed a nonsignificantly elevated risk.

A single record-linkage morbidity study reported an increased risk of borderline significance for *melanoma* among male, but not female, textile workers.

One mortality study in the USA showed a significantly increased risk for cancer of *connective tissue* among white female textile workers. A study based on national statistics in the UK showed no increase in risk for cancer at this site.

One case–control study showed no association between cancer of the *renal pelvis and ureter* and work in the textile industry; another case control study showed no association between cancer of the *kidney* and work in the textile industry.

A single cancer registry study showed a significant association between the incidence of *intracranial gliomas* in women and employment in the wool industry.

One Dutch case–control study of lymphocytic leukaemia showed a risk of borderline significance among *children* whose mothers had been employed in the textile industry during pregnancy.

### 4.4 Other relevant data

A study of spontaneous abortions in Finland showed a moderately increased risk among mothers employed as spinners, fabric inspectors and weavers. A study in Canada gave no evidence of an increased risk of prematurity or low birth weight in babies of women employed in the textile industry. An analysis of birth records in the USA found an increased risk for fetal death among offspring of women employed in the textile industry.

### 4.5 Evaluation[1]

There is *limited evidence* that working in the textile manufacturing industry entails a carcinogenic risk.

This evaluation is based mainly on findings of bladder cancer among dyers (possibly due to exposure to dyes) and among weavers (possibly due to exposure to dusts from fibres and yarns) and of cancer of the nasal cavity among weavers (possibly due to exposure to dusts from fibres and yarns) and among other textile workers.

Working in the textile manufacturing industry entails exposures that are *possibly carcinogenic to humans (Group 2B)*.

# 5. References

Acheson, E.D., Cowdell, R.H. & Rang, E. (1972) Adenocarcinoma of the nasal cavity and sinuses in England and Wales. *Br. J. ind. Med.*, 29, 21–30

Acheson, E.D., Cowdell, R.H. & Rang, E. (1981) Nasal cancer in England and Wales: an occupational survey. *Br. J. ind. Med.*, 38, 218–224

American Conference of Governmental Industrial Hygienists (1989) *TLVs, Threshold Limit Values and Biological Exposure Indices for 1988–1989*, Cincinnati, OH, p. 16

---

[1]This evaluation applies to exposures in the textile manufacturing industry that exclude the manufacture of asbestos textiles (IARC, 1977, 1987) and mule spinning with exposure to mineral oils (IARC, 1984, 1987). For description of the italicized terms and criteria for making the evaluation, see Preamble, pp. 25–29.

Anthony, H.M. & Thomas, G.M. (1970) Tumors of the urinary bladder: an analysis of the occupations of 1,030 patients in Leeds, England. *J. natl Cancer Inst.*, 45, 879–895

Antweiler, H. (1960) Observations about a histamine liberating substance in cotton dust. *Ann. occup. Hyg.*, 1, 152–156

Ashley, D.J.B. (1967) The distribution of lung cancer and bronchitis in England and Wales. *Br. J. Cancer*, 21, 243–259

Ashley, D.J.B. (1969) Environmental factors in the aetiology of lung cancer and bronchitis. *Br. J. prev. soc. Med.*, 23, 258–262

Bateman, E.G. (1978) *Toxic Material Handling in the Textile Drug Room*, MA Thesis, Chapel Hill, NC, University of North Carolina

Bernard, S.M., Cartwright, R.A., Darwin, C.M., Richards, I.D.G., Roberts, B., O'Brien, C.O. & Bird, C.C. (1987) Hodgkin's disease: case control epidemiological study in Yorkshire. *Br. J. Cancer*, 55, 85–90

Blair, A. & Fraumeni, J.F., Jr (1978) Geographic patterns of prostate cancer in the United States. *J. natl Cancer Inst.*, 61, 1379–1384

Blot, W.J. & Fraumeni, J.F., Jr (1977) Geographic patterns of oral cancer in the United States: etiologic implications. *J. chronic Dis.*, 30, 745–757

Bogle, M. (1977) *Textile Dyes, Finishes and Auxiliaries*, New York, Garland Publishing, pp. 125–128

Brinton, L.A., Blot, W.J., Stone, B.J. & Fraumeni, J.F., Jr (1977) A death certificate analysis of nasal cancer among furniture workers in North Carolina. *Cancer Res.*, 37, 3473–3474

Brinton, L.A., Blot, W.J., Becker, J.A., Winn, D.M., Browder, J.P., Farmer, J.C., Jr & Fraumeni, J.F., Jr (1984) A case–control study of cancer of the nasal cavity and paranasal sinuses. *Am. J. Epidemiol.*, 119, 896–906

Brinton, L.A., Blot, W.J. & Fraumeni, J.F., Jr (1985) Nasal cancer in the textile and clothing industries. *Br. J. ind. Med.*, 42, 469–474

Bross, I.D.J., Viadana, E. & Houten, L. (1978) Occupational cancer in men exposed to dust and other environmental hazards. *Arch. environ. Health*, 33, 300–307

Buck, M.G., Schachter, E.N., Fick, R.B., Merrill, W.W., Cooper, J.A.D., Jr, Keirns, J.J., Oliver, J. & Wall, J.H. (1986) Biologic activity of purified cotton bract extracts in man and guinea pig. *Environ. Health Perspect.*, 66, 37–44

Buiatti, E., Baccetti, S., Cecchi, F., Tomassini, A. & Dolara, P. (1979) Evidence of increased lung cancer rate among textile workers. *Med. Lav.*, 1, 21–23

Bukayev, P.T. (1984) *General Technology of Cotton Manufacturing*, Moscow, MIR Publishers

Burch, J.D., Howe, G.R., Miller, A.B. & Semenciw, R. (1981) Tobacco, alcohol, asbestos and nickel in the etiology of cancer of the larynx: a case–control study. *J. natl Cancer Inst.*, 67, 1219–1224

Cartwright, R. (1982) Occupational bladder cancer and cigarette smoking in West Yorkshire. *Scand. J. Work Environ. Health, Suppl.* 1, 79–82

Castellan, R.M., Olenchock, S.A., Hankinson, J.L., Millner, P.D., Cocke, J.B., Bragg, C.K., Perkins, H.H., Jr & Jacobs, R.R. (1984) Acute bronchoconstriction by cotton dust: dose-related responses to endotoxin and other dust factors. *Ann. intern. Med.*, 101, 157–163

Castellan, R.M., Olenchock, S.A., Kinsley, K.B. & Hankinson, J.L. (1987) Inhaled endotoxin and decreased spirometric values. An exposure–response relation for cotton dust. *New Engl. J. Med.*, 317, 605–610

Christiani, D.C., Eisen, E.A., Wegman, D.H., Ye, T.T., Lu, P.-L., Gong, Z.-C. & Dai, H.-L. (1986) Respiratory disease in cotton textile workers in the People's Republic of China. I. Respiratory symptoms. *Scand. J. Work Environ. Health*, 12, 40–45

Cinkotai, F.F. & Whitaker, C.J. (1978) Airborne bacteria and the prevalence of byssinotic symptoms in 21 cotton spinning mills in Lancashire. *Ann. occup. Hyg.*, 21, 239–250

Cinkotai, F.F., Sharpe, T.C. & Gibbs, A.C.C. (1984) Circadian rhythms in peak expiratory flow rate in workers exposed to cotton dust. *Thorax, 39*, 759–765

Clarke, E.A. & Anliker, R. (1980) Organic dyes and pigments. In: Hutzinger, O., ed., *The Handbook of Environmental Chemistry*, Vol. 3, Part A, *Anthropogenic Compounds*, Heidelberg, Springer, pp. 181–215

Claude, J.C., Frentzel-Beyme, R.R. & Kunze, E. (1988) Occupation and risk of cancer of the lower urinary tract among men: a case–control study. *Int. J. Cancer, 41*, 371–379

Coggon, D., Pannett, B., Osmond, C. & Acheson, E.D. (1986a) A survey of cancer and occupation in young and middle aged men. I. Cancers of the respiratory tract. *Br. J. ind. Med., 43*, 332–338

Coggon, D., Pannett, B., Osmond, C. & Acheson, E.D. (1986b) A survey of cancer and occupation in young and middle aged men. II. Non-respiratory cancers. *Br. J. ind. Med., 43*, 381–386

Commission of the European Communities (1988) *Industrial Production. Quarterly Statistics (Theme 4, Series B)*, Luxembourg, Eurostat, pp. 95–97

Cook, W.A., ed. (1987) *Occupational Exposure Limits – Worldwide*, Washington DC, American Industrial Hygiene Association

Corisco, C.G., Quesada, J.M.L., Albadalejo, D.T., González, J.J.M. & Rozas, F.G. (1987) Bladder urothelioma: epidemiological case–control study in the area of Madrid (Sp.). *Rev. clín. Esp., 180*, 352–356

Decouflé, P., Stanislawczyk, K., Houten, L., Bross, I.D.J. & Viadana, E. (1978) *A Retrospective Survey of Cancer in Relation to Occupation*, Cincinnati, OH, National Institute for Occupational Safety and Health

Delzell, E. & Grufferman, S. (1983) Cancer and other causes of death among female textile workers, 1976–78. *J. natl Cancer Inst., 71*, 735–740

De Rosa, E., Bartolucci, G.B., Brighenti, F., Toffolo, D. & Sigon, M. (1984) Vegetable dust pollution in the textile industry. Comparison between various sampling methods. *Ann. occup. Hyg., 28*, 341–346

Deutsche Forschungsgemeinschaft (German Research Society) (1988) *Maximale Arbeitsplatzkonzentrationen und Biologische Arbeitsstofftoleranzwerte 1988* (Maximal Concentrations at the Work Place and Biological Tolerance Values for Working Materials 1988) (*Report No. XXIV*), Weinheim, Verlagsgesellschaft, p. 20

Dubrow, R. & Gute, D.M. (1988) Cause-specific mortality among male textile workers in Rhode Island. *Am. J. ind. Med., 13*, 439–454

Ellakkani, M.A., Alarie, Y.C., Weyel, D.A., Mazumdar, S. & Karol, M.H. (1984) Pulmonary reactions to inhaled cotton dust: an animal model for byssinosis. *Toxicol. appl. Pharmacol., 74*, 267–284

Ellakkani, M.A., Alarie, Y.C., Weyel, D.A. & Karol, M.H. (1985) Concentration-dependent respiratory response of guinea pigs to a single exposure of cotton dust. *Toxicol. appl. Pharmacol., 80*, 357–366

Ellakkani, M.A., Alarie, Y.C., Weyel, D.A. & Karol, M.H. (1987) Chronic pulmonary effects in guinea pigs from prolonged inhalation of cotton dust. *Toxicol. appl. Pharmacol., 88*, 354–369

Enterline, P.E., Sykora, J.L., Keleti, G. & Lange, J.H. (1985) Endotoxins, cotton dust, and cancer. *Lancet, ii*, 934–935

Flanders, W.D., Cann, C.I., Rothman, K.J. & Fried, M.P. (1984) Work-related risk factors for laryngeal cancer. *Am. J. Epidemiol., 119*, 23–32

Gonzáles, C.A., Riboli, E. & Lopez-Abente, G. (1988) Bladder cancer among workers in the textile industry: results of a Spanish case–control study. *Am. J. ind. Med., 14*, 673–680

Gonzáles, C.A., López-Abente, G., Errezola, M., Escolar, A., Riboli, E., Izarzugaza, I. & Nebot, M. (1989) Occupation and bladder cancer in Spain. A multi-centre case–control study. *Int. J. Epidemiol., 18*, 569–577

Goodson, A.L., Jr (1984) Formaldehyde and the textile industry. *Text. Chem. Color.*, *16*, 15-18

Gupta, M.N. (1969) Review of byssinosis in India. *Med. Res.*, *57*, 1776-1789

Guralnick, L. (1963) *Mortality by Occupation and Cause of Death Among Men 20 to 64 Years of Age: United States, 1950 (Vital Statistics – Special Reports, Vol. 53, No. 3)*, Washington DC, US Department of Health, Education, and Welfare

Hammad, Y.Y., Dharmarajan, V. & Weill, H. (1981) Sampling of cotton dust for epidemiologic investigations. *Chest*, *79*, 108S-113S

Harrington, J.M., Blot, W.J., Hoover, R.N., Housworth, W.J., Heath, C.W., Jr & Fraumeni, J.F., Jr (1978) Lung cancer in coastal Georgia: a death certificate analysis of occupation: brief communication. *J. natl Cancer Inst.*, *60*, 295-298

Hatch, K.L. & Maibach, H.I. (1985) Textile fiber dermatitis. *Contact Dermatitis*, *12*, 1-11

Hatch, K.L. & Maibach, H.I. (1986) Textile chemical finish dermatitis. *Contact Dermatitis*, *14*, 1-13

Henderson, V. & Enterline, P.E. (1973) An unusual mortality experience in cotton textile workers. *J. occup. Med.*, *15*, 717-719

Hoar, S.K. & Blair, A. (1984) Death certificate case-control study of cancers of the prostate and colon and employment in the textile industry. *Arch. environ. Health*, *39*, 280-283

Hobson, J.L. (1974) *Towards a Healthy Working Environment*, London, Health and Safety Executive

Hurwitz, M.D. (1987) The evolution of permanent press. *Text. Chem. Color.*, *19*, 13-23

IARC (1974) *IARC Monographs on the Evaluation of Carcinogenic Risk of chemicals to Man*, Vol. 4, *Some Aromatic Amines, Hydrazine and Related Substances, N-Nitroso Compounds and Miscellaneous Alkylating Agents*, Lyon, pp. 57-64

IARC (1977) *IARC Monographs on the Evaluation of Carcinogenic Risk of Chemicals to Man*, Vol. 14, *Asbestos*, Lyon

IARC (1979a) *IARC Monographs on the Evaluation of the Carcinogenic Risk of chemicals to Humans*, Vol. 20, *Some Halogenated Hydrocarbons*, Lyon, pp. 575-588

IARC (1979b) *IARC Monographs on the Evaluation of the Carcinogenic Risk of Chemicals to Humans*, Vol. 20, *Some Halogenated Hydrocarbons*, Lyon, pp. 545-572

IARC (1979c) *IARC Monographs on the Evaluation of the Carcinogenic Risk of Chemicals to Humans*, Vol. 20, *Some Halogenated Hydrocarbons*, Lyon, pp. 491-514

IARC (1982) *IARC Monographs on the Evaluation of the Carcinogenic Risk of Chemicals to Humans*, Vol. 29, *Some Industrial Chemicals and Dyestuffs*, Lyon, pp. 345-389

IARC (1984) *IARC Monographs on the Evaluation of the Carcinogenic Risk of chemicals to Humans*, Vol. 33, *Polynuclear Aromatic Compounds, Part 2, Carbon Blacks, Mineral Oils and Some Nitroarenes*, Lyon, pp. 87-168

IARC (1985) *IARC Monographs on the Evaluation of the Carcinogenic Risk of Chemicals to Humans*, Vol. 36, *Allyl Compounds, Aldehydes, Epoxides and Peroxides*, Lyon, pp. 285-314

IARC (1987a) *IARC Monographs on the Evaluation of Carcinogenic Risks to Humans*, Suppl. 7, *Overall Evaluations of Carcinogenicity: An Updating of* IARC Monographs *Volumes 1 to 42*, Lyon, pp. 125-126

IARC (1987b) *IARC Monographs on the Evaluation of Carcinogenic Risks to Humans*, Suppl. 7, *Overall Evaluations of Carcinogenicity: An Updating of* IARC Monographs *Volumes 1 to 42*, Lyon, pp. 211-216

IARC (1987c) *IARC Monographs on the Evaluation of Carcinogenic Risks to Humans*, Suppl. 7, *Overall Evaluations of Carcinogenicity: An Updating of* IARC Monographs *Volumes 1 to 42*, Lyon, pp. 123-125

IARC (1987d) *IARC Monographs on the Evaluation of Carcinogenic Risks to Humans*, Suppl. 7, *Overall Evaluations of Carcinogenicity: An Updating of* IARC Monographs *Volumes 1 to 42*, Lyon, pp. 364–366

IARC (1987e) *IARC Monographs on the Evaluation of Carcinogenic Risks to Humans*, Suppl. 7, *Overall Evaluations of Carcinogenicity: An Updating of* IARC Monographs *Volumes 1 to 42*, Lyon, pp. 355–357

International Labour Office (1988) *Yearbook of Labour Statistics, 1988*, Geneva

Jensen, O.M., Wahrendorf, J., Knudsen, J.B. & Sorensen, B.L. (1987) The Copenhagen case-referent study on bladder cancer. Risks among drivers, painters and certain other occupations. *Scand. J. Work Environ. Health*, 13, 129–134

Jensen, O.M., Knudsen, J.B., McLaughlin, J.K. & Sørensen, B.L. (1988) The Copenhagen case–control study of renal pelvis and ureter cancer: role of smoking and occupational exposures. *Int. J. Cancer*, 41, 557–561

Johnson, C.M., Hanson, M.N. & Rohrbach, M.S. (1986) Endothelial cell cytotoxicity of cotton bracts tannin and aqueous cotton bracts extract: tannin is the predominant cytotoxin present in aqueous cotton bracts extract. *Environ. Health Perspect.*, 66, 97–104

Jones, R.N., Diem, J.E., Glindmeyer, H., Dharmarajan, V., Hammad, Y.Y., Carr, J. & Weill, H. (1979) Mill effect and dose–response relationships in byssinosis. *Br. J. ind. Med.*, 36, 305–313

Keenlyside, R.A. & Elliott, L. (1981) *Health Hazard Evaluation Report. Rock Hill Printing and Finishing Company, Rock Hill, NC (Report No. HHE 80–192–828)*, Cincinnati, OH, National Institute for Occupational Safety and Health

Kennaway, N.M. & Kennaway, E.L. (1936) A study of the incidence of cancer of the lung and larynx. *J. Hyg.*, 36, 236–267

Kennedy, S.M., Christiani, D.C., Eisen, E.A., Wegman, D.H., Greaves, I.A., Olenchock, S.A., Ye, T.-T. & Lu, P.-L. (1987) Cotton dust and endotoxin exposure–response relationships in cotton textile workers. *Am. Rev. respir. Dis.*, 135, 194–200

Kieć-Świerczyńska, M. (1982) Occupational contact dermatitis in the workers employed in production of Texas textiles. *Dermatosen*, 30, 41–43

Krol, J.A. (1985) The global outlook on marketing and research. In: *Annual World Conference, World Textiles: Investment, Innovation, Invention, May 9–14, 1985* (Paper No. 18), Manchester, UK, The Textile Institute

Kutz, S.A., Mentnech, M.S., Mull, J.C., Olenchock, S.A. & Major, P.C. (1980) Acute experimental pulmonary responses to cardroom cotton dust. *Environ. environ. Health*, 35, 205–210

Levin, L.I., Goa, Y.-T., Blot, W.J., Zheng, W. & Fraumeni, J.F., Jr (1987) Decreased risk of lung cancer in the cotton textile industry of Shanghai. *Cancer Res.*, 47, 5777–5781

Levin, L.I., Zheng, W., Blot, W.J., Gao, Y.-T. & Fraumeni, J.F., Jr (1988) Occupation and lung cancer in Shanghai: a case–control study. *Br. J. ind. Med.*, 45, 450–458

Lindbohm, M.-L., Hemminki, K. & Kyyrönen, P. (1984) Parental occupational exposure and spontaneous abortions in Finland. *Am. J. Epidemiol.*, 120, 370–378

Logan, W.P.D., ed. (1982) *Cancer Mortality by Occupation and Social Class* (IARC Scientific Publications No. 36), Lyon, IARC

Love, R.G., Smith, T.A., Gurr, D., Sovtan, C.A., Scarisbrick, D.A. & Seaton, A. (1988) Respiratory and allergic symptoms in wool textile workers. *Br. J. ind. Med.*, 45, 727–741

Maffi, L. & Vineis, P. (1986) Occupation and bladder cancer in females. *Med. Lav.*, 77, 511–514

Magnani, C., Coggon, D., Osmond, C. & Acheson, E.D. (1987) Occupation and five cancers: a case–control study using death certificates. *Br. J. ind. Med.*, 44, 769–776

Makushkina, V.K. (1983) Clinico-morphological changes in the skin of female workers of textile industry processing flax (Russ.). *Vestn. Dermatol. Venerol.*, 59, 57–60

Malker, H.S.R., McLaughlin, J.K., Blot, W.J., Weiner, J.A., Malker, B.K., Ericsson, J.L.E. & Stone, B.J. (1986a) Nasal cancer and occupation in Sweden, 1961-1979. *Am. J. ind. Med.*, 9, 477-485

Malker, H.S.R., McLaughlin, J.K., Malker, B.K., Stone, B.J., Weiner, J.A., Ericsson, J.L.E. & Blot, W.J. (1986b) Biliary tract cancer and occupation in Sweden. *Br. J. ind. Med.*, 43, 257-262

Malker, H.S.R., McLaughlin, J.K., Silverman, D.T., Ericsson, J.L.E., Stone, B.J., Weiner, J.A., Malker, B.K. & Blot, W.J. (1987) Occupational risks for bladder cancer among men in Sweden. *Cancer Res.*, 47, 6763-6766

Malmberg, P. (1985) *Bomullsdamm. Kriterieredokument för Gränsvärden* (Cotton Dust. Criteria Document for Limit Values) (*Arbete och Hälsa 1985:30*), Stockholm, Arbetarskyddsverket

Marsh, J.T. (1962) *Self-smoothing Fabrics*, London, Chapman and Hall, p. 64

Marvin, J.H. (1973) *Textile Processing*, Vol. I, Columbia, SC, State Department of Education

Mathur, N.K., Mathur, A. & Banerjee, K. (1985) Contact dermatitis in tie and dye industry workers. *Contact Dermatitis*, 12, 38-41

McDonald, A.D., McDonald, J.C., Armstrong, B., Cherry, N.M., Nolin, A.D. & Robert, D. (1988) Prematurity and work in pregnancy. *Br. J. ind. Med.*, 45, 56-62

McLaughlin, J.K., Malker, H.S.R., Blot, W.J., Malker, B.K., Stone, B.J., Weiner, J.A., Ericsson, J.L.E. & Fraumeni, J.F., Jr (1987) Occupational risks for intracranial gliomas in Sweden. *J. natl Cancer Inst.*, 78, 253-257

Meal, P.F., Cocker, J., Wilson, H.K. & Gilmour, J.M. (1981) Search for benzidine and its metabolites in urine of workers weighing benzidine-derived dyes. *Br. J. ind. Med.*, 38, 191-193

Menck, H.R. & Henderson, B.E. (1976) Occupational differences in rates of lung cancer. *J. occup. Med.*, 18, 797-801

Merchant, J.A. & Ortmeyer, C. (1981) Mortality of employees of two cotton mills in North Carolina. *Chest*, 79 (*Suppl.*), 6S-11S

Milne, K.L., Sandler, D.P., Everson, R.B. & Brown, S.M. (1983) Lung cancer and occupation in Alameda County: a death certificate case-control study. *Am. J. ind. Med.*, 4, 565-575

Morrison, A.S., Ahlbom, A., Verhoek, W.G., Aoki, K., Leck, I., Ohno, Y. & Obata, K. (1985) Occupation and bladder cancer in Boston, USA, Manchester, UK, and Nagoya, Japan. *J. Epidemiol. Community Health*, 39, 294-300

Moss, E. (1976) Oral and pharyngeal cancer in textile workers. *Ann. N.Y. Acad. Sci.*, 271, 301-307

Moss, E. & Lee, W.R. (1974) Occurrence of oral and pharyngeal cancers in textile workers. *Br. J. ind. Med.*, 31, 224-232

Munn, A. & Smagghe, G. (1983) Dyes and dyestuffs. In: Parmeggiani, L., ed., *ILO Encyclopaedia of Occupational Safety and Health*, 3rd ed., Vol. I, Geneva, International Labour Office, pp. 699-701

Najem, G.R., Louria, D.B., Seebode, J.J., Thind, I.S., Prusakowski, J.M., Ambrose, R.B. & Fernicola, A.R. (1982) Life time occupation, smoking, caffeine, saccharine, hair dyes and bladder carcinogenesis. *Int. J. Epidemiol.*, 11, 212-217

National Cancer Institute (1985a) *Monographs on Human Exposure to Chemicals in the Workplace: Diphenyl*, Bethesda, MD

National Cancer Institute (1985b) *Monographs on Human Exposure to Chemicals in the Workplace: Tetrachloroethylene*, Bethesda, MD

National Institute for Occupational Safety and Health (1977) *National Occupational Hazard Survey, 1972-74*, Cincinnati, OH

National Institute for Occupational Safety and Health (1978) *Current Intelligence Bulletin 24. Direct Blue 6, Direct Black 38, Direct Brown 95* (*DHEW (NIOSH) Publ. No. 78-148*), Cincinnati, OH

National Institute for Occupational Safety and Health (1980) *NIOSH Technical Report: Carcinogenicity and Metabolism of Azo Dyes, Especially Those Derived from Benzidine*, Cincinnati, OH, US Department of Health and Human Services, pp. 1-5

National Institute for Occupational Safeth and Health (1981) *The Dyeing and Finishing of Textiles (Report No. 3)*, Vol. 1, Cincinnati, OH

National Institute for Occupational Safety and Health (1988) NIOSH recommendations for occupational safety and health standards 1988. *Morb. Mort. Wkly Rep.*, 37 (S.7), 1-29

Neefus, J.D., Lumsden, J.C. & Jones, M.T. Jr (1977) Cotton dust sampling. II. Vertical elutriation. *Am. ind. Hyg. Assoc. J.*, 38, 394-400

Newhouse, M.L. (1978) Mortality study of bleachers and dyers. *Ann. occup. Hyg.*, 21, 293-296

Ng, T.P. (1986) A case-referent study of cancer of the nasal cavity and sinuses in Hong Kong. *Int. J. Epidemiol.*, 15, 171-175

Niyogi, A.K. (1983) Dyeing industry. In: Parmeggiani, L., ed., *ILO Encyclopaedia of Occupational Safety and Health*, 3rd ed., Vol. I, Geneva, International Labour Office, pp. 697-699

Nousiainen, P. (1988) *Chemical Flame Retardation Mechanisms of Viscose-Polyester Fabrics (VTT Publications 45)*, Espoo, Technical Research Centre of Finland, pp. 9-10

Nousiainen, P. & Sundquist, J. (1979) *Kemialliset Haittatekijät Tekstiiliteo Llisuudessa Työilman Epäpuhtandet* (Harmful Chemicals in the Textile Industry. Impurities in Workplace Air) (*Information Bull. 16*), Tampere, State Technical Research Centre

Noweir, M.H. (1975) Epidemiologic studies in cotton and flax industries. In: Ayer, H., ed., *Cotton Dust, Proceedings of a Topical Symposium*, Cincinnati, OH, American Conference of Governmental Industrial Hygienists

O'Brien, T.R. & Decouflé, P. (1988) Cancer mortality among northern Georgia carpet and textile workers. *Am. J. ind. Med.*, 14, 15-24

Office of Population Censuses and Surveys (1958) *Occupational Mortality. The Registrar-General's Decennial Supplement 1951*, London, Her Majesty's Stationery Office

Office of Population Censuses and Surveys (1971) *Occupational Mortality. The Registrar-General's Decennial Supplement 1961*, London, Her Majesty's Stationery Office

Office of Population Censuses and Surveys (1978) *Occupational Mortality. The Registrar-General's Decennial Supplement 1970-72*, London, Her Majesty's Stationery Office

Office of Population Censuses and Surveys (1986) *Occupational Mortality. The Registrar-General's Decennial Supplement 1979-80, 1982-83*, London, Her Majesty's Stationery Office

Ohi, G. & Wegman, D.H. (1978) Transcutaneous ethylene glycol monomethyl ether poisoning in the work setting. *J. occup. Med.*, 20, 675-676

Olenchock, S.A., Mull, J.C. & Jones, W.G. (1983) Endotoxins in cotton: washing effects and size distribution. *Am. J. ind. Med.*, 4, 515-521

Olsen, J.H. (1988) Occupational risks of sinonasal cancer in Denmark. *Br. J. ind. Med.*, 45, 329-335

Olsen, J.H. & Jensen, O.M. (1987) Occupation and risk of cancer in Denmark. An analysis of 93 810 cancer cases, 1970-1979. *Scand. J. Work Environ. Health*, 13 (Suppl. 1), 1-91

Olsen, J. & Sabroe, S. (1984) Occupational causes of laryngeal cancer. *J. Epidemiol. Community Health*, 38, 117-121

Ong, S.G., Lam, T.H., Wong, C.M., Ma, P.L., Lam, S.K. & O'Kelly, F.J. (1985) Byssinosis in Hong Kong. *Br. J. ind. Med.*, 42, 449-502

Özesmi, M., Aslan, H., Hillerdal, G., Rylander, R., Özesmi, C. & Baris, Y.I. (1987) Byssinosis in carpet weavers exposed to wool contaminated with endotoxins. *Br. J. ind. Med.*, 44, 479-483

Paci, E., Buiatti, E. & Geddes, M. (1987) A case-referent study of lung tumors in non-asbestos textile workers. *Am. J. ind. Med.*, 11, 267-273

Peters, R.H. (1975) *Textile Chemistry*, Vol. III, *The Physical Chemistry of Dyeing*, Amsterdam, Elsevier, p. 1

Priha, E., Vuorinen, R., Schimberg, R. & Ahonen, I. (1988) *Tekstiilien Viimeistysaineet* (Textile Finishing Agents) (*Series No. 65*), Helsinki, Institute of Occupational Health

Quinn, A.E. (1983) Textile industry. In: Parmeggiani, L., ed., *ILO Encyclopaedia of Occupational Safety and Health*, 3rd ed., Vol. I, Geneva, International Labour Office, pp. 2167-2169

Registrar General (1897) *Supplement to 55th Annual Report for England and Wales, 1891*, Part 2, London, Her Majesty's Stationery Office

Registrar General (1908) *Supplement to 65th Annual Report for England and Wales, 1901*, Part 2, London, His Majesty's Stationery Office

Registrar General (1923) *Supplement to 75th Annual Report for England and Wales, 1910-1912*, Part IV, London, His Majesty's Stationery Office

Registrar General (1927) *Decennial Supplement, England and Wales for 1921*, Part II, London, His Majesty's Stationery Office

Registrar General (1938) *Decennial Supplement, England and Wales for 1931*, Part IIa, London, His Majesty's Stationery Office

Reinhard, M. & Tronnier, H. (1970) Toxic skin lesions caused by dyeing synthetic fibres (Ger.). *Berufsdermatosen*, *18*, 220-227

Reisch, M.S. (1988) Better times ahead for US dye producers. *Chem. Eng. News*, 25 July, 7-14

Risch, H.A., Burch, J.D., Miller, A.B., Hill, G.B., Steele, R. & Howe, G.R. (1988) Occupational factors and the incidence of cancer of the bladder in Canada. *Br. J. ind. Med.*, *45*, 361-367

Roman, E., Beral, V. & Inskip, H. (1985) Occupational mortality among women in England and Wales. *Br. med. J.*, *291*, 194-196

Rosén, G., Bergström, B. & Ekholm, U. (1984) *Formaldehydexponering på Arbetsplaster i Sverige* (Formaldehyde Exposure in Workplaces in Sweden) (*Arbete och Hälsa 1984:50*), Stockholm, Arbetarskyddsverket

Roush, G.C., Walrath, J., Stayner, L.T., Kaplan, S.A., Flannery, J.T. & Blair, A. (1987) Nasopharyngeal cancer, sinonasal cancer and occupations related to formaldehyde: a case-control study. *J. natl Cancer Inst.*, *79*, 1221-1224

Rylander, R. (1987) The role of endotoxin for reactions after exposure to cotton dust. *Am. J. ind. Med.*, *12*, 687-697

Rylander, R. & Morey, P. (1982) Airborne endotoxin in industries processing vegetable fibers. *Am. ind. Hyg. Assoc. J.*, *43*, 811-812

Rylander, R. & Snella, M.-C. (1976) Acute inhalation toxicity of cotton plant dusts. *Br. J. ind. Med.*, *33*, 175-180

Rylander, R., Haglund, P. & Lundholm, M. (1985) Endotoxin in cotton dust and respiratory function decrement among cotton workers in an experimental cardroom. *Am. Rev. respir. Dis.*, *131*, 209-213

Rylander, R., Schilling, R.S.F., Pickering, C.A.C., Rooke, G.B., Dempsey, A.N. & Jacobs, R.R. (1987) Effects after acute and chronic exposure to cotton dust: the Manchester criteria. *Br. J. ind. Med.*, *44*, 577-579

Schilling, R. & Goodman, N. (1951) Cardiovascular disease in cotton workers. Part 1. *Br. J. ind. Med.*, *8*, 77-90

Schimberg, R.W. & Vuorinen, R. (1986) Exposure to dyes in the textile and clothing industries (Abstract). *Nord. Arbejdsmiljømøde*, *35*, 210-211

Schoenberg, J.B., Stemhagen, A., Mogielnicki, A.P., Altman, R., Abe, T. & Mason, T.J. (1984) Case-control study of bladder cancer in New Jersey. I. Occupational exposures in white males. *J. natl Cancer Inst.*, *72*, 973-981

Schumacher, M.C. & Delzell, E. (1988) A death-certificate case-control study of non-Hodgkin's lymphoma and occupation in men in North Carolina. *Am. J. ind. Med.*, *13*, 317-330

Siemiatycki, J., Richardson, L., Gérin, M., Goldberg, M., Dewar, R., Désy, M., Campbell, S. & Wacholder, S. (1986) Associations between several sites of cancer and nine organic dusts: results from an hypothesis-generating case-control study in Montreal, 1979-1983. *Am. J. Epidemiol.*, *123*, 235-249

Silverman, D.T., Hoover, R.N., Albert, S. & Graff, K.M. (1983) Occupation and cancer of the lower urinary tract in Detroit. *J. natl Cancer Inst.*, *70*, 237-245

Sokolova, E.M. (1972) The causes of occupational dermatoses in textile factories (Russ.). *Vestn. Dermatol. Venerol.*, *46*, 40-43

Takam, J. & Nemery, B. (1988) Byssinosis in a textile factory in Cameroun: a preliminary study. *Br. J. ind. Med.*, *45*, 803-809

Thomson, T.A., Edwards, J.H., Al-Zubaidy, T.S., Brown, R.C., Poole, A. & Nicholls, P.J. (1986) In vitro release of arachidonic acid and in vitro responses to respirable fractions of cotton dust. *Environ. Health Perspect.*, *66*, 87-90

Tola, S., Tenho, M., Korkala, M.-L. & Järvinen, E. (1980) Cancer of the urinary bladder in Finland. Association with occupation. *Int. Arch. occup. environ. Health*, *46*, 43-51

Travis, A.S. (1988) William Henry Perkin: a teenage chemist discovers how to make the first synthetic dye from coal tar. *Text. Chem. Color.*, *20*, 13-18

United Nations (1987) *Industrial Statistics Yearbook 1985*, Vol. II, New York, pp. 236-237

Vail, S.L. (1983) Finishing. In: Mark, H.F., Othmer, D.F., Overberger, T.G., Seaborg, G.T. & Grayson, M., eds, *Kirk-Othmer Encyclopedia of Chemical Technology*, Vol. 22, 3rd ed., New York, John Wiley & Sons, pp. 769-802

Valić, F. & Žuškin, E. (1971) Effects of hemp dust exposure on nonsmoking female textile workers. *Arch. environ. Health*, *23*, 359-364

Van Steensel-Moll, H.A., Valkenburg, H.A. & Van Zanen, G.E. (1985) Childhood leukemia and parental occupation. A register-based case-control study. *Am. J. Epidemiol.*, *121*, 216-224

Vaughan, T.L., Daling, J.R. & Starzyk, P.M. (1984) Fetal death and maternal occupation. An analysis of birth records in the State of Washington. *J. occup. Med.*, *26*, 676-678

Versluys, J.J. (1949) Cancer and occupation in the Netherlands. *Br. J. Cancer*, *3*, 161-185

Vineis, P. & Magnani, C. (1985) Occupation and bladder cancer in males: a case-control study. *Int. J. Cancer*, *35*, 599-606

Vobecky, J., Devroede, G., Lacaille, J. & Watier, A. (1978) An occupational group with a high risk of large bowel cancer. *Gastroenterology*, *75*, 221-223

Vobecky, J., Caro, J. & Devroede, G. (1983) A case-control study of risk factors for large bowel carcinoma. *Cancer*, *51*, 1958-1963

Vobecky, J., Devroede, G. & Caro, J. (1984) Risk of large-bowel cancer in synthetic fiber manufacture. *Cancer*, *54*, 2537-2542

Walker, R.F., Eidson, G. & Hatcher, J.D. (1975) Influence of cotton dust inhalation on free lung cells in rats and guinea pigs. *Lab. Invest.*, *33*, 28-32

Ward, E. (1984) *Formaldehyde. Interim Exposure Report*, Washington DC, US Environmental Protection Agency

Whitaker, C.J., Moss, E., Lee, W.R. & Cunliffe, S. (1979) Oral and pharyngeal cancer in the North-west and West Yorkshire regions of England, and occupation. *Br. J. ind. Med.*, *36*, 292-298

Williams, R.R., Stegens, N.L. & Goldsmith, J.R. (1977) Associations of cancer site and type with occupation and industry from the Third National Cancer Survey Interview. *J. natl Cancer Inst.*, *59*, 1147-1185

Winn, D.M., Blot, W.J., Shy, C.M., Pickle, L.W., Toledo, A. & Fraumeni, J.F., Jr (1981) Snuff dipping and oral cancer among women in the southern United States. *New Engl. J. Med.*, *304*, 745-749

Winn, D.M., Blot, W.J., Shy, C.M. & Fraumeni, J.F, Jr (1982) Occupation and oral cancer among women in the South. *Am. J. ind. Med.*, *3*, 161-167

Witek, T.J., Jr, Gundel, R.H., Wegner, C.D., Schachter, E.N. & Buck, M.G. (1988) Acute pulmonary response to cotton bract extract in monkeys: lung function and effects of mediator modifying compounds. *Lung*, *166*, 25-31

World Health Organization (1983) *Recommended Health-based Occupational Limits for Selected Vegetable Dusts (WHO tech. Rep. Ser. No. 684)*, Geneva

Wynder, E.L., Onerdonk, J. & Mantel, N. (1963) An epidemiological investigation of cancer of the bladder. *Cancer*, *16*, 1388-1407

Žuskin, E., Valić, F. & Bouhuys, A. (1976) Effect of wool dust on respiratory function. *Am. Rev. respir. Dis.*, *114*, 705-709

# GLOSSARY

Some of the terms used in the text, diagrams and tables are defined below; others are defined in the text (see, e.g., p. 221).

| | |
|---|---|
| Beaming | The primary operation in making a **warp**, in which fibre ends are wound onto a cylinder (**beam**) |
| Blowing | Process by which revolving beaters and exhaust fans remove motes and dust from compressed cotton |
| Carding | Process of cleaning, opening and paralleling fibres |
| Drawing | Operations by which a continuous strand of fibre (formed after **carding** or combing) is blended, levelled and reduced to **roving** |
| Drug room | Area of **dye house** where dyes are stored and weighed |
| Dye house | Dyeing department of a textile factory |
| Elutriator | Appliance for washing or sizing very fine powders in an upward current of water or air |
| Filling | (1) Used in Canada and the USA to denote **weft** yarns<br>(2) Size added to cloth |
| Finishing | Treatment (mainly chemical) to enhance properties of fabrics and textiles; usually includes impregnantion, drying and curing |
| Hackling | Process of combing beaten flax to parallel long fibres and to remove short fibres and impurities |
| Opening | Action of separating closely packed fibres from each other at an early stage in the processing of raw material into yarn |
| Picking | Removing extraneous matter (e.g., outstanding hairs or tufts) from the face of a fabric and delivering the thick sheet of fibres for further processing |
| Piecing | Finishing lengths of woollen fabric by subjecting them to pressure |
| Roving | A continuous strand of fibres drawn to a diameter suitable for **twisting** into yarn |

| | |
|---|---|
| **Slashing** | Coating **warp** yarn with size, drying it and rewinding it onto a weaver's **beam** |
| **Spooling** | Winding yarn onto a bobbin |
| **Stripper and grinder** | Person who sharpens the cutting edges in **carding** machines in revolving carborundum rollers then resets the machine |
| **Twisting** | Process carried out to improve yarn strength and uniformity; spiral disposition of a yarn, usually as a result of relative rotation of the extremities |
| **Warp** | Total number of yarns wound onto the weaver's **beam** to constitute the lengthwise threads in a piece of cloth |
| **Warping** | Arranging threads in long lengths parallel to one another preparatory to further processing |
| **Weft** | Threads across the width of a fabric |
| **Willow** | Old term for **willey** |
| **Willey** | A revolving machine of a conical or cylindrical shape armed internally with spikes for opening and cleaning wool, cotton and flax |
| **Winding** | Process in which yarn is transferred onto **spools** |

# SUMMARY OF FINAL EVALUATIONS

| Agent | Degree of evidence for carcinogenicity | | Overall evaluation |
|---|---|---|---|
| | Humans | Animals | |
| *Agents and groups of agents* | | | |
| Chlorendic acid | No data | Sufficient | Possibly carcinogenic (2B) |
| Decabromodiphenyl oxide | No data | Limited | Not classifiable (3) |
| Dimethyl hydrogen phosphite | No data | Limited | Not classifiable (3) |
| Tetrakis(hydroxymethyl) phosphonium salts | No data | Inadequate | Not classifiable (3) |
| Tris(2-chloroethyl) phosphate | No data | Inadequate | Not classifiable (3) |
| para-Chloro-ortho-toluidine and its strong acid salts | | | Probably carcinogenic (2A) |
|    para-Chloro-ortho-toluidine | Limited | | |
|    para-Chloro-ortho-toluidine hydrochloride | | Sufficient | |
| Disperse Blue 1 | No data | Sufficient | Possibly carcinogenic (2B) |
| Disperse Yellow 3 | No data | Limited | Not classifiable (3) |
| Vat Yellow 4 | No data | Limited | Not classifiable (3) |
| 5-Nitro-ortho-toluidine | No data | Limited | Not classifiable (3) |
| Nitrilotriacetic acid and its salts | No data | | Possibly carcinogenic (2B) |
|    Nitrilotriacetic acid and its sodium salts | | Sufficient | |
| *Mixtures* | | | |
| Chlorinated paraffins | No data | | |
|    Chlorinated paraffins of average carbon–chain length $C_{12}$ and average degree of chlorination approximately 60% | | | Possibly carcinogenic (2B) |
|    A commercial chlorinated paraffin product of average carbon–chain length $C_{12}$ and average degree of chlorination 60% | | Sufficient | |
|    A commercial chlorinated paraffin product of average carbon–chain length $C_{23}$ and average degree of chlorination 43% | | Limited | |
| *Exposure circumstances* | | | |
| Working in the textile manufacturing industry | Limited | | Exposures possibly carcinogenic (2B) |

# APPENDIX 1
# ACTIVITY PROFILES FOR GENETIC AND RELATED EFFECTS

*Methods*

The x-axis of the activity profile (Waters *et al.*, 1987, 1988) represents the bioassays in phylogenetic sequence by endpoint, and the values on the y-axis represent the logarithmically transformed lowest effective doses (LED) and highest ineffective doses (HID) tested. The term 'dose', as used in this report, does not take into consideration length of treatment or exposure and may therefore be considered synonymous with concentration. In practice, the concentrations used in all the in-vitro tests were converted to µg/ml, and those for in-vivo tests were expressed as mg/kg bw. Because dose units are plotted on a log scale, differences in molecular weights of compounds do not, in most cases, greatly influence comparisons of their activity profiles. Conventions for dose conversions are given below.

Profile-line height (the magnitude of each bar) is a function of the LED or HID, which is associated with the characteristics of each individual test system – such as population size, cell–cycle kinetics and metabolic competence. Thus, the detection limit of each test system is different, and, across a given activity profile, responses will vary substantially. No attempt is made to adjust or relate responses in one test system to those of another.

Line heights are derived as follows: for negative test results, the highest dose tested without appreciable toxicity is defined as the HID. If there was evidence of extreme toxicity, the next highest dose is used. A single dose tested with a negative result is considered to be equivalent to the HID. Similarly, for positive results, the LED is recorded. If the original data were analysed statistically by the author, the dose recorded is that at which the response was significant ($p < 0.05$). If the available data were not analysed statistically, the dose required to produce an effect is estimated as follows: when a dose–related positive response is observed with two or more doses, the lower of the doses is taken as the LED; a single dose resulting in a positive response is considered to be equivalent to the LED.

In order to accommodate both the wide range of doses encountered and positive and negative responses on a continuous scale, doses are transformed logarithmically, so that effective (LED) and ineffective (HID) doses are represented by positive and negative numbers, respectively. The response, or logarithmic dose unit ($LDU_{ij}$), for a given test system $i$ and chemical $j$ *is* represented by the expressions

$$LDU_{ij} = -\log_{10}(\text{dose}), \text{ for HID values; } LDU \leq 0$$

and (1)

$$LDU_{ij} = -\log_{10}(\text{dose} \times 10^{-5}), \text{ for LED values; } LDU \geq 0.$$

These simple relationships define a dose range of 0 to −5 logarithmic units for ineffective doses (1–100 000 μg/ml or mg/kg bw) and 0 to +8 logarithmic units for effective doses (100 000–0.001 μg/ml or mg/kg bw). A scale illustrating the LDU values is shown in Figure 1. Negative responses at doses less than 1 μg/ml (mg/kg bw) are set equal to 1. Effectively, an LED value ≥100 000 or an HID value ≤1 produces an LDU = 0; no quantitative information is gained from such extreme values. The dotted lines at the levels of log dose units 1 and −1 define a 'zone of uncertainty' in which positive results are reported at such high doses (between 10 000 and 100 000 μg/ml or mg/kg bw) or negative results are reported at such low dose levels (1 to 10 μg/ml or mg/kg bw) as to call into question the adequacy of the test.

**Fig. 1. Scale of log dose units used on the y-axis of activity profiles**

| Positive (μg/ml or mg/kg bw) | | Log dose units | |
|---|---|---|---|
| 0.001 | ............................................. | 8 | ---- |
| 0.01 | ............................................. | 7 | -- |
| 0.1 | ............................................. | 6 | -- |
| 1.0 | ............................................. | 5 | -- |
| 10 | ............................................. | 4 | -- |
| 100 | ............................................. | 3 | -- |
| 1000 | ............................................. | 2 | -- |
| 10 000 | ............................................. | 1 | -- |
| 100 000 | ............... 1 .................... | 0 | ---- |
| | ............... 10 .................... | −1 | -- |
| | ............... 100 .................... | −2 | -- |
| | ............... 1000 .................... | −3 | -- |
| | ............... 10 000 .................... | −4 | -- |
| | ............... 100 000 .................... | −5 | ---- |
| | Negative (μg/ml or mg/kg bw) | | |

LED and HID are expressed as μg/ml or mg/kg bw.

In practice, an activity profile is computer generated. A data entry programme is used to store abstracted data from published reports. A sequential file (in ASCII) is created for each compound, and a record within that file consists of the name and Chemical Abstracts Service number of the compound, a three-letter code for the test system (see below), the qualitative test result (with and without an exogenous metabolic system), dose (LED or HID), citation number and additional source information. An abbreviated citation for each publication is stored in a segment of a record accessing both the test data file and the citation file. During processing of the data file, an average of the logarithmic values of the data subset is calculated, and the length of the profile line represents this average value. All dose values are plotted for each profile line, regardless of whether results are positive or negative. Results obtained in the absence of an exogenous metabolic system are indicated by a bar (−), and results obtained in the presence of an exogenous metabolic system are indicated by an upward-directed arrow (↑). When all results for a given assay are either positive or negative, the mean of the LDU values is plotted as a solid line; when conflicting data are reported for the same assay (i.e., both positive and negative results), the majority data are shown by a solid line and the minority data by a dashed line (drawn to the extreme conflicting response). In the few cases in which the numbers of positive and negative results are equal, the solid line is drawn in the positive direction and the maximal negative response is indicated with a dashed line.

Profile lines are identified by three-letter code words representing the commonly used tests. Code words for most of the test systems in current use in genetic toxicology were defined for the US Environmental Protection Agency's GENE-TOX Program (Waters, 1979; Waters & Auletta, 1981). For IARC Monographs Supplement 6, Volume 44 and subsequent volumes, including this publication, codes were redefined in a manner that should facilitate inclusion of additional tests. If a test system is not defined precisely, a general code is used that best defines the category of the test. Naming conventions are described below.

Data listings are presented with each activity profile and include endpoint and test codes, a short test code definition, results [either with (M) or without (NM) an exogenous activation system], the associated LED or HID value and a short citation. Test codes are organized phylogenetically and by endpoint from left to right across each activity profile and from top to bottom of the corresponding data listing. Endpoints are defined as follows: A, aneuploidy; C, chromosomal aberrations; D, DNA damage; F, assays of body fluids; G, gene mutation; H, host-mediated assays; I, inhibition of intercellular communication; M, micronuclei; P, sperm morphology; R, mitotic recombination or gene conversion; S, sister chromatid exchange; and T, cell transformation.

*Dose conversions for activity profiles*

Doses are converted to µg/ml for in-vitro tests and to mg/kg bw per day for in-vivo experiments.

1. In-vitro test systems

    (a) Weight/volume converts directly to µg/ml.

    (b) Molar (M) concentration x molecular weight = mg/ml = $10^3$ µg/ml; mM concentration x molecular weight = µg/ml.

    (c) Soluble solids expressed as % concentration are assumed to be in units of mass per volume (i.e., 1% = 0.01 g/ml = 10 000 µg/ml; also, 1 ppm = 1 µg/ml).

    (d) Liquids and gases expressed as % concentration are assumed to be given in units of volume per volume. Liquids are converted to weight per volume using the density (D) of the solution (D = g/ml). Gases are converted from volume to mass using the ideal gas law, PV = nRT. For exposure at 20–37°C at standard atmospheric pressure, 1% (v/v) = 0.4 µg/ml x molecular weight of the gas. Also, 1 ppm (v/v) = 4 x $10^{-5}$ µg/ml x molecular weight.

    (e) In microbial plate tests, it is usual for the doses to be reported as weight/plate, whereas concentrations are required to enter data on the activity profile chart. While remaining cognisant of the errors involved in the process, it is assumed that a 2-ml volume of top agar is delivered to each plate and that the test substance remains in solution within it; concentrations are derived from the reported weight/plate values by dividing by this arbitrary volume. For spot tests, a 1-ml volume is used in the calculation.

(f) Conversion of particulate concentrations given in μg/cm$^2$ are based on the area (A) of the dish and the volume of medium per dish; i.e., for a 100-mm dish: A = $\pi R^2$ = $\pi \times (5\text{ cm})^2$ = 78.5 cm$^2$. If the volume of medium is 10 ml, then 78.5 cm$^2$ = 10 ml and 1 cm$^2$ = 0.13 ml.

2. In-vitro systems using in-vivo activation

For the body fluid-urine (BF-) test, the concentration used is the dose (in mg/kg bw) of the compound administered to test animals or patients.

3. In-vivo test systems

(a) Doses are converted to mg/kg bw per day of exposure, assuming 100% absorption. Standard values are used for each sex and species of rodent, including body weight and average intake per day, as reported by Gold *et al.* (1984). For example, in a test using male mice fed 50 ppm of the agent in the diet, the standard food intake per day is 12% of body weight, and the conversion is dose = 50 ppm × 12% = 6 mg/kg bw per day.

Standard values used for humans are: weight – males, 70 kg; females, 55 kg; surface area, 1.7 m$^2$; inhalation rate, 20 l/min for light work, 30 l/min for mild exercise.

(b) When reported, the dose at the target site is used. For example, doses given in studies of lymphocytes of humans exposed *in vivo* are the measured blood concentrations in μg/ml.

*Codes for test systems*

For specific nonmammalian test systems, the first two letters of the three-symbol code word define the test organism (e.g., SA- for *Salmonella typhimurium*, EC- for *Escherichia coli*). If the species is not known, the convention used is -S-. The third symbol may be used to define the tester strain (e.g., SA8 for *S. typhimurium* TA1538, ECW for *E. coli* WP2*uvr*A). When strain designation is not indicated, the third letter is used to define the specific genetic endpoint under investigation (e.g., --D for differential toxicity, --F for forward mutation, --G for gene conversion or genetic crossing-over, --N for aneuploidy, --R for reverse mutation, --U for unscheduled DNA synthesis). The third letter may also be used to define the general endpoint under investigation when a more complete definition is not possible or relevant (e.g., --M for mutation, --C for chromosomal aberration).

For mammalian test systems, the first letter of the three-letter code word defines the genetic endpoint under investigation: A-- for aneuploidy, B-- for binding, C-- for chromosomal aberration, D-- for DNA strand breaks, G-- for gene mutation, I-- for inhibition of intercellular communication, M-- for micronucleus formation, R-- for DNA repair, S-- for sister chromatid exchange, T-- for cell transformation and U-- for unscheduled DNA synthesis.

# APPENDIX 1

For animal (i.e., non-human) test systems *in vitro*, when the cell type is not specified, the code letters –IA are used. For such assays *in vivo*, when the animal species is not specified, the code letters –VA are used. Commonly used animal species are identified by the third letter (e.g., --C for Chinese hamster, --M for mouse, --R for rat, --S for Syrian hamster).

For test systems using human cells *in vitro*, when the cell type is not specified, the code letters –IH are used. For assays on humans *in vivo*, when the cell type is not specified, the code letters –VH are used. Otherwise, the second letter specifies the cell type under investigation (e.g., –BH for bone marrow, –LH for lymphocytes).

Some other specific coding conventions used for mammalian systems are as follows: BF– for body fluids, HM– for host-mediated, --L for leucocytes or lymphocytes *in vitro* (–AL, animals; –HL, humans), –L– for leucocytes *in vivo* (–LA, animals; –LH, humans), --T for transformed cells.

Note that these are examples of major conventions used to define the assay code words. The alphabetized listing of codes must be examined to confirm a specific code word. As might be expected from the limitation to three symbols, some codes do not fit the naming conventions precisely. In a few cases, test systems are defined by first-letter code words, for example: MST, mouse spot test; SLP, mouse specific locus test, postspermatogonia; SLO, mouse specific locus test, other stages; DLM, dominant lethal test in mice; DLR, dominant lethal test in rats; MHT, mouse heritable translocation test.

The genetic activity profiles and listings that follow were prepared in collaboration with Environmental Health Research and Testing Inc. (EHRT) under contract to the US Environmental Protection Agency; EHRT also determined the doses used. The references cited in each genetic activity profile listing can be found in the list of references in the appropriate monograph.

*References*

Garrett, N.E., Stack, H.F., Gross, M.R. & Waters, M.D. (1984) An analysis of the spectra of genetic activity produced by known or suspected human carcinogens. *Mutat. Res., 134,* 89–111

Gold, L.S., Sawyer, C.B., Magaw, R., Backman, G.M., de Veciana, M., Levinson, R., Hooper, N.K., Havender, W.R., Bernstein, L., Peto, R., Pike, M.C. & Ames, B.N. (1984) A carcinogenic potency database of the standardized results of animal bioassays. *Environ. Health Perspect., 58,* 9–319

Waters, M.D. (1979) *The GENE-TOX program.* In: Hsie, A.W., O'Neill, J.P. & McElheny, V.K., eds, *Mammalian Cell Mutagenesis: The Maturation of Test Systems (Banbury Report 2),* Cold Spring Harbor, NY, CHS Press, pp. 449–467

Waters, M.D. & Auletta, A. (1981) The GENE-TOX program: genetic activity evaluation. *J. chem. Inf. comput. Sci., 21,* 35–38

Waters, M.D., Stack, H.F., Brady, A.L., Lohman, P.H.M., Haroun, L. & Vainio, H. (1987) Appendix 1: Activity profiles for genetic and related tests. In: *IARC Monographs on the Evaluation of the Carcinogenic Risk of Chemicals to Humans,* Suppl. 6, *Genetic and Related Effects: An Update of Selected IARC Monographs from Volumes 1 to 42,* Lyon, IARC, pp. 687–696

Waters, M.D., Stack, H.F., Brady, A.L., Lohman, P.H.M., Haroun, L. & Vainio, H. (1988) Use of computerized data listings and activity profiles of genetic and related effects in the review of 195 compounds. *Mutat. Res., 205,* 295–312

CHLORENDIC ACID

| END POINT | TEST CODE | TEST SYSTEM | RESULTS NM M | DOSE (LED OR HID) | REFERENCE |
|---|---|---|---|---|---|
| G | SA0 | S. TYPHIMURIUM TA100, REVERSE MUTATION | - - | 3845.0000 | NTP, 1987 |
| G | SA5 | S. TYPHIMURIUM TA1535, REVERSE MUTATION | - - | 3845.0000 | NTP, 1987 |
| G | SA7 | S. TYPHIMURIUM TA1537, REVERSE MUTATION | - - | 3845.0000 | NTP, 1987 |
| G | SA9 | S. TYPHIMURIUM TA98, REVERSE MUTATION | - - | 3845.0000 | NTP, 1987 |
| G | G5T | MUTATION, L5178Y CELLS, TK LOCUS | + 0 | 1700.0000 | NTP, 1987 |

# APPENDIX 1

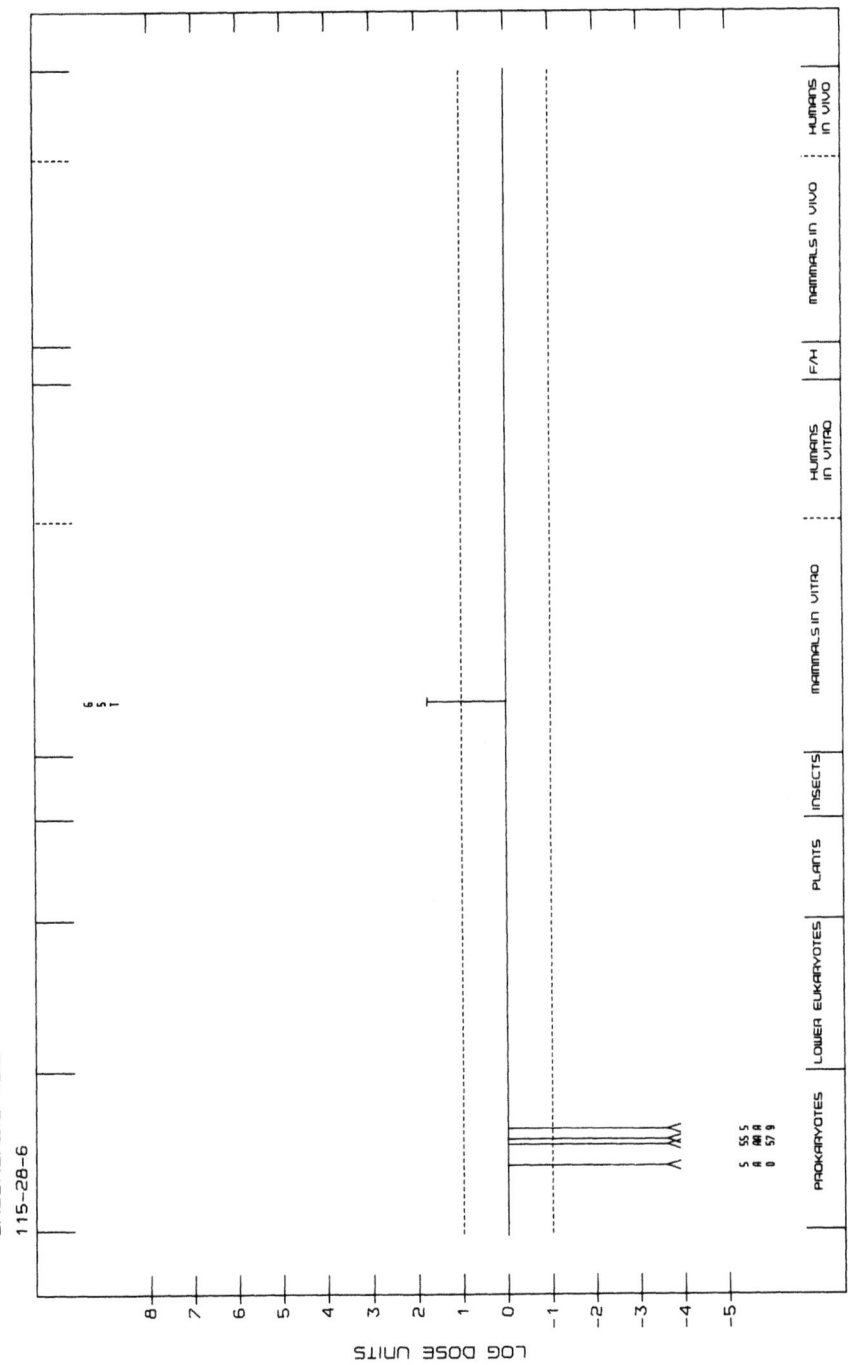

CHLORINATED PARAFFINS

| END POINT | TEST CODE | TEST SYSTEM | RESULTS NM M | DOSE (LED OR HID) | REFERENCE |
|---|---|---|---|---|---|
| G | SA0 | S. TYPHIMURIUM TA100, REVERSE MUTATION | - - | 1250.0000 | BIRTLEY ET AL., 1980 |
| G | SA0 | S. TYPHIMURIUM TA100, REVERSE MUTATION | - - | 2300.0000 | MEIJER ET AL., 1981 |
| G | SA0 | S. TYPHIMURIUM TA100, REVERSE MUTATION | - - | 1667.0000 | NTPa, 1986 |
| G | SA0 | S. TYPHIMURIUM TA100, REVERSE MUTATION | - - | 5000.0000 | NTPb, 1986 |
| G | SA5 | S. TYPHIMURIUM TA1535, REVERSE MUTATION | - - | 1250.0000 | BIRTLEY ET AL., 1980 |
| G | SA5 | S. TYPHIMURIUM TA1535, REVERSE MUTATION | - - | 1667.0000 | NTPa, 1986 |
| G | SA5 | S. TYPHIMURIUM TA1535, REVERSE MUTATION | - - | 5000.0000 | NTPb, 1986 |
| G | SA7 | S. TYPHIMURIUM TA1537, REVERSE MUTATION | - - | 2300.0000 | MEIJER ET AL., 1981 |
| G | SA8 | S. TYPHIMURIUM TA1538, REVERSE MUTATION | - - | 1250.0000 | BIRTLEY ET AL., 1980 |
| G | SA9 | S. TYPHIMURIUM TA98, REVERSE MUTATION | - - | 1250.0000 | BIRTLEY ET AL., 1980 |
| G | SA9 | S. TYPHIMURIUM TA98, REVERSE MUTATION | - - | 2300.0000 | MEIJER ET AL., 1981 |
| G | SA9 | S. TYPHIMURIUM TA98, REVERSE MUTATION | - - | 1667.0000 | NTPa, 1986 |
| G | SA9 | S. TYPHIMURIUM TA98, REVERSE MUTATION | - - | 5000.0000 | NTPb, 1986 |
| G | SAS | S. TYPHIMURIUM (OTHER), REVERSE MUTATION | - - | 1667.0000 | NTPa, 1986 |
| G | SAS | S. TYPHIMURIUM (OTHER), REVERSE MUTATION | - - | 5000.0000 | NTPb, 1986 |

# APPENDIX 1

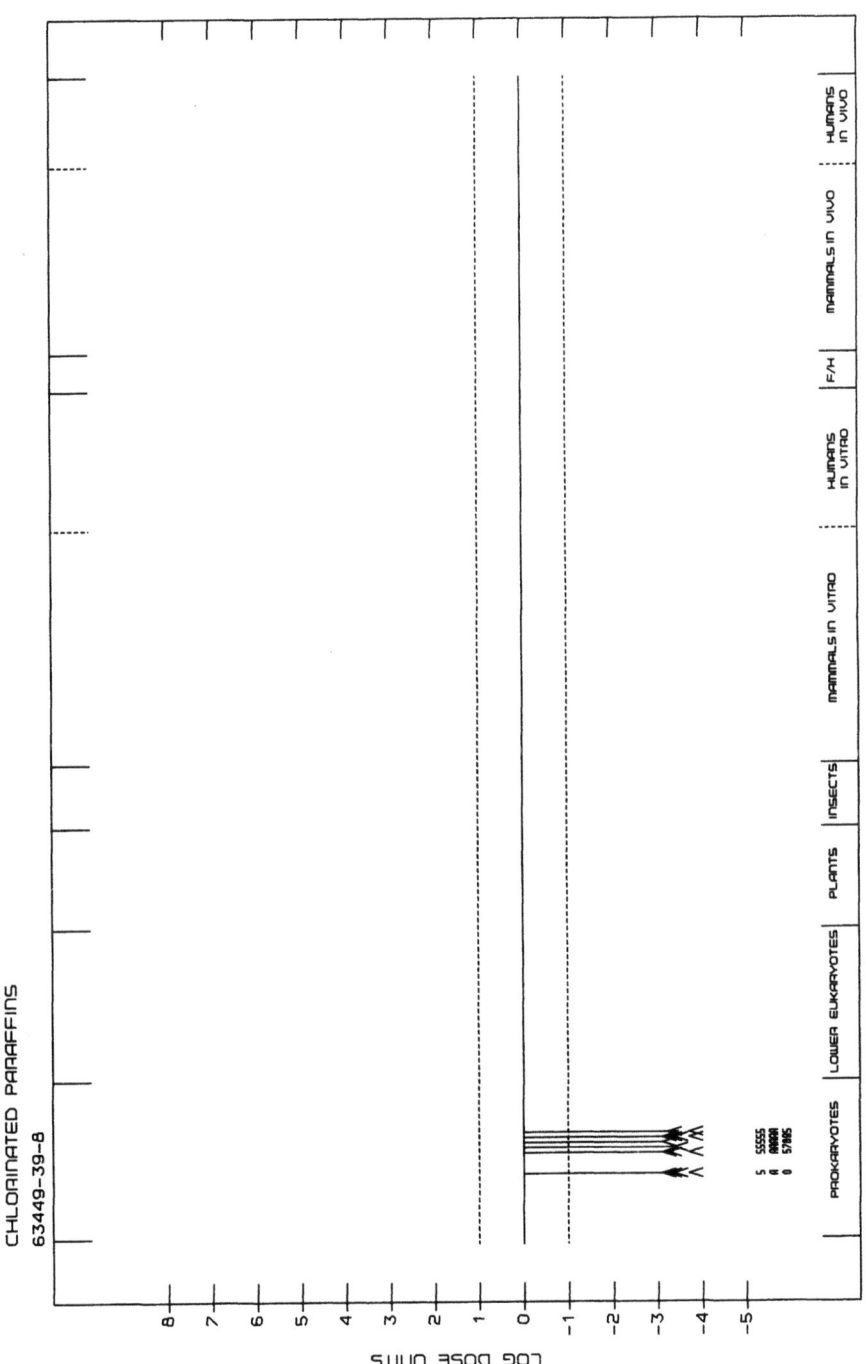

## DECABROMODIPHENYL OXIDE

| END POINT | TEST CODE | TEST SYSTEM | RESULTS NM M | DOSE (LED OR HID) | REFERENCE |
|---|---|---|---|---|---|
| G | SA0 | S. TYPHIMURIUM TA100, REVERSE MUTATION | - - | 5000.0000 | NTP, 1986 |
| G | SA5 | S. TYPHIMURIUM TA1535, REVERSE MUTATION | - - | 5000.0000 | NTP, 1986 |
| G | SA7 | S. TYPHIMURIUM TA1537, REVERSE MUTATION | - - | 5000.0000 | NTP, 1986 |
| G | SA9 | S. TYPHIMURIUM TA98, REVERSE MUTATION | - - | 5000.0000 | NTP, 1986 |
| G | G5T | MUTATION, L5178Y CELLS, TK LOCUS | - - | 10.0000 | NTP, 1986 |
| S | SIC | SCE, CHINESE HAMSTER CELLS IN VITRO | - - | 500.0000 | NTP, 1986 |
| C | CIC | CHROM ABERR, CHINESE HAMSTER CELLS IN VITRO | - - | 500.0000 | NTP, 1986 |

# APPENDIX 1

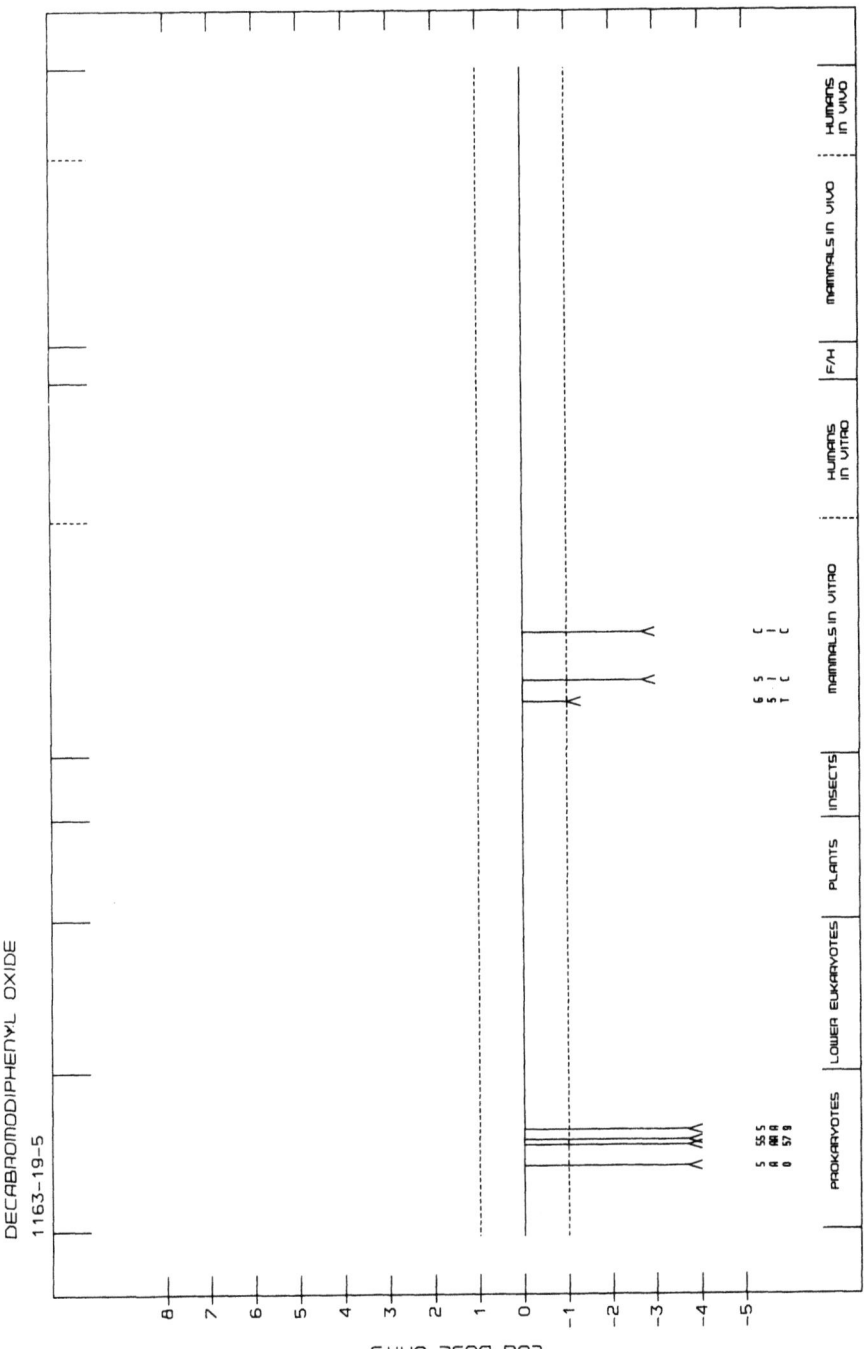

DIMETHYL HYDROGEN PHOSPHITE

| END POINT | TEST CODE | TEST SYSTEM | RESULTS NM M | DOSE (LED OR HID) | REFERENCE |
|---|---|---|---|---|---|
| G | SA0 | S. TYPHIMURIUM TA100, REVERSE MUTATION | – | 5000.0000 | NTP, 1985 |
| G | SA5 | S. TYPHIMURIUM TA1535, REVERSE MUTATION | – | 5000.0000 | NTP, 1985 |
| G | SA7 | S. TYPHIMURIUM TA1537, REVERSE MUTATION | – | 5000.0000 | NTP, 1985 |
| G | SA9 | S. TYPHIMURIUM TA98, REVERSE MUTATION | – | 5000.0000 | NTP, 1985 |
| G | DMX | D. MELANOGASTER, SEX-LINKED RECESSIVES | – 0 | 1500.0000 | NTP, 1985 |
| G | G5T | MUTATION, L5178Y CELLS, TK LOCUS | – + | 2100.0000 | MCGREGOR ET AL., 1988 |
| S | SIC | SCE, CHINESE HAMSTER CELLS IN VITRO | + + | 250.0000 | TENNANT ET AL., 1987b |
| C | CIC | CHROM ABERR, CHINESE HAMSTER CELLS IN VITRO | + + | 1600.0000 | TENNANT ET AL., 1987b |

# APPENDIX 1

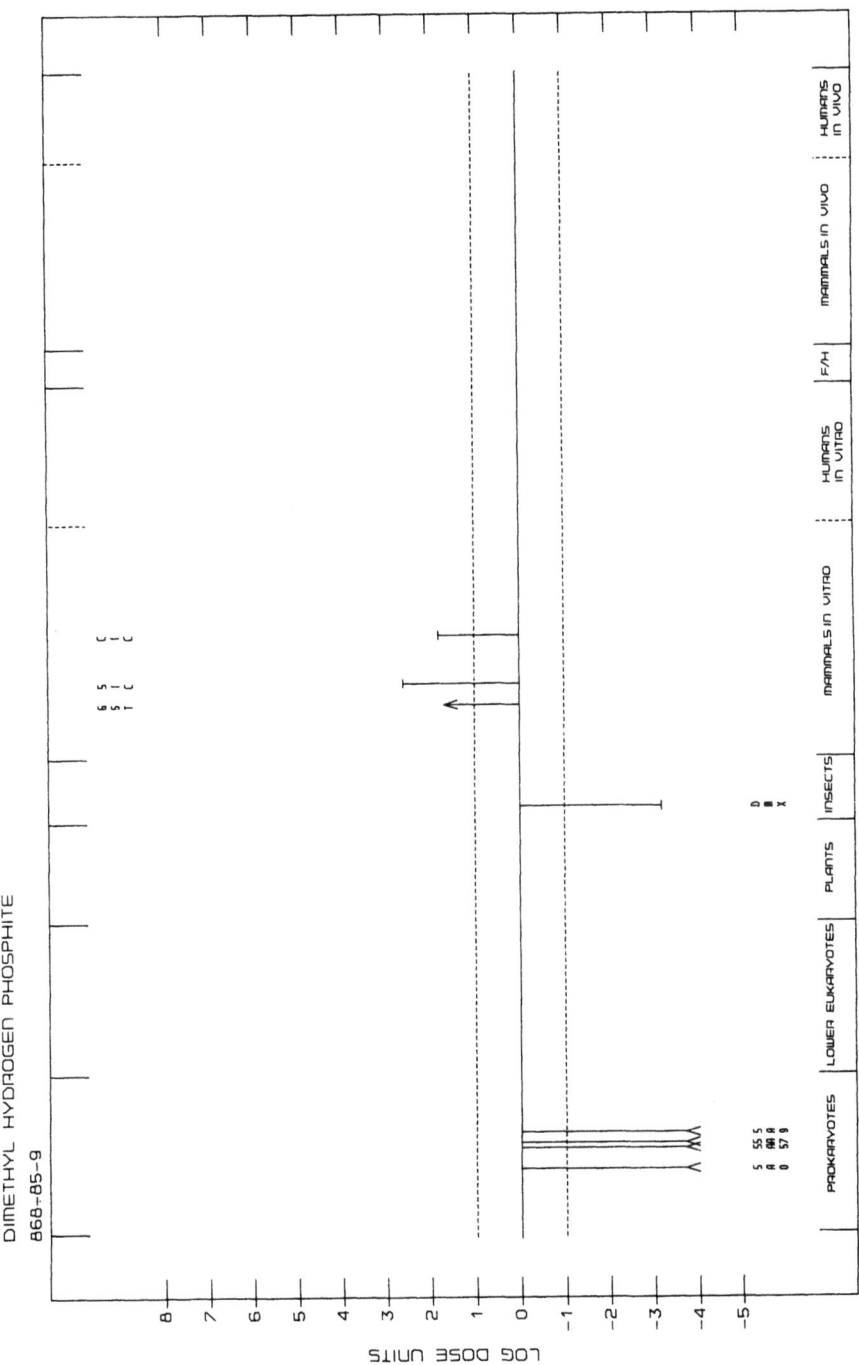

THPS

| END POINT | TEST CODE | TEST SYSTEM | RESULTS NM M | DOSE (LED OR HID) | REFERENCE |
|---|---|---|---|---|---|
| G | SA0 | S. TYPHIMURIUM TA100, REVERSE MUTATION | – | 50.0000 | CONNOR ET AL., 1980 |
| G | SA0 | S. TYPHIMURIUM TA100, REVERSE MUTATION | – | 50.0000 | MACGREGOR ET AL., 1980 |
| G | SA5 | S. TYPHIMURIUM TA1535, REVERSE MUTATION | – | 50.0000 | CONNOR ET AL., 1980 |
| G | SA5 | S. TYPHIMURIUM TA1535, REVERSE MUTATION | – | 5.0000 | MACGREGOR ET AL., 1980 |
| G | SA7 | S. TYPHIMURIUM TA1537, REVERSE MUTATION | – | 50.0000 | CONNOR ET AL., 1980 |
| G | SA7 | S. TYPHIMURIUM TA1537, REVERSE MUTATION | – | 5.0000 | MACGREGOR ET AL., 1980 |
| G | SA8 | S. TYPHIMURIUM TA1538, REVERSE MUTATION | – | 50.0000 | CONNOR ET AL., 1980 |
| G | SA9 | S. TYPHIMURIUM TA98, REVERSE MUTATION | – | 50.0000 | CONNOR ET AL., 1980 |
| G | SA9 | S. TYPHIMURIUM TA98, REVERSE MUTATION | – | 50.0000 | MACGREGOR ET AL., 1980 |
| G | G5T | MUTATION, L5178Y CELLS, TK LOCUS | + 0 | 5.0000 | NTP, 1987 |
| F | BFA | ANIMAL BODY FLUIDS, MICROBIAL MUTAGENICITY | – 0 | 1000.0000 | CONNOR ET AL., 1980 |
| M | MVM | MICRONUCLEUS TEST, MICE IN VIVO | – 0 | 1000.0000 | CONNOR ET AL., 1980 |
| C | CBA | CHROM ABERR, ANIMAL BONE MARROW IN VIVO | (+) 0 | 10.0000 | CONNOR ET AL., 1980 |

# APPENDIX 1

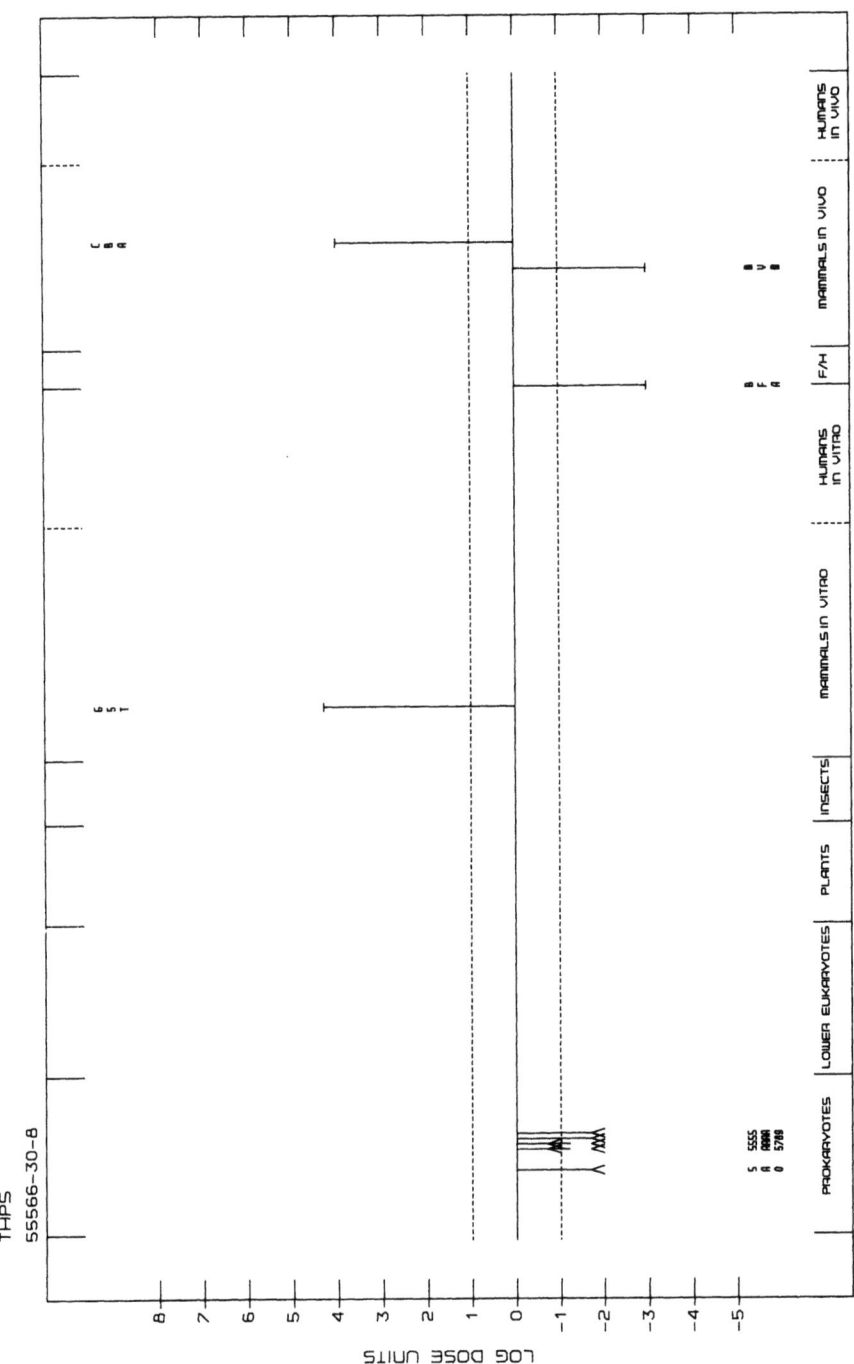

THPC

| END POINT | TEST CODE | TEST SYSTEM | RESULTS NM M | DOSE (LED OR HID) | REFERENCE |
|---|---|---|---|---|---|
| G | SA0 | S. TYPHIMURIUM TA100, REVERSE MUTATION | – | 50.0000 | MACGREGOR ET AL., 1980 |
| G | SA0 | S. TYPHIMURIUM TA100, REVERSE MUTATION | – | 17.0000 | NTP, 1987 |
| G | SA5 | S. TYPHIMURIUM TA1535, REVERSE MUTATION | – | 50.0000 | MACGREGOR ET AL., 1980 |
| G | SA5 | S. TYPHIMURIUM TA1535, REVERSE MUTATION | – | 17.0000 | NTP, 1987 |
| G | SA7 | S. TYPHIMURIUM TA1537, REVERSE MUTATION | – | 50.0000 | MACGREGOR ET AL., 1980 |
| G | SA7 | S. TYPHIMURIUM TA1537, REVERSE MUTATION | – | 17.0000 | NTP, 1987 |
| G | SA9 | S. TYPHIMURIUM TA98, REVERSE MUTATION | – | 50.0000 | MACGREGOR ET AL., 1980 |
| G | SA9 | S. TYPHIMURIUM TA98, REVERSE MUTATION | – | 17.0000 | NTP, 1987 |
| G | G5T | MUTATION, L5178Y CELLS, TK LOCUS | + 0 | 5.0000 | NTP, 1987 |
| S | SIC | SCE, CHINESE HAMSTER CELLS IN VITRO | + + | 15.0000 | NTP, 1987 |
| S | SIC | SCE, CHINESE HAMSTER CELLS IN VITRO | + + | 20.0000 | LOVEDAY ET AL., 1989 |
| C | CIC | CHROM ABERR, CHINESE HAMSTER CELLS IN VITRO | + + | 30.0000 | NTP, 1987 |
| C | CIC | CHROM ABERR, CHINESE HAMSTER CELLS IN VITRO | + 0 | 19.0000 | SASAKI ET AL., 1980 |
| C | CIC | CHROM ABERR, CHINESE HAMSTER CELLS IN VITRO | + ? | 30.0000 | LOVEDAY ET AL., 1989 |
| C | CIC | CHROM ABERR, CHINESE HAMSTER CELLS IN VITRO | + 0 | 30.0000 | ISHIDATE (ED), 1983 |

# APPENDIX 1

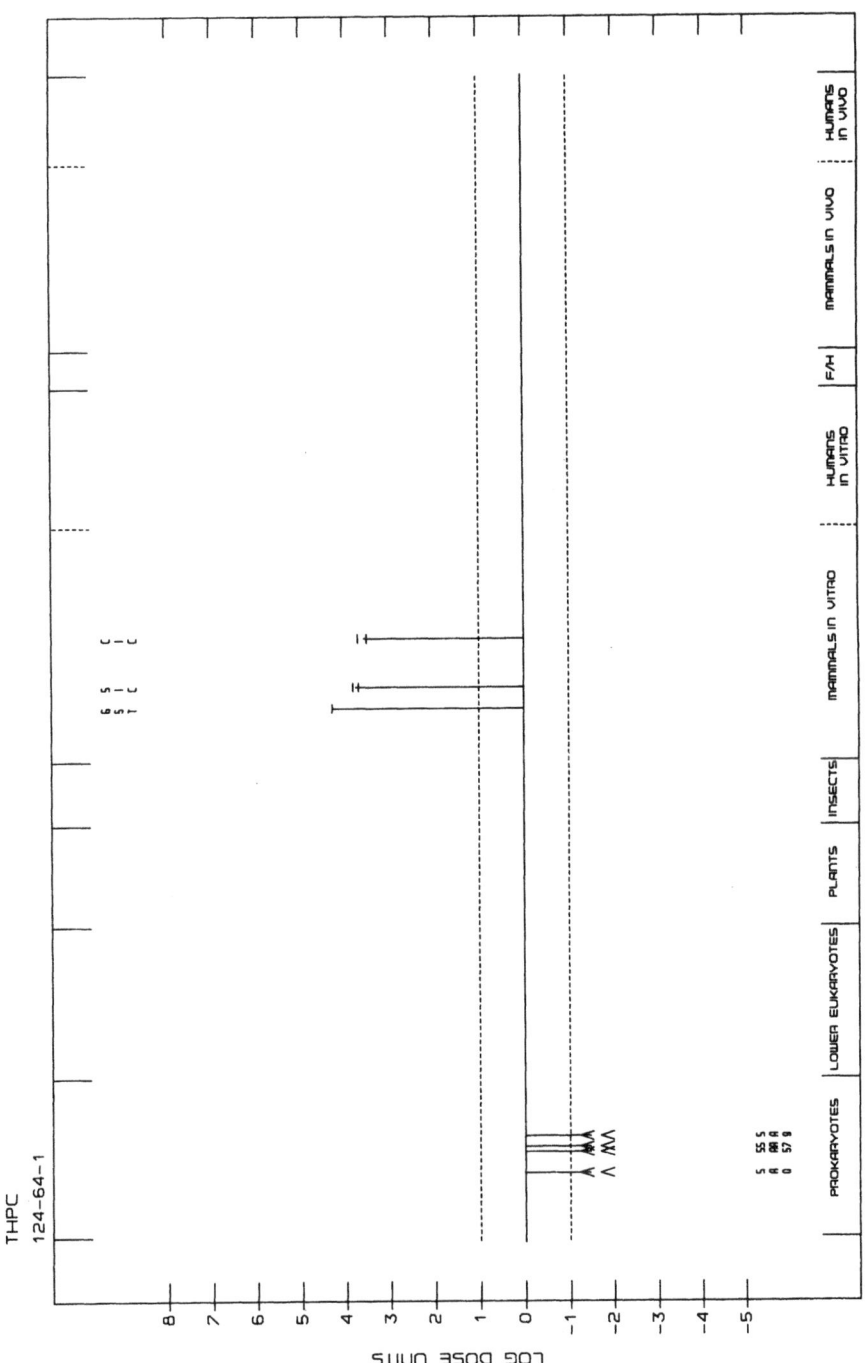

TRIS(2-CHLOROETHYL) PHOSPHATE

| END POINT | TEST CODE | TEST SYSTEM | RESULTS NM M | DOSE (LED OR HID) | REFERENCE |
|---|---|---|---|---|---|
| G | SA0 | S. TYPHIMURIUM TA100, REVERSE MUTATION | – – | 6950.0000 | PRIVAL ET AL., 1977 |
| G | SA0 | S. TYPHIMURIUM TA100, REVERSE MUTATION | – (+) | 1427.0000 | NAKAMURA ET AL., 1979 |
| G | SA0 | S. TYPHIMURIUM TA100, REVERSE MUTATION | – – | 500.0000 | HAWORTH ET AL., 1983 |
| G | SA5 | S. TYPHIMURIUM TA1535, REVERSE MUTATION | – – | 6950.0000 | PRIVAL ET AL., 1977 |
| G | SA5 | S. TYPHIMURIUM TA1535, REVERSE MUTATION | – + | 143.0000 | NAKAMURA ET AL., 1979 |
| G | SA5 | S. TYPHIMURIUM TA1535, REVERSE MUTATION | – – | 500.0000 | HAWORTH ET AL., 1983 |
| G | SA7 | S. TYPHIMURIUM TA1537, REVERSE MUTATION | – – | 500.0000 | HAWORTH ET AL., 1983 |
| G | SA8 | S. TYPHIMURIUM TA1538, REVERSE MUTATION | – – | 6950.0000 | PRIVAL ET AL., 1977 |
| G | SA9 | S. TYPHIMURIUM TA98, REVERSE MUTATION | – – | 500.0000 | HAWORTH ET AL., 1983 |
| G | G9H | MUTATION, CHL V79 CELLS, HPRT | – – | 2000.0000 | SALA ET AL., 1982 |
| S | SIC | SCE, CHINESE HAMSTER CELLS IN VITRO | + + | 700.0000 | SALA ET AL., 1982 |
| T | TCM | CELL TRANSFORMATION, C3H10T1/2 CELLS | – (+) | 900.0000 | SALA ET AL., 1982 |
| T | TCS | CELL TRANSFORMATION, SHE, CLONAL ASSAY | + 0 | 400.0000 | SALA ET AL., 1982 |
| M | MVM | MICRONUCLEUS TEST, MICE IN VIVO | ? 0 | 250.0000 | SALA ET AL., 1982 |
| C | DLR | DOMINANT LETHAL TEST, RATS | + 0 | 0.5000 | SHEPEL'SKAIA & DYSHGINEVICH, 1981 |

# APPENDIX 1

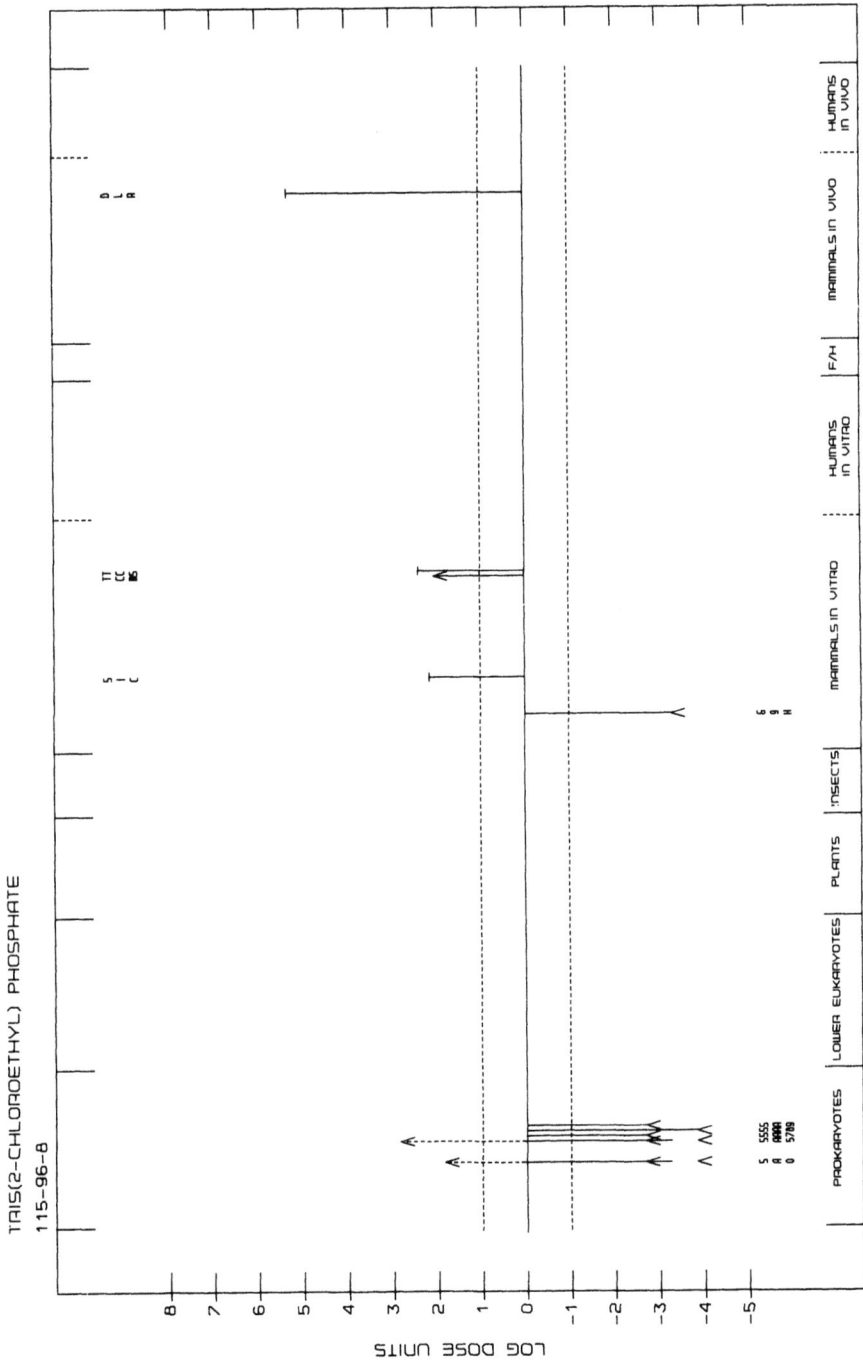

p-CHLORO-o-TOLUIDINE

| END POINT | TEST CODE | TEST SYSTEM | RESULTS NM M | | DOSE (LED OR HID) | REFERENCE |
|---|---|---|---|---|---|---|
| D | SAD | S. TYPHIMURIUM, DIFFERENTIAL TOXICITY | + | 0 | 250.0000 | RASHID ET AL., 1984 |
| D | ERD | E. COLI REC, DIFFERENTIAL TOXICITY | - | 0 | 2000.0000 | RASHID ET AL., 1984 |
| G | SA0 | S. TYPHIMURIUM TA100, REVERSE MUTATION | + | | 7.0000 | ZIMMER ET AL., 1980 |
| G | SA0 | S. TYPHIMURIUM TA100, REVERSE MUTATION | - | | 167.0000 | HAWORTH ET AL., 1983 |
| G | SA0 | S. TYPHIMURIUM TA100, REVERSE MUTATION | - | 0 | 163.0000 | RASHID ET AL., 1984 |
| G | SA5 | S. TYPHIMURIUM TA1535, REVERSE MUTATION | - | | 500.0000 | HAWORTH ET AL., 1983 |
| G | SA5 | S. TYPHIMURIUM TA1535, REVERSE MUTATION | + | 0 | 163.0000 | RASHID ET AL., 1984 |
| G | SA7 | S. TYPHIMURIUM TA1537, REVERSE MUTATION | - | | 100.0000 | ZIMMER ET AL., 1980 |
| G | SA7 | S. TYPHIMURIUM TA1537, REVERSE MUTATION | - | | 167.0000 | HAWORTH ET AL., 1983 |
| G | SA7 | S. TYPHIMURIUM TA1537, REVERSE MUTATION | - | 0 | 163.0000 | RASHID ET AL., 1984 |
| G | SA8 | S. TYPHIMURIUM TA1538, REVERSE MUTATION | - | 0 | 163.0000 | RASHID ET AL., 1984 |
| G | SA9 | S. TYPHIMURIUM TA98, REVERSE MUTATION | - | | 100.0000 | ZIMMER ET AL., 1980 |
| G | SA9 | S. TYPHIMURIUM TA98, REVERSE MUTATION | - | | 167.0000 | HAWORTH ET AL., 1983 |
| G | SA9 | S. TYPHIMURIUM TA98, REVERSE MUTATION | - | 0 | 163.0000 | RASHID ET AL., 1984 |
| G | ECW | E. COLI WP2 UVRA, REVERSE MUTATION | - | | 1000.0000 | RASHID ET AL., 1984 |
| G | EC2 | E. COLI WP2, REVERSE MUTATION | - | | 1000.0000 | RASHID ET AL., 1984 |
| G | ECR | E. COLI (OTHER), REVERSE MUTATION | - | | 1000.0000 | RASHID ET AL., 1984 |
| D | DIA | STRAND BREAKS/X-LINKS, ANIMAL CELLS IN VITRO | (+) | 0 | 425.0000 | ZIMMER ET AL., 1980 |
| S | SIC | SCE, CHINESE HAMSTER CELLS IN VITRO | + | + | 50.0000 | GALLOWAY ET AL., 1987 |
| C | CIC | CHROM ABERR, CHINESE HAMSTER CELLS IN VITRO | - | + | 400.0000 | GALLOWAY ET AL., 1987 |
| G | MST | MOUSE SPOT TEST | + | 0 | 100.0000 | LANG, 1984 |
| C | MHT | MOUSE HERITABLE TRANSLOCATION TEST | - | 0 | 200.0000 | LANG & ADLER, 1982 |
| D | BVD | BINDING TO DNA, ANIMALS IN VIVO | + | 0 | 25.0000 | BENTLEY ET AL., 1986 |
| D | BVP | BINDING TO RNA/PROTEIN, ANIMALS IN VIVO | + | 0 | 25.0000 | BENTLEY ET AL., 1986 |

# APPENDIX 1

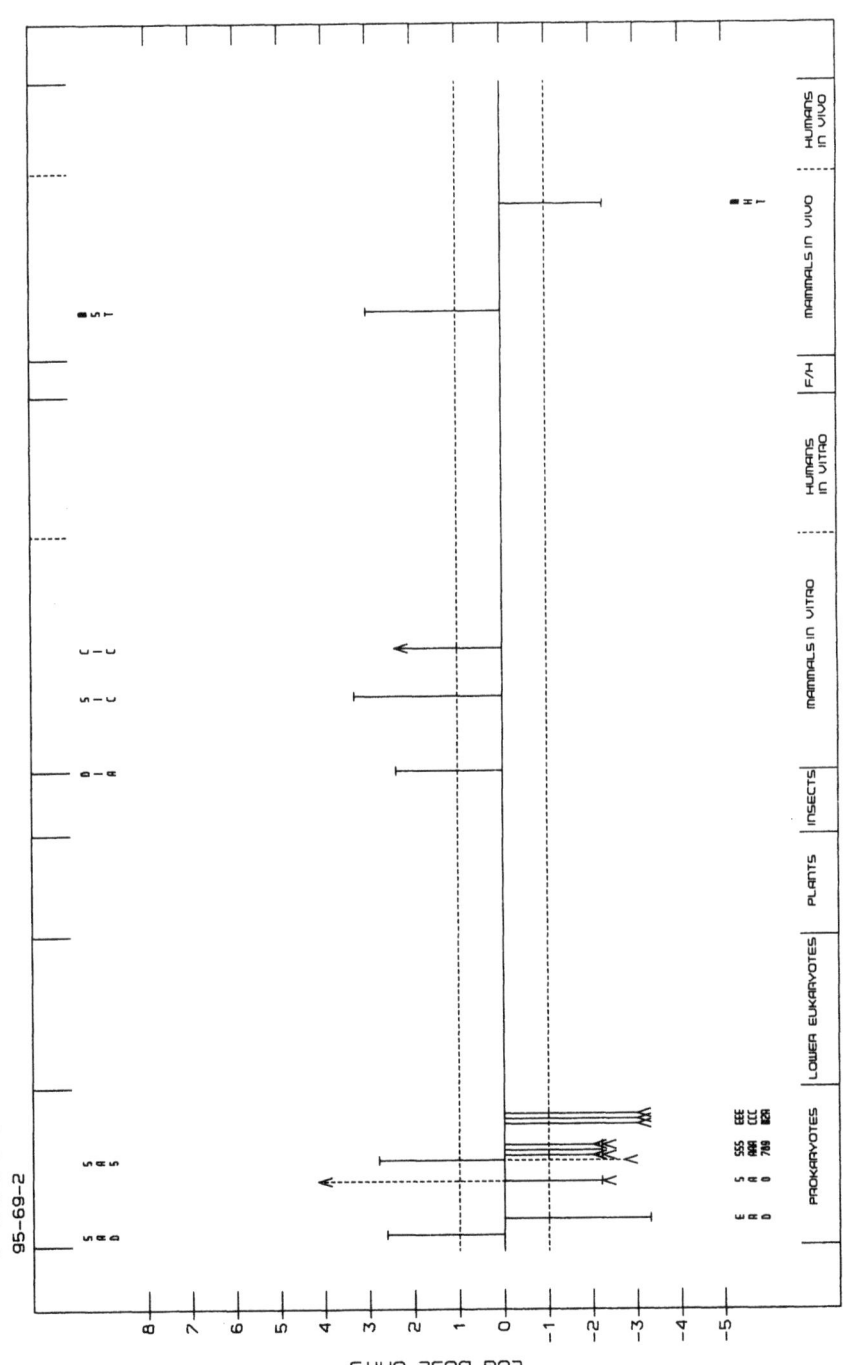

DISPERSE BLUE 1

| END POINT | TEST CODE | TEST SYSTEM | RESULTS NM M | DOSE (LED OR HID) | REFERENCE |
|---|---|---|---|---|---|
| G | SA0 | S. TYPHIMURIUM TA100, REVERSE MUTATION | – | 1000.0000 | BROWN & BROWN, 1976 |
| G | SA0 | S. TYPHIMURIUM TA100, REVERSE MUTATION | – | 1000.0000 | NTP, 1986 |
| G | SA5 | S. TYPHIMURIUM TA1535, REVERSE MUTATION | – | 1000.0000 | BROWN & BROWN, 1976 |
| G | SA5 | S. TYPHIMURIUM TA1535, REVERSE MUTATION | – + | 1000.0000 | NTP, 1986 |
| G | SA7 | S. TYPHIMURIUM TA1537, REVERSE MUTATION | (+) (+) | 50.0000 | BROWN & BROWN, 1976 |
| G | SA8 | S. TYPHIMURIUM TA1538, REVERSE MUTATION | – – | 1000.0000 | BROWN & BROWN, 1976 |
| G | SA9 | S. TYPHIMURIUM TA98, REVERSE MUTATION | – – | 1000.0000 | BROWN & BROWN, 1976 |
| G | SA9 | S. TYPHIMURIUM TA98, REVERSE MUTATION | + + | 50.0000 | NTP, 1986 |
| G | SAS | S. TYPHIMURIUM (OTHER), REVERSE MUTATION | + – | 5.0000 | NTP, 1986 |

# APPENDIX 1

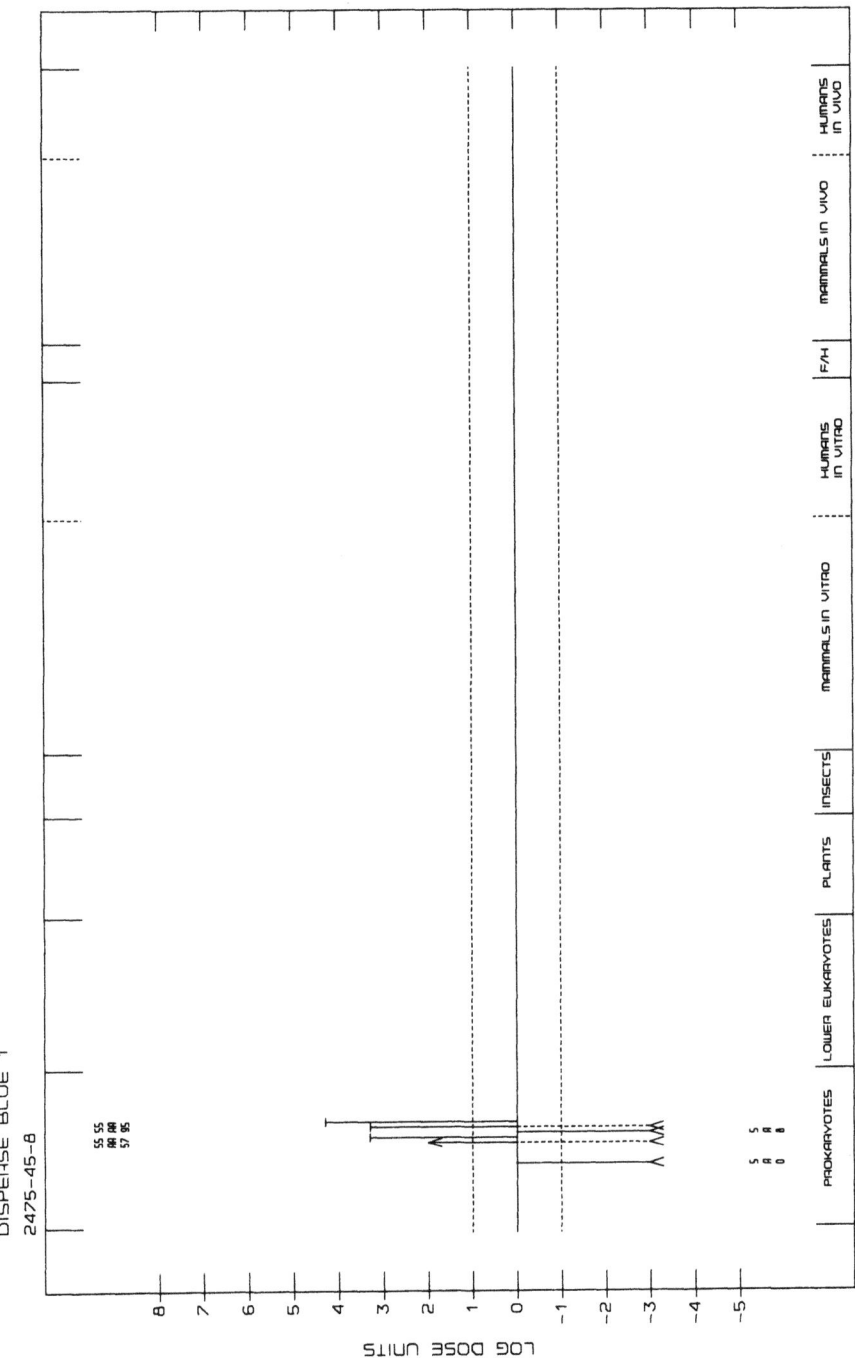

DISPERSE YELLOW 3

| END POINT | TEST CODE | TEST SYSTEM | RESULTS NM M | DOSE (LED OR HID) | REFERENCE |
|---|---|---|---|---|---|
| G | SA0 | S. TYPHIMURIUM TA100, REVERSE MUTATION | - + | 167.0000 | CAMERON ET AL., 1987 |
| G | SA0 | S. TYPHIMURIUM TA100, REVERSE MUTATION | + + | 17.0000 | ZEIGER ET AL., 1988 |
| G | SA5 | S. TYPHIMURIUM TA1535, REVERSE MUTATION | - - | 5000.0000 | CAMERON ET AL., 1987 |
| G | SA5 | S. TYPHIMURIUM TA1535, REVERSE MUTATION | - - | 500.0000 | ZEIGER ET AL., 1988 |
| G | SA7 | S. TYPHIMURIUM TA1537, REVERSE MUTATION | + + | 167.0000 | CAMERON ET AL., 1987 |
| G | SA8 | S. TYPHIMURIUM TA1538, REVERSE MUTATION | + + | 167.0000 | CAMERON ET AL., 1987 |
| G | SA9 | S. TYPHIMURIUM TA98, REVERSE MUTATION | + + | 167.0000 | CAMERON ET AL., 1987 |
| G | SA9 | S. TYPHIMURIUM TA98, REVERSE MUTATION | + + | 5.0000 | ZEIGER ET AL., 1988 |
| G | SAS | S. TYPHIMURIUM (OTHER), REVERSE MUTATION | + + | 5.0000 | ZEIGER ET AL., 1988 |
| G | G5T | MUTATION, L5178Y CELLS, TK LOCUS | + | 10.0000 | MCGREGOR ET AL., 1988 |
| G | G5T | MUTATION, L5178Y CELLS, TK LOCUS | (+) - | 229.0000 | CAMERON ET AL., 1987 |
| S | SIC | SCE, CHINESE HAMSTER CELLS IN VITRO | + 0 | 5.0000 | TENNANT ET AL., 1987b |
| C | CIC | CHROM ABERR, CHINESE HAMSTER CELLS IN VITRO | - 0 | 1500.0000 | TENNANT ET AL., 1987b |

# APPENDIX 1

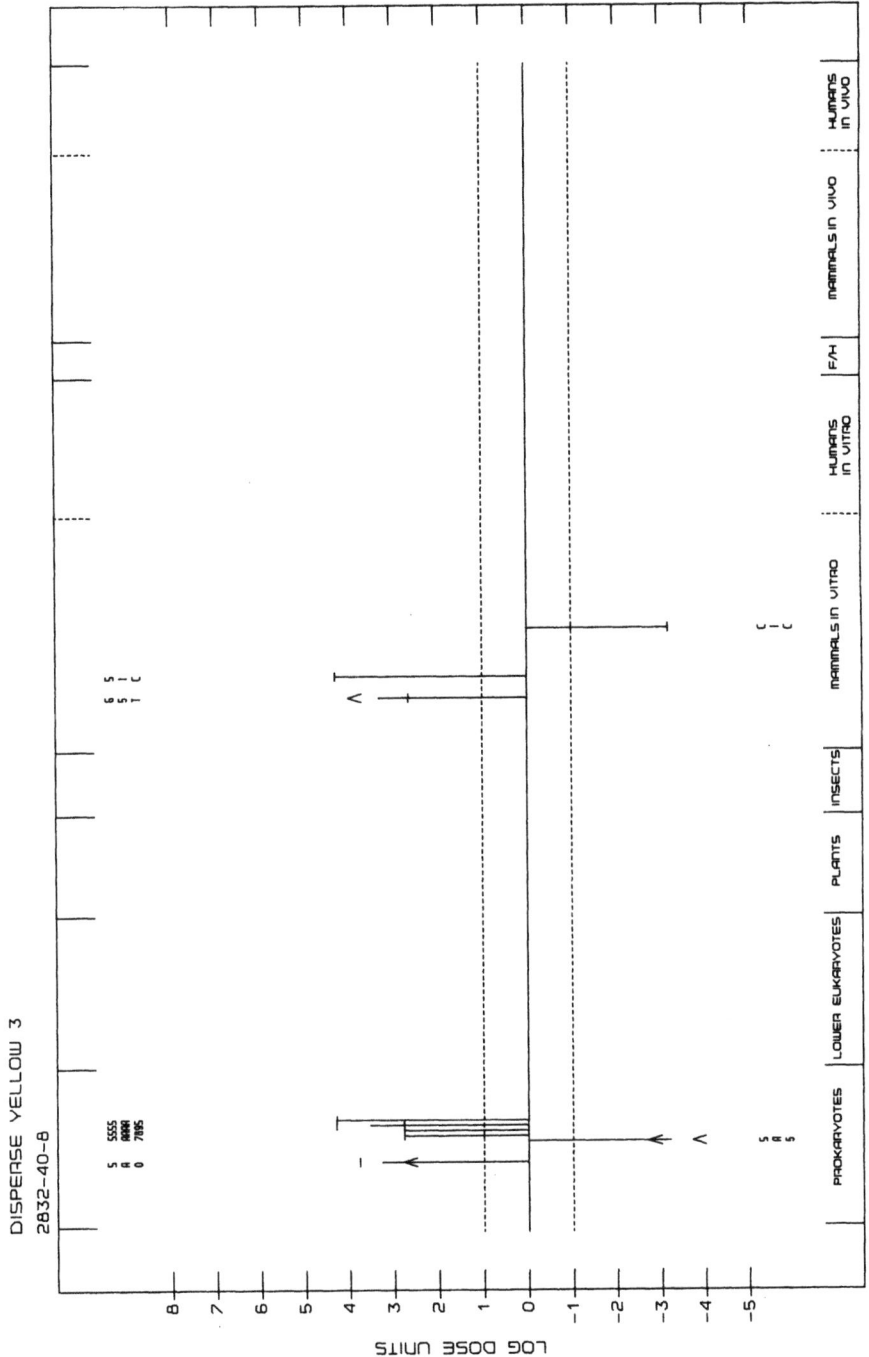

VAT YELLOW 4

| END POINT | TEST CODE | TEST SYSTEM | RESULTS NM M | DOSE (LED OR HID) | REFERENCE |
|---|---|---|---|---|---|
| G | SA0 | S. TYPHIMURIUM TA100, REVERSE MUTATION | - - | 5000.0000 | ZEIGER ET AL., 1987 |
| G | SA5 | S. TYPHIMURIUM TA1535, REVERSE MUTATION | - - | 5000.0000 | ZEIGER ET AL., 1987 |
| G | SA7 | S. TYPHIMURIUM TA1537, REVERSE MUTATION | - - | 5000.0000 | ZEIGER ET AL., 1987 |
| G | SA9 | S. TYPHIMURIUM TA98, REVERSE MUTATION | - - | 5000.0000 | ZEIGER ET AL., 1987 |

# APPENDIX 1

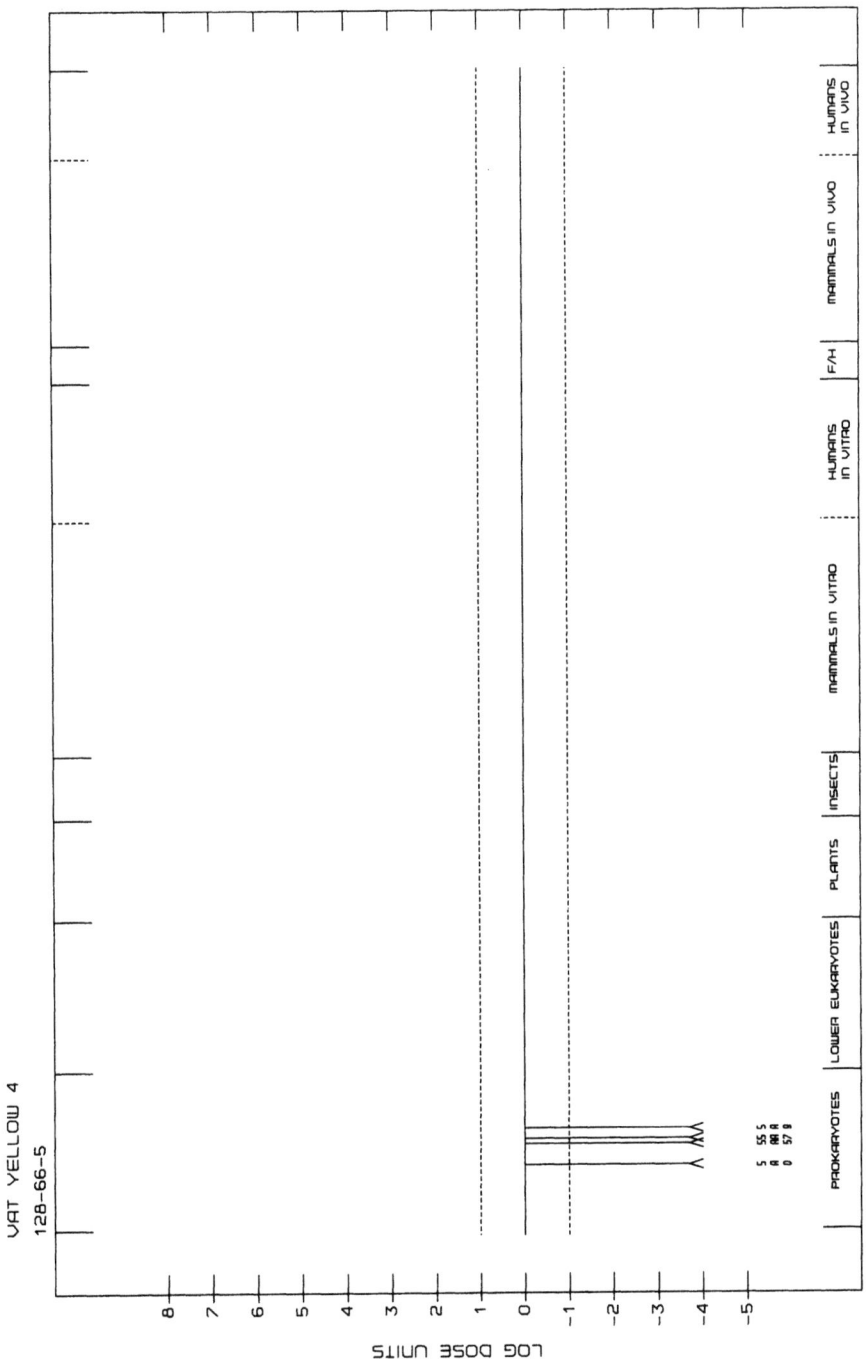

5-NITRO-O-TOLUIDINE

| END POINT | TEST CODE | TEST SYSTEM | RESULTS NM M | DOSE (LED OR HID) | REFERENCE |
|---|---|---|---|---|---|
| G | SA0 | S. TYPHIMURIUM TA100, REVERSE MUTATION | + + | 0.0000 | SPANGGORD ET AL., 1982b |
| G | SA0 | S. TYPHIMURIUM TA100, REVERSE MUTATION | + + | 167.0000 | DUNKEL ET AL., 1985 |
| G | SA5 | S. TYPHIMURIUM TA1535, REVERSE MUTATION | + - | 0.0000 | SPANGGORD ET AL., 1982b |
| G | SA5 | S. TYPHIMURIUM TA1535, REVERSE MUTATION | + + | 167.0000 | DUNKEL ET AL., 1985 |
| G | SA7 | S. TYPHIMURIUM TA1537, REVERSE MUTATION | + + | 0.0000 | SPANGGORD ET AL., 1982b |
| G | SA7 | S. TYPHIMURIUM TA1537, REVERSE MUTATION | + + | 50.0000 | DUNKEL ET AL., 1985 |
| G | SA8 | S. TYPHIMURIUM TA1538, REVERSE MUTATION | + + | 0.0000 | SPANGGORD ET AL., 1982b |
| G | SA8 | S. TYPHIMURIUM TA1538, REVERSE MUTATION | + + | 17.0000 | DUNKEL ET AL., 1985 |
| G | SA9 | S. TYPHIMURIUM TA98, REVERSE MUTATION | + + | 0.0000 | SPANGGORD ET AL., 1982b |
| G | SA9 | S. TYPHIMURIUM TA98, REVERSE MUTATION | + + | 50.0000 | DUNKEL ET AL., 1985 |
| G | SA9 | S. TYPHIMURIUM TA98, REVERSE MUTATION | + + | 500.0000 | COUCH ET AL., 1987 |
| G | EC2 | E. COLI WP2, REVERSE MUTATION | - - | 1667.0000 | DUNKEL ET AL., 1985 |

# APPENDIX 1

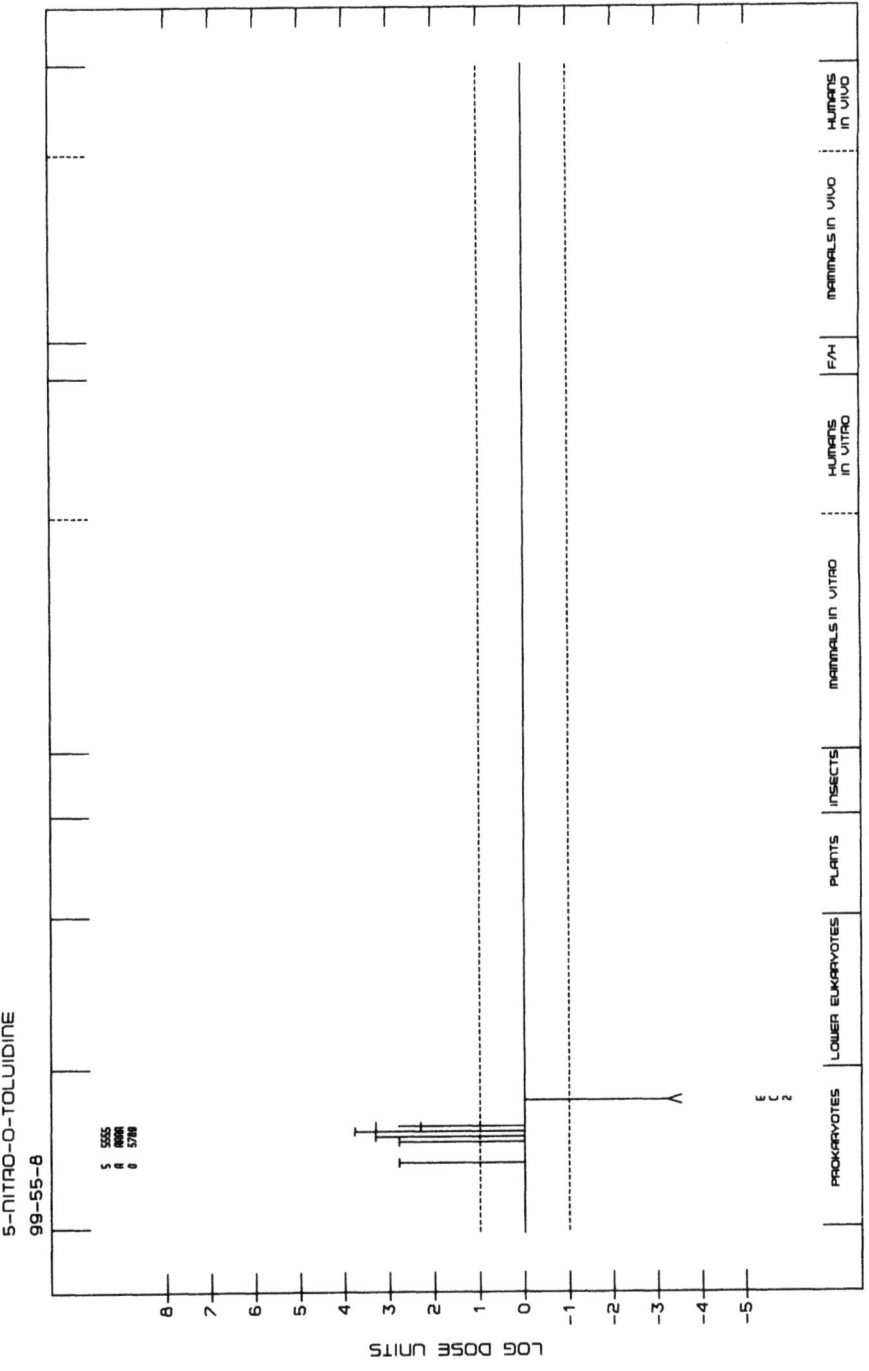

NITRILOTRIACETIC ACID

| END POINT | TEST CODE | TEST SYSTEM | RESULTS NM M | DOSE (LED OR HID) | REFERENCE |
|---|---|---|---|---|---|
| G | EC2 | E. COLI WP2, REVERSE MUTATION | − 0 | 4000.0000 | ZETTERBERG, 1970 |
| G | SCF | S. CEREVISIAE, FORWARD MUTATION | − 0 | 4000.0000 | ZETTERBERG, 1970 |
| G | SCR | S. CEREVISIAE, REVERSE MUTATION | − 0 | 4000.0000 | ZETTERBERG, 1970 |
| G | SZR | S. POMBE, REVERSE MUTATION | − 0 | 4000.0000 | ZETTERBERG, 1970 |
| G | DMX | D. MELANOGASTER, SEX-LINKED RECESSIVES | − 0 | 1911.0000 | KRAMERS, 1976 |
| G | DMX | D. MELANOGASTER, SEX-LINKED RECESSIVES | − 0 | 4000.0000 | WOODRUFF ET AL., 1985 |
| C | DML | D. MELANOGASTER, DOMINANT LETHALS | − 0 | 0.0000 | KRAMERS, 1976 |
| A | DMN | D. MELANOGASTER, ANEUPLOIDY | + 0 | 9557.0000 | COSTA ET AL., 1988a |
| A | DMN | D. MELANOGASTER, ANEUPLOIDY | + 0 | 4000.0000 | RAMEL & MAGNUSSON, 1979 |
| S | SIC | SCE, CHINESE HAMSTER CELLS IN VITRO | − − | 5.0000 | LOVEDAY ET AL., 1989 |
| C | CIC | CHROM ABERR, CHINESE HAMSTER CELLS IN VITRO | − − | 5.0000 | LOVEDAY ET AL., 1989 |
| C | DLM | DOMINANT LETHAL TEST, MICE | − 0 | 125.0000 | EPSTEIN ET AL., 1972 |
| A | AVA | ANEUPLOIDY, ANIMAL CELLS IN VIVO | + 0 | 275.0000 | COSTA ET AL., 1988a |

# APPENDIX 1

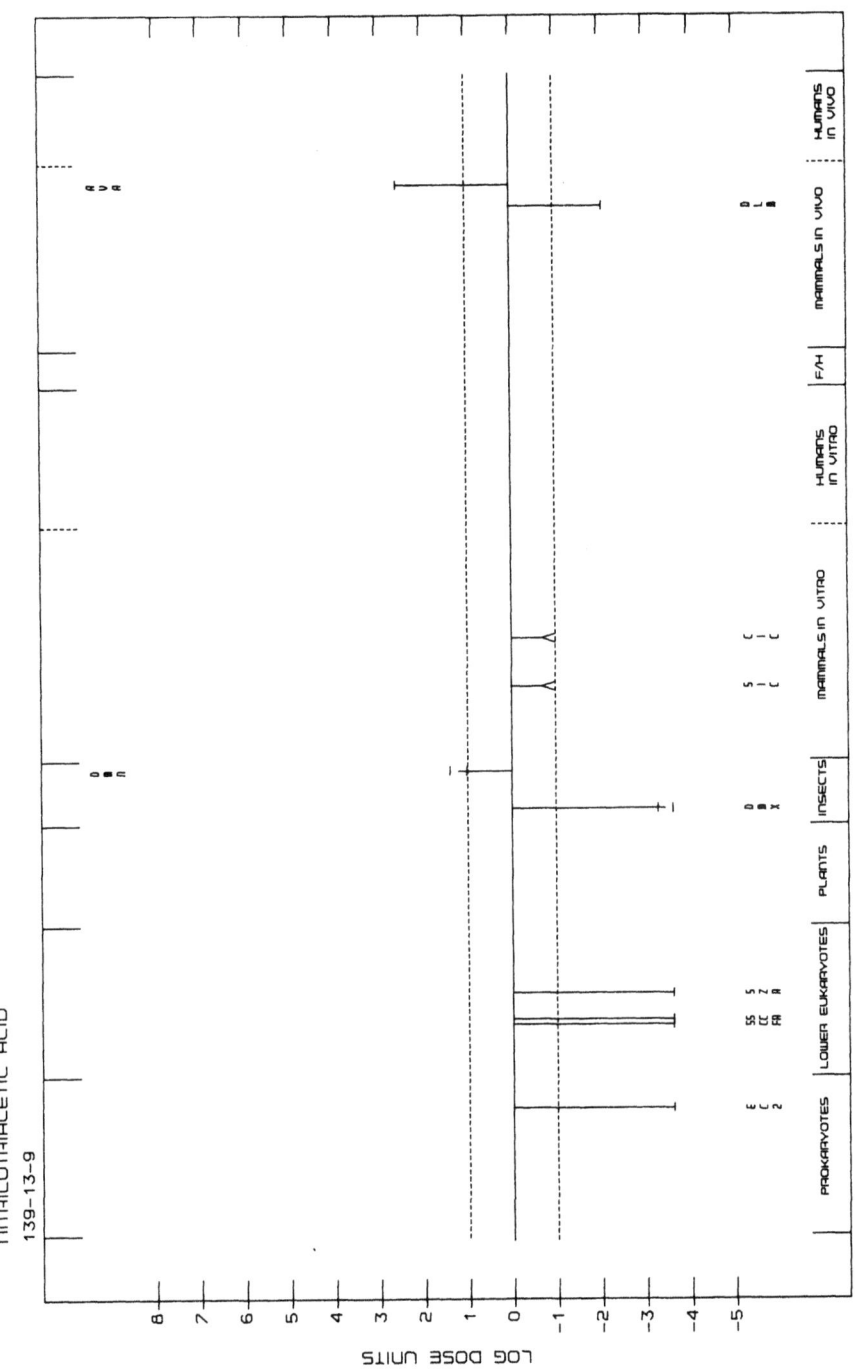

NITRILOTRIACETIC ACID 3NA SALT

| END POINT | TEST CODE | TEST SYSTEM | RESULTS NM | RESULTS M | DOSE (LED OR HID) | REFERENCE |
|---|---|---|---|---|---|---|
| D | PRB | PROPHAGE, INDUCT/SOS/STRAND BREAKS/X-LINKS | – | – | 0.0000 | VENIER ET AL., 1987 |
| D | ERD | E. COLI REC, DIFFERENTIAL TOXICITY | + | + | 250.0000 | VENIER ET AL., 1987 |
| G | SA0 | S. TYPHIMURIUM TA100, REVERSE MUTATION | – | | 435.0000 | LOPRIENO ET AL., 1985 |
| G | SA0 | S. TYPHIMURIUM TA100, REVERSE MUTATION | – | | 5000.0000 | DUNKEL ET AL., 1985 |
| G | SA0 | S. TYPHIMURIUM TA100, REVERSE MUTATION | – | | 435.0000 | VENIER ET AL., 1987 |
| G | SA5 | S. TYPHIMURIUM TA1535, REVERSE MUTATION | – | | 435.0000 | LOPRIENO ET AL., 1985 |
| G | SA5 | S. TYPHIMURIUM TA1535, REVERSE MUTATION | – | | 5000.0000 | DUNKEL ET AL., 1985 |
| G | SA7 | S. TYPHIMURIUM TA1537, REVERSE MUTATION | – | | 435.0000 | LOPRIENO ET AL., 1985 |
| G | SA7 | S. TYPHIMURIUM TA1537, REVERSE MUTATION | – | | 5000.0000 | DUNKEL ET AL., 1985 |
| G | SA8 | S. TYPHIMURIUM TA1538, REVERSE MUTATION | – | | 435.0000 | LOPRIENO ET AL., 1985 |
| G | SA8 | S. TYPHIMURIUM TA1538, REVERSE MUTATION | – | | 5000.0000 | DUNKEL ET AL., 1985 |
| G | SA9 | S. TYPHIMURIUM TA98, REVERSE MUTATION | – | | 435.0000 | LOPRIENO ET AL., 1985 |
| G | SA9 | S. TYPHIMURIUM TA98, REVERSE MUTATION | – | | 5000.0000 | DUNKEL ET AL., 1985 |
| G | ECW | E. COLI WP2 UVRA, REVERSE MUTATION | – | | 100000.0000 | VENIER ET AL., 1987 |
| R | SCG | S. CEREVISIAE, GENE CONVERSION | 0 | | 40.0000 | LOPRIENO ET AL., 1985 |
| R | ANG | A. NIDULANS, CROSSING-OVER | 0 | | 10930.0000 | CREBELLI ET AL., 1986 |
| G | SZF | S. POMBE, FORWARD MUTATION | – | | 40.0000 | LOPRIENO ET AL., 1985 |
| G | ANF | A. NIDULANS, FORWARD MUTATION | 0 | | 18510.0000 | CREBELLI ET AL., 1986 |
| A | ANN | A. NIDULANS, ANEUPLOIDY | 0 | | 10930.0000 | CREBELLI ET AL., 1986 |
| M | PLI | PLANTS (OTHER), MICRONUCLEI | + | | 550.0000 | DE MARCO ET AL., 1986 |
| C | VFC | VICIA FABA, CHROM ABERR | + | | 1375.0000 | KIHLMAN & STURELID, 1970 |
| D | URP | UDS, RAT PRIMARY HEPATOCYTES | 0 | | 1000.0000 | WILLIAMS ET AL., 1982 |
| G | G9H | MUTATION, CHL V79 CELLS, HPRT | 0 | | 1.5000 | CELOTTI ET AL., 1987 |
| G | G5T | MUTATION, L5178Y CELLS, TK LOCUS | – | | 2350.0000 | MITCHELL ET AL., 1985 |
| S | SIC | SCE, CHINESE HAMSTER CELLS IN VITRO | 0 | | 1.9000 | LOPRIENO ET AL., 1985 |
| S | SIC | SCE, CHINESE HAMSTER CELLS IN VITRO | – | | 1.0000 | VENIER ET AL., 1985 |
| S | SIC | SCE, CHINESE HAMSTER CELLS IN VITRO | 0 | | 275.0000 | VED BRAT & WILLIAMS, 1984 |
| S | SIC | SCE, CHINESE HAMSTER CELLS IN VITRO | 0 | | 514.0000 | MONTALDI ET AL., 1985 |
| S | SIM | SCE, MOUSE CELLS IN VITRO | – | | 257.0000 | MONTALDI ET AL., 1985 |

# APPENDIX 1

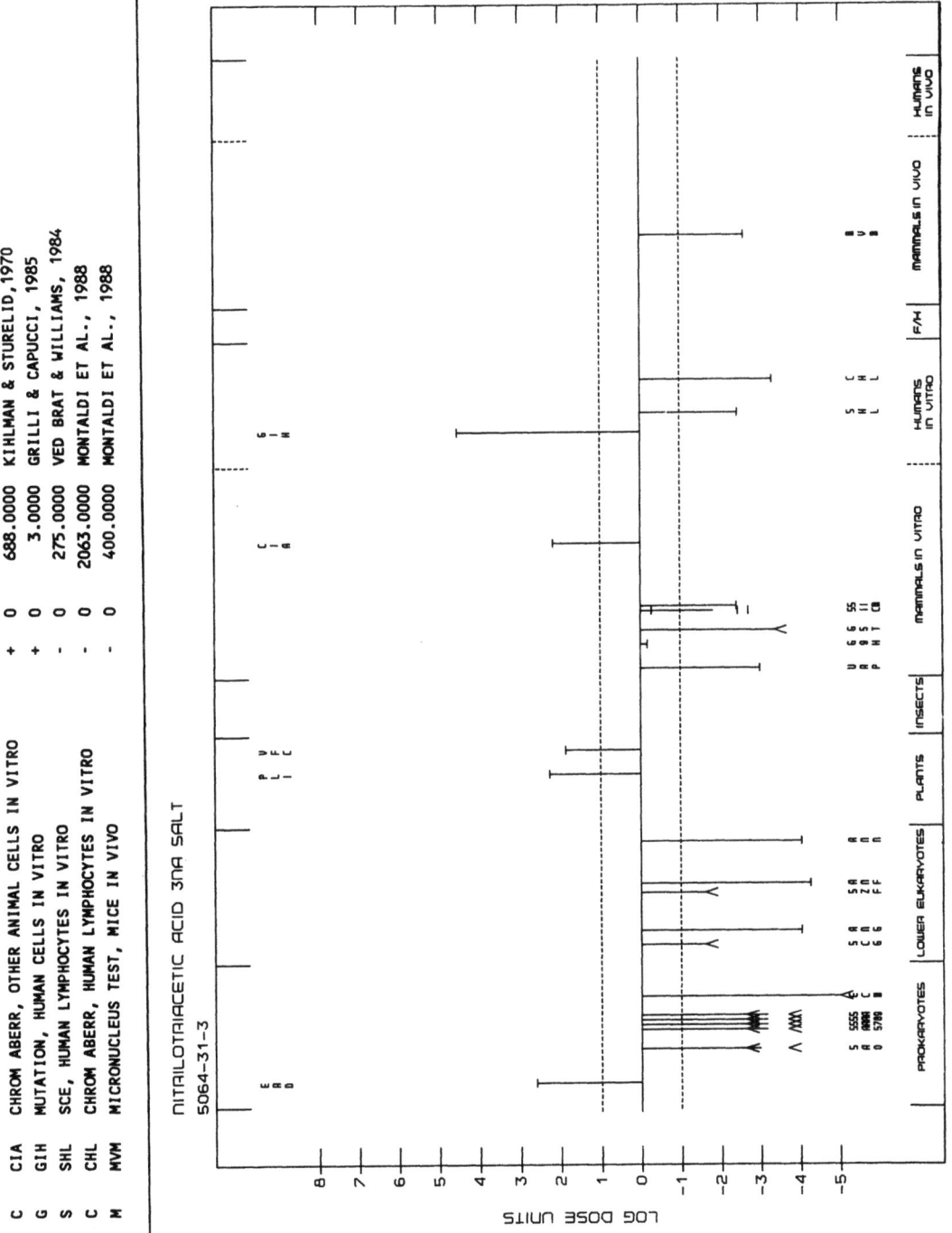

# CUMULATIVE CROSS INDEX TO *IARC MONOGRAPHS* ON THE EVALUATION OF CARCINOGENIC RISKS TO HUMANS

The volume, page and year are given. References to corrigenda are given in parentheses.

## A

| | |
|---|---|
| A-α-C | *40*, 245 (1986); *Suppl. 7*, 56 (1987) |
| Acetaldehyde | *36*, 101 (1985) (*corr. 42*, 263); *Suppl. 7*, 77 (1987) |
| Acetaldehyde formylmethylhydrazone (*see* Gyromitrin) | |
| Acetamide | *7*, 197 (1974); *Suppl. 7*, 389 (1987) |
| Acridine orange | *16*, 145 (1978); *Suppl. 7*, 56 (1987) |
| Acriflavinium chloride | *13*, 31 (1977); *Suppl. 7*, 56 (1987) |
| Acrolein | *19*, 479 (1979); *36*, 133 (1985); *Suppl. 7*, 78 (1987); |
| Acrylamide | *39*, 41 (1986); *Suppl. 7*, 56 (1987) |
| Acrylic acid | *19*, 47 (1979); *Suppl. 7*, 56 (1987) |
| Acrylic fibres | *19*, 86 (1979); *Suppl. 7*, 56 (1987) |
| Acrylonitrile | *19*, 73 (1979); *Suppl. 7*, 79 (1987) |
| Acrylonitrile-butadiene-styrene copolymers | *19*, 91 (1979); *Suppl. 7*, 56 (1987) |
| Actinolite (*see* Asbestos) | |
| Actinomycins | *10*, 29 (1976) (*corr. 42*, 255); *Suppl. 7*, 80 (1987) |
| Adriamycin | *10*, 43 (1976); *Suppl. 7*, 82 (1987) |
| AF-2 | *31*, 47 (1983); *Suppl. 7*, 56 (1987) |
| Aflatoxins | *1*, 145 (1972) (*corr. 42*, 251); *10*, 51 (1976); *Suppl. 7*, 83 (1987) |
| Aflatoxin B$_1$ (*see* Aflatoxins) | |
| Aflatoxin B$_2$ (*see* Aflatoxins) | |
| Aflatoxin G$_1$ (*see* Aflatoxins) | |
| Aflatoxin G$_2$ (*see* Aflatoxins) | |
| Aflatoxin M$_1$ (*see* Aflatoxins) | |
| Agaritine | *31*, 63 (1983); *Suppl. 7*, 56 (1987) |
| Alcohol drinking | *44* |
| Aldrin | *5*, 25 (1974); *Suppl. 7*, 88 (1987) |
| Allyl chloride | *36*, 39 (1985); *Suppl. 7*, 56 (1987) |

| | |
|---|---|
| Allyl isothiocyanate | *36*, 55 (1985); *Suppl. 7*, 56 (1987) |
| Allyl isovalerate | *36*, 69 (1985); *Suppl. 7*, 56 (1987) |
| Aluminium production | *34*, 37 (1984); *Suppl. 7*, 89 (1987) |
| Amaranth | *8*, 41 (1975); *Suppl. 7*, 56 (1987) |
| 5-Aminoacenaphthene | *16*, 243 (1978); *Suppl. 7*, 56 (1987) |
| 2-Aminoanthraquinone | *27*, 191 (1982); *Suppl. 7*, 56 (1987) |
| *para*-Aminoazobenzene | *8*, 53 (1975); *Suppl. 7*, 390 (1987) |
| *ortho*-Aminoazotoluene | *8*, 61 (1975) (*corr. 42*, 254); *Suppl. 7*, 56 (1987) |
| *para*-Aminobenzoic acid | *16*, 249 (1978); *Suppl. 7*, 56 (1987) |
| 4-Aminobiphenyl | *1*, 74 (1972) (*corr. 42*, 251); *Suppl. 7*, 91 (1987) |
| 2-Amino-3,4-dimethylimidazo[4,5-*f*]quinoline (*see* MeIQ) | |
| 2-Amino-3,8-dimethylimidazo[4,5-*f*]quinoxaline (*see* MeIQx) | |
| 3-Amino-1,4-dimethyl-5*H*-pyrido[4,3-*b*]indole (*see* Trp-P-1) | |
| 2-Aminodipyrido[1,2-*a*:3′,2′-*d*]imidazole (*see* Glu-P-2) | |
| 1-Amino-2-methylanthraquinone | *27*, 199 (1982); *Suppl. 7*, 57 (1987) |
| 2-Amino-3-methylimidazo[4,5-*f*]quinoline (*see* IQ) | |
| 2-Amino-6-methyldipyrido[1,2-*a*:3′,2′-*d*]-imidazole (*see* Glu-P-1) | |
| 2-Amino-3-methyl-9*H*-pyrido[2,3-*b*]indole (*see* MeA-α-C) | |
| 3-Amino-1-methyl-5*H*-pyrido[4,3-*b*]indole (*see* Trp-P-2) | |
| 2-Amino-5-(5-nitro-2-furyl)-1,3,4-thiadiazole | *7*, 143 (1974); *Suppl. 7*, 57 (1987) |
| 4-Amino-2-nitrophenol | *16*, 43 (1978); *Suppl.7*, 57 (1987) |
| 2-Amino-5-nitrothiazole | *31*, 71 (1983); *Suppl. 7*, 57 (1987) |
| 2-Amino-9*H*-pyrido[2,3-*b*]indole [*see* A-α-C] | |
| 11-Aminoundecanoic acid | *39*, 239 (1986); *Suppl. 7*, 57 (1987) |
| Amitrole | *7*, 31 (1974); *41*, 293 (1986) *Suppl. 7*, 92 (1987) |
| Ammonium potassium selenide (*see* Selenium and selenium compounds) | |
| Amorphous silica (*see also* Silica) | *Suppl. 7*, 341 (1987) |
| Amosite (*see* Asbestos) | |
| Anabolic steroids (*see* Androgenic (anabolic) steroids) | |
| Anaesthetics, volatile | *11*, 285 (1976); *Suppl. 7*, 93 (1987) |
| Analgesic mixtures containing phenacetin (*see also* Phenacetin) | *Suppl. 7*, 310 (1987) |
| Androgenic (anabolic) steroids | *Suppl. 7*, 96 (1987) |
| Angelicin and some synthetic derivatives (*see also* Angelicins) | *40*, 291 (1986) |
| Angelicin plus ultraviolet radiation (*see also* Angelicin and some synthetic derivatives) | *Suppl. 7*, 57 (1987) |
| Angelicins | *Suppl. 7*, 57 (1987) |
| Aniline | *4*, 27 (1974) (*corr. 42*, 252); *27*, 39 (1982); *Suppl. 7*, 99 (1987) |
| *ortho*-Anisidine | *27*, 63 (1982); *Suppl. 7*, 57 (1987) |
| *para*-Anisidine | *27*, 65 (1982); *Suppl. 7*, 57 (1987) |
| Anthanthrene | *32*, 95 (1983); *Suppl. 7*, 57 (1987) |

Anthophyllite (*see* Asbestos)
Anthracene                                          *32*, 105 (1983); *Suppl. 7*, 57 (1987)
Anthranilic acid                                    *16*, 265 (1978); *Suppl. 7*, 57 (1987)
Antimony trioxide                                   *47*, 291 (1989)
Antimony trisulfide                                 *47*, 291 (1989)
ANTU (*see* 1-Naphthylthiourea)

Apholate                                            *9*, 31 (1975); *Suppl. 7*, 57 (1987)
Aramite®                                            *5*, 39 (1974); *Suppl. 7*, 57 (1987)
Areca nut (*see* Betel quid)
Arsanilic acid (*see* Arsenic and arsenic compounds)
Arsenic and arsenic compounds                       *1*, 41 (1972); *2*, 48 (1973);
                                                    *23*, 39 (1980); *Suppl. 7*, 100 (1987)

Arsenic pentoxide (*see* Arsenic and arsenic compounds)
Arsenic sulphide (*see* Arsenic and arsenic compounds)
Arsenic trioxide (*see* Arsenic and arsenic compounds)
Arsine (*see* Arsenic and arsenic compounds)
Asbestos                                            *2*, 17 (1973) (*corr. 42*, 252);
                                                    *14* (1977) (*corr. 42*, 256); Suppl. 7,
                                                    106 (1987) (*corr. 45*, 283)
Attapulgite                                         *42*, 159 (1987); *Suppl. 7*, 117 (1987)
Auramine (technical-grade)                          *1*, 69 (1972) (*corr. 42*, 251); *Suppl.
                                                    7*, 118 (1987)
Auramine, manufacture of (*see also* Auramine, technical-grade)  *Suppl. 7*, 118 (1987)
Aurothioglucose                                     *13*, 39 (1977); *Suppl. 7*, 57 (1987)
5-Azacytidine                                       *26*, 37 (1981); *Suppl. 7*, 57 (1987)
Azaserine                                           *10*, 73 (1976) (*corr. 42*, 255);
                                                    *Suppl. 7*, 57 (1987)
Azathioprine                                        *26*, 47 (1981); *Suppl. 7*, 119 (1987)
Aziridine                                           *9*, 37 (1975); *Suppl. 7*, 58 (1987)
2-(1-Aziridinyl)ethanol                             *9*, 47 (1975); *Suppl. 7*, 58 (1987)
Aziridyl benzoquinone                               *9*, 51 (1975); *Suppl. 7*, 58 (1987)
Azobenzene                                          *8*, 75 (1975); *Suppl. 7*, 58 (1987)

# B

Barium chromate (*see* Chromium and chromium compounds)
Basic chromic sulphate (*see* Chromium and chromium compounds)
BCNU (*see* Bischloroethyl nitrosourea)
Benz[*a*]acridine                                   *32*, 123 (1983); *Suppl. 7*, 58 (1987)
Benz[*c*]acridine                                   *3*, 241 (1973); *32*, 129 (1983);
                                                    *Suppl. 7*, 58 (1987)
Benzal chloride (*see also* α-Chlorinated toluenes)  *29*, 65 (1982); *Suppl. 7*, 148 (1987)
Benz[*a*]anthracene                                 *3*, 45 (1973); *32*, 135 (1983);
                                                    *Suppl. 7*, 58 (1987)

| | |
|---|---|
| Benzene | 7, 203 (1974) (*corr.* 42, 254); 29, 93, 391 (1982); *Suppl.* 7, 120 (1987) |
| Benzidine | 1, 80 (1972); 29, 149, 391 (1982); *Suppl.* 7, 123 (1987) |
| Benzidine-based dyes | *Suppl.* 7, 125 (1987) |
| Benzo[*b*]fluoranthene | 3, 69 (1973); 32, 147 (1983); *Suppl.* 7, 58 (1987) |
| Benzo[*j*]fluoranthene | 3, 82 (1973); 32, 155 (1983); *Suppl.* 7, 58 (1987) |
| Benzo[*k*]fluoranthene | 32, 163 (1983); *Suppl.* 7, 58 (1987) |
| Benzo[*ghi*]fluoranthene | 32, 171 (1983); *Suppl.* 7, 58 (1987) |
| Benzo[*a*]fluorene | 32, 177 (1983); *Suppl.* 7, 58 (1987) |
| Benzo[*b*]fluorene | 32, 183 (1983); *Suppl.* 7, 58 (1987) |
| Benzo[*c*]fluorene | 32, 189 (1983); *Suppl.* 7, 58 (1987) |
| Benzo[*ghi*]perylene | 32, 195 (1983); *Suppl.* 7, 58 (1987) |
| Benzo[*c*]phenanthrene | 32, 205 (1983); *Suppl.* 7, 58 (1987) |
| Benzo[*a*]pyrene | 3, 91 (1973); 32, 211 (1983); *Suppl.* 7, 58 (1987) |
| Benzo[*e*]pyrene | 3, 137 (1973); 32, 225 (1983); *Suppl.* 7, 58 (1987) |
| *para*-Benzoquinone dioxime | 29, 185 (1982); *Suppl.* 7, 58 (1987) |
| Benzotrichloride (*see also* α-Chlorinated toluenes) | 29, 73 (1982); *Suppl.* 7, 148 (1987) |
| Benzoyl chloride | 29, 83 (1982) (*corr.* 42, 261); *Suppl.* 7, 126 (1987) |
| Benzoyl peroxide | 36, 267 (1985); *Suppl.* 7, 58 (1987) |
| Benzyl acetate | 40, 109 (1986); *Suppl.* 7, 58 (1987) |
| Benzyl chloride (*see also* α-Chlorinated toluenes) | 11, 217 (1976) (*corr.* 42, 256); 29, 49 (1982); *Suppl.* 7, 148 (1987) |
| Benzyl violet 4B | 16, 153 (1978); *Suppl.* 7, 58 (1987) |
| Bertrandite (*see* Beryllium and beryllium compounds) | |
| Beryllium and beryllium compounds | 1, 17 (1972); 23, 143 (1980) (*corr.* 42, 260); *Suppl.* 7, 127 (1987) |

Beryllium acetate (*see* Beryllium and beryllium compounds)
Beryllium acetate, basic (*see* Beryllium and beryllium compounds)
Beryllium–aluminium alloy (*see* Beryllium and beryllium compounds)
Beryllium carbonate (*see* Beryllium and beryllium compounds)
Beryllium chloride (*see* Beryllium and beryllium compounds)
Beryllium–copper alloy (*see* Beryllium and beryllium compounds)
Beryllium–copper–cobalt alloy (*see* Beryllium and beryllium compounds)
Beryllium fluoride (*see* Beryllium and beryllium compounds)
Beryllium hydroxide (*see* Beryllium and beryllium compounds)
Beryllium–nickel alloy (*see* Beryllium and beryllium compounds)
Beryllium oxide (*see* Beryllium and beryllium compounds)
Beryllium phosphate (*see* Beryllium and beryllium compounds)

Beryllium silicate (see Beryllium and beryllium compounds)
Beryllium sulphate (see Beryllium and beryllium compounds)
Beryl ore (see Beryllium and beryllium compounds)
Betel quid                                                                37, 141 (1985); Suppl. 7, 128 (1987)
Betel-quid chewing (see Betel quid)
BHA (see Butylated hydroxyanisole)
BHT (see Butylated hydroxytoluene)
Bis(1-aziridinyl)morpholinophosphine sulphide                             9, 55 (1975); Suppl. 7, 58 (1987)
Bis(2-chloroethyl)ether                                                   9, 117 (1975); Suppl. 7, 58 (1987)
N,N-Bis(2-chloroethyl)-2-naphthylamine                                    4, 119 (1974) (corr. 42, 253); Suppl. 7, 130 (1987)
Bischloroethyl nitrosourea (see also Chloroethyl nitrosoureas)            26, 79 (1981); Suppl. 7, 150 (1987)
1,2-Bis(chloromethoxy)ethane                                              15, 31 (1977); Suppl. 7, 58 (1987)
1,4-Bis(chloromethoxymethyl)benzene                                       15, 37 (1977); Suppl. 7, 58 (1987)
Bis(chloromethyl)ether                                                    4, 231 (1974) (corr. 42, 253); Suppl. 7, 131 (1987)
Bis(2-chloro-1-methylethyl)ether                                          41, 149 (1986); Suppl. 7, 59 (1987)
Bis(2,3-epoxycyclopentyl)ether                                            47, 231 (1989)
Bitumens                                                                  35, 39 (1985); Suppl. 7, 133 (1987)
Bleomycins                                                                26, 97 (1981); Suppl. 7, 134 (1987)
Blue VRS                                                                  16, 163 (1978); Suppl. 7, 59 (1987)
Boot and shoe manufacture and repair                                      25, 249 (1981); Suppl. 7, 232 (1987)
Bracken fern                                                              40, 47 (1986); Suppl. 7, 135 (1987)
Brilliant Blue FCF                                                        16, 171 (1978) (corr. 42, 257); Suppl. 7, 59 (1987)
1,3-Butadiene                                                             39, 155 (1986) (corr. 42, 264); Suppl. 7, 136 (1987)
1,4-Butanediol dimethanesulphonate                                        4, 247 (1974); Suppl. 7, 137 (1987)
n-Butyl acrylate                                                          39, 67 (1986); Suppl. 7, 59 (1987)
Butylated hydroxyanisole                                                  40, 123 (1986); Suppl. 7, 59 (1987)
Butylated hydroxytoluene                                                  40, 161 (1986); Suppl. 7, 59 (1987)
Butyl benzyl phthalate                                                    29, 193 (1982) (corr. 42, 261); Suppl. 7, 59 (1987)
β-Butyrolactone                                                           11, 225 (1976); Suppl. 7, 59 (1987)
γ-Butyrolactone                                                           11, 231 (1976); Suppl. 7, 59 (1987)

# C

Cabinet-making (see Furniture and cabinet-making)
Cadmium acetate (see Cadmium and cadmium compounds)
Cadmium and cadmium compounds                                             2, 74 (1973); 11, 39 (1976) (corr. 42, 255); Suppl. 7, 139 (1987)
Cadmium chloride (see Cadmium and cadmium compounds)
Cadmium oxide (see Cadmium and cadmium compounds)

Cadmium sulphate (*see* Cadmium and cadmium compounds)
Cadmium sulphide (*see* Cadmium and cadmium compounds)
Calcium arsenate (*see* Arsenic and arsenic compounds)
Calcium chromate (*see* Chromium and chromium compounds)
Calcium cyclamate (*see* Cyclamates)
Calcium saccharin (*see* Saccharin)

| | |
|---|---|
| Cantharidin | *10*, 79 (1976); *Suppl. 7*, 59 (1987) |
| Caprolactam | *19*, 115 (1979) (*corr. 42*, 258); *39*, 247 (1986) *(corr. 42*, 264); *Suppl. 7*, 390 (1987) |
| Captan | *30*, 295 (1983); *Suppl. 7*, 59 (1987) |
| Carbaryl | *12*, 37 (1976); *Suppl. 7*, 59 (1987) |
| Carbazole | *32*, 239 (1983); *Suppl. 7*, 59 (1987) |
| 3-Carbethoxypsoralen | *40*, 317 (1986); *Suppl. 7*, 59 (1987) |
| Carbon blacks | *3*, 22 (1973); *33*, 35 (1984); *Suppl. 7*, 142 (1987) |
| Carbon tetrachloride | *1*, 53 (1972); *20*, 371 (1979); *Suppl. 7*, 143 (1987) |
| Carmoisine | *8*, 83 (1975); *Suppl. 7*, 59 (1987) |
| Carpentry and joinery | *25*, 139 (1981); *Suppl. 7*, 378 (1987) |
| Carrageenan | *10*, 181 (1976) (*corr. 42*, 255); *31*, 79 (1983); *Suppl. 7*, 59 (1987) |
| Catechol | *15*, 155 (1977); *Suppl. 7*, 59 (1987) |

CCNU (*see* 1-(2-Chloroethyl)-3-cyclohexyl-1-nitrosourea)
Ceramic fibres (*see* Man-made mineral fibres)
Chemotherapy, combined, including alkylating agents
    (*see* MOPP and other combined chemotherapy including
    alkylating agents)

| | |
|---|---|
| Chlorambucil | *9*, 125 (1975); *26*, 115 (1981); *Suppl. 7*, 144 (1987) |
| Chloramphenicol | *10*, 85 (1976); *Suppl. 7*, 145 (1987) |
| Chlorendic acid | *48*, 45 (1990) |
| Chlordane (*see also* Chlordane/Heptachlor) | *20*, 45 (1979) (*corr. 42*, 258) |
| Chlordane/Heptachlor | *Suppl. 7*, 146 (1987) |
| Chlordecone | *20*, 67 (1979); *Suppl. 7*, 59 (1987) |
| Chlordimeform | *30*, 61 (1983); *Suppl. 7*, 59 (1987) |
| Chlorinated dibenzodioxins (other than TCDD) | *15*, 41 (1977); *Suppl. 7*, 59 (1987) |
| Chlorinated paraffins | *48*, 55 (1990) |
| α-Chlorinated toluenes | *Suppl. 7*, 148 (1987) |
| Chlormadinone acetate (*see also* Progestins; Combined oral contraceptives) | *6*, 149 (1974); *21*, 365 (1979) |

Chlornaphazine (*see* *N,N*-Bis(2-chloroethyl)-2-naphthylamine)

| | |
|---|---|
| Chlorobenzilate | *5*, 75 (1974); *30*, 73 (1983); *Suppl. 7*, 60 (1987) |
| Chlorodifluoromethane | *41*, 237 (1986); *Suppl. 7*, 149 (1987) |

| | |
|---|---|
| 1-(2-Chloroethyl)-3-cyclohexyl-1-nitrosourea (*see also* Chloroethyl nitrosoureas) | *26*, 137 (1981) (*corr. 42*, 260); *Suppl. 7*, 150 (1987) |
| 1-(2-Chloroethyl)-3-(4-methylcyclohexyl)-1-nitrosourea (*see also* Chloroethyl nitrosoureas) | *Suppl. 7*, 150 (1987) |
| Chloroethyl nitrosoureas | *Suppl. 7*, 150 (1987) |
| Chlorofluoromethane | *41*, 229 (1986); *Suppl. 7*, 60 (1987) |
| Chloroform | *1*, 61 (1972); *20*, 401 (1979); *Suppl. 7*, 152 (1987) |
| Chloromethyl methyl ether (technical-grade) (*see also* Bis(chloromethyl)ether) | *4*, 239 (1974) |
| (4-Chloro-2-methylphenoxy)acetic acid (*see* MCPA) | |
| Chlorophenols | *Suppl. 7*, 154 (1987) |
| Chlorophenols (occupational exposures to) | *41*, 319 (1986) |
| Chlorophenoxy herbicides | *Suppl. 7*, 156 (1987) |
| Chlorophenoxy herbicides (occupational exposures to) | *41*, 357 (1986) |
| 4-Chloro-*ortho*-phenylenediamine | *27*, 81 (1982); *Suppl. 7*, 60 (1987) |
| 4-Chloro-*meta*-phenylenediamine | *27*, 82 (1982); *Suppl. 7*, 60 (1987) |
| Chloroprene | *19*, 131 (1979); *Suppl. 7*, 160 (1987) |
| Chloropropham | *12*, 55 (1976); *Suppl. 7*, 60 (1987) |
| Chloroquine | *13*, 47 (1977); *Suppl. 7*, 60 (1987) |
| Chlorothalonil | *30*, 319 (1983); *Suppl. 7*, 60 (1987) |
| *para*-Chloro-*ortho*-toluidine and its strong acid salts (*see also* Chlordimeform) | *16*, 277 (1978); *30*, 65 (1983); *Suppl. 7*, 60 (1987); *48*, 123 (1990) |
| Chlorotrianisene (*see also* Nonsteroidal oestrogens) | *21*, 139 (1979) |
| 2-Chloro-1,1,1-trifluoroethane | *41*, 253 (1986); *Suppl. 7*, 60 (1987) |
| Cholesterol | *10*, 99 (1976); *31*, 95 (1983); *Suppl. 7*, 161 (1987) |
| Chromic acetate (*see* Chromium and chromium compounds) | |
| Chromic chloride (*see* Chromium and chromium compounds) | |
| Chromic oxide (*see* Chromium and chromium compounds) | |
| Chromic phosphate (*see* Chromium and chromium compounds) | |
| Chromite ore (*see* Chromium and chromium compounds) | |
| Chromium and chromium compounds | *2*, 100 (1973); *23*, 205 (1980); *Suppl. 7*, 165 (1987) |
| Chromium carbonyl (*see* Chromium and chromium compounds) | |
| Chromium potassium sulphate (*see* Chromium and chromium compounds) | |
| Chromium sulphate (*see* Chromium and chromium compounds) | |
| Chromium trioxide (*see* Chromium and chromium compounds) | |
| Chrysene | *3*, 159 (1973); *32*, 247 (1983); *Suppl. 7*, 60 (1987) |
| Chrysoidine | *8*, 91 (1975); *Suppl. 7*, 169 (1987) |
| Chrysotile (*see* Asbestos) | |
| CI Disperse Yellow 3 | *8*, 97 (1975); *Suppl. 7*, 60 (1987) |

| | |
|---|---|
| Cinnamyl anthranilate | *16*, 287 (1978); *31*, 133 (1983); *Suppl. 7*, 60 (1987) |
| Cisplatin | *26*, 151 (1981); *Suppl. 7*, 170 (1987) |
| Citrinin | *40*, 67 (1986); *Suppl. 7*, 60 (1987) |
| Citrus Red No. 2 | *8*, 101 (1975) (*corr. 42*, 254); *Suppl. 7*, 60 (1987) |
| Clofibrate | *24*, 39 (1980); *Suppl. 7*, 171 (1987) |
| Clomiphene citrate | *21*, 551 (1979); *Suppl. 7*, 172 (1987) |
| Coal gasification | *34*, 65 (1984); *Suppl. 7*, 173 (1987) |
| Coal-tar pitches (*see also* Coal-tars) | *Suppl. 7*, 174 (1987) |
| Coal-tars | *35*, 83 (1985); *Suppl. 7*, 175 (1987) |
| Cobalt–chromium alloy (*see* Chromium and chromium compounds) | |
| Coke production | *34*, 101 (1984); *Suppl. 7*, 176 (1987) |
| Combined oral contraceptives (*see also* Oestrogens, progestins and combinations) | *Suppl. 7*, 297 (1987) |
| Conjugated oestrogens (*see also* Steroidal oestrogens) | *21*, 147 (1979) |
| Contraceptives, oral (*see* Combined oral contraceptives; Sequential oral contraceptives) | |
| Copper 8-hydroxyquinoline | *15*, 103 (1977); *Suppl. 7*, 61 (1987) |
| Coronene | *32*, 263 (1983); *Suppl. 7*, 61 (1987) |
| Coumarin | *10*, 113 (1976); *Suppl. 7*, 61 (1987) |
| Creosotes (*see also* Coal-tars) | *Suppl. 7*, 177 (1987) |
| *meta*-Cresidine | *27*, 91 (1982); *Suppl. 7*, 61 (1987) |
| *para*-Cresidine | *27*, 92 (1982); *Suppl. 7*, 61 (1987) |
| Crocidolite (*see* Asbestos) | |
| Crude oil | *45*, 119 (1989) |
| Crystalline silica (*see also* Silica) | *Suppl. 7*, 341 (1987) |
| Cycasin | *1*, 157 (1972) (*corr. 42*, 251); *10*, 121 (1976); *Suppl. 7*, 61 (1987) |
| Cyclamates | *22*, 55 (1980); *Suppl. 7*, 178 (1987) |
| Cyclamic acid (*see* Cyclamates) | |
| Cyclochlorotine | *10*, 139 (1976); *Suppl. 7*, 61 (1987) |
| Cyclohexanone | *47*, 157 (1989) |
| Cyclohexylamine (*see* Cyclamates) | |
| Cyclopenta[*cd*]pyrene | *32*, 269 (1983); *Suppl. 7*, 61 (1987) |
| Cyclopropane (*see* Anaesthetics, volatile) | |
| Cyclophosphamide | *9*, 135 (1975); *26*, 165 (1981); *Suppl. 7*, 182 (1987) |

# D

| | |
|---|---|
| 2,4-D (*see also* Chlorophenoxy herbicides; Chlorophenoxy herbicides, occupational exposures to) | *15*, 111 (1977) |
| Dacarbazine | *26*, 203 (1981); *Suppl. 7*, 184 (1987) |

| | |
|---|---|
| D & C Red No. 9 | 8, 107 (1975); Suppl. 7, 61 (1987) |
| Dapsone | 24, 59 (1980); Suppl. 7, 185 (1987) |
| Daunomycin | 10, 145 (1976); Suppl. 7, 61 (1987) |
| DDD (see DDT) | |
| DDE (see DDT) | |
| DDT | 5, 83 (1974) (corr. 42, 253); Suppl. 7, 186 (1987) |
| Decabromodiphenyl oxide | 48, 73 (1990) |
| Diacetylaminoazotoluene | 8, 113 (1975); Suppl. 7, 61 (1987) |
| N,N'-Diacetylbenzidine | 16, 293 (1978); Suppl. 7, 61 (1987) |
| Diallate | 12, 69 (1976); 30, 235 (1983); Suppl. 7, 61 (1987) |
| 2,4-Diaminoanisole | 16, 51 (1978); 27, 103 (1982); Suppl. 7, 61 (1987) |
| 4,4'-Diaminodiphenyl ether | 16, 301 (1978); 29, 203 (1982); Suppl. 7, 61 (1987) |
| 1,2-Diamino-4-nitrobenzene | 16, 63 (1978); Suppl. 7, 61 (1987) |
| 1,4-Diamino-2-nitrobenzene | 16, 73 (1978); Suppl. 7, 61 (1987) |
| 2,6-Diamino-3-(phenylazo)pyridine (see Phenazopyridine hydrochloride) | |
| 2,4-Diaminotoluene (see also Toluene diisocyanates) | 16, 83 (1978); Suppl. 7, 61 (1987) |
| 2,5-Diaminotoluene (see also Toluene diisocyanates) | 16, 97 (1978); Suppl. 7, 61 (1987) |
| ortho-Dianisidine (see 3,3'-Dimethoxybenzidine) | |
| Diazepam | 13, 57 (1977); Suppl. 7, 189 (1987) |
| Diazomethane | 7, 223 (1974); Suppl. 7, 61 (1987) |
| Dibenz[a,h]acridine | 3, 247 (1973); 32, 277 (1983); Suppl. 7, 61 (1987) |
| Dibenz[a,j]acridine | 3, 254 (1973); 32, 283 (1983); Suppl. 7, 61 (1987) |
| Dibenz[a,c]anthracene | 32, 289 (1983) (corr. 42, 262); Suppl. 7, 61 (1987) |
| Dibenz[a,h]anthracene | 3, 178 (1973) (corr. 43, 261); 32, 299 (1983); Suppl. 7, 61 (1987) |
| Dibenz[a,j]anthracene | 32, 309 (1983); Suppl. 7, 61 (1987) |
| 7H-Dibenzo[c,g]carbazole | 3, 260 (1973); 32, 315 (1983); Suppl. 7, 61 (1987) |
| Dibenzodioxins, chlorinated (other than TCDD) (see Chlorinated dibenzodioxins (other than TCDD)) | |
| Dibenzo[a,e]fluoranthene | 32, 321 (1983); Suppl. 7, 61 (1987) |
| Dibenzo[h,rst]pentaphene | 3, 197 (1973); Suppl. 7, 62 (1987) |
| Dibenzo[a,e]pyrene | 3, 201 (1973); 32, 327 (1983); Suppl. 7, 62 (1987) |
| Dibenzo[a,h]pyrene | 3, 207 (1973); 32, 331 (1983); Suppl. 7, 62 (1987) |

| | |
|---|---|
| Dibenzo[*a,i*]pyrene | *3*, 215 (1973); *32*, 337 (1983); *Suppl.* 7, 62 (1987) |
| Dibenzo[*a,l*]pyrene | *3*, 224 (1973); *32*, 343 (1983); *Suppl.* 7, 62 (1987) |
| 1,2-Dibromo-3-chloropropane | *15*, 139 (1977); *20*, 83 (1979); *Suppl.* 7, 191 (1987) |
| Dichloroacetylene | *39*, 369 (1986); *Suppl.* 7, 62 (1987) |
| *ortho*-Dichlorobenzene | *7*, 231 (1974); *29*, 213 (1982); *Suppl.* 7, 192 (1987) |
| *para*-Dichlorobenzene | *7*, 231 (1974); *29*, 215 (1982); *Suppl.* 7, 192 (1987) |
| 3,3′-Dichlorobenzidine | *4*, 49 (1974); *29*, 239 (1982); *Suppl.* 7, 193 (1987) |
| *trans*-1,4-Dichlorobutene | *15*, 149 (1977); *Suppl.* 7, 62 (1987) |
| 3,3′-Dichloro-4,4′-diaminodiphenyl ether | *16*, 309 (1978); *Suppl.* 7, 62 (1987) |
| 1,2-Dichloroethane | *20*, 429 (1979); *Suppl.* 7, 62 (1987) |
| Dichloromethane | *20*, 449 (1979); *41*, 43 (1986); *Suppl.* 7, 194 (1987) |
| 2,4-Dichlorophenol (*see* Chlorophenols; Chlorophenols, occupational exposures to) | |
| (2,4-Dichlorophenoxy)acetic acid (*see* 2,4-D) | |
| 2,6-Dichloro-*para*-phenylenediamine | *39*, 325 (1986); *Suppl.* 7, 62 (1987) |
| 1,2-Dichloropropane | *41*, 131 (1986); *Suppl.* 7, 62 (1987) |
| 1,3-Dichloropropene (technical-grade) | *41*, 113 (1986); *Suppl.* 7, 195 (1987) |
| Dichlorvos | *20*, 97 (1979); *Suppl.* 7, 62 (1987) |
| Dicofol | *30*, 87 (1983); *Suppl.* 7, 62 (1987) |
| Dicyclohexylamine (*see* Cyclamates) | |
| Dieldrin | *5*, 125 (1974); *Suppl.* 7, 196 (1987) |
| Dienoestrol (*see also* Nonsteroidal oestrogens) | *21*, 161 (1979) |
| Diepoxybutane | *11*, 115 (1976) (*corr.* 42, 255); *Suppl.* 7, 62 (1987) |
| Diesel and gasoline engine exhausts | *46*, 41 (1989) |
| Diesel fuels | *45*, 219 (1989) (*corr.* 47, 505) |
| Diethyl ether (*see* Anaesthetics, volatile) | |
| Di(2-ethylhexyl)adipate | *29*, 257 (1982); *Suppl.* 7, 62 (1987) |
| Di(2-ethylhexyl)phthalate | *29*, 269 (1982) (*corr.* 42, 261); *Suppl.* 7, 62 (1987) |
| 1,2-Diethylhydrazine | *4*, 153 (1974); *Suppl.* 7, 62 (1987) |
| Diethylstilboestrol | *6*, 55 (1974); *21*, 173 (1979) (*corr.* 42, 259); *Suppl.* 7, 273 (1987) |
| Diethylstilboestrol dipropionate (*see* Diethylstilboestrol) | |
| Diethyl sulphate | *4*, 277 (1974); *Suppl.* 7, 198 (1987) |
| Diglycidyl resorcinol ether | *11*, 125 (1976); *36*, 181 (1985); *Suppl.* 7, 62 (1987) |

| | |
|---|---|
| Dihydrosafrole | *1*, 170 (1972); *10*, 233 (1976); *Suppl. 7*, 62 (1987) |
| Dihydroxybenzenes (*see* Catechol; Hydroquinone; Resorcinol) | |
| Dihydroxymethylfuratrizine | *24*, 77 (1980); *Suppl. 7*, 62 (1987) |
| Dimethisterone (*see also* Progestins; Sequential oral contraceptives) | *6*, 167 (1974); *21*, 377 (1979) |
| Dimethoxane | *15*, 177 (1977); *Suppl. 7*, 62 (1987) |
| 3,3'-Dimethoxybenzidine | *4*, 41 (1974); *Suppl. 7*, 198 (1987) |
| 3,3'-Dimethoxybenzidine-4,4'-diisocyanate | *39*, 279 (1986); *Suppl. 7*, 62 (1987) |
| *para*-Dimethylaminoazobenzene | *8*, 125 (1975); *Suppl. 7*, 62 (1987) |
| *para*-Dimethylaminoazobenzenediazo sodium sulphonate | *8*, 147 (1975); *Suppl. 7*, 62 (1987) |
| *trans*-2-[(Dimethylamino)methylimino]-5-[2-(5-nitro-2-furyl)-vinyl]-1,3,4-oxadiazole | *7*, 147 (1974) (*corr. 42*, 253); *Suppl. 7*, 62 (1987) |
| 4,4'-Dimethylangelicin plus ultraviolet radiation (*see also* Angelicin and some synthetic derivatives) | *Suppl. 7*, 57 (1987) |
| 4,5'-Dimethylangelicin plus ultraviolet radiation (*see also* Angelicin and some synthetic derivatives) | *Suppl. 7*, 57 (1987) |
| Dimethylarsinic acid (*see* Arsenic and arsenic compounds) | |
| 3,3'-Dimethylbenzidine | *1*, 87 (1972); *Suppl. 7*, 62 (1987) |
| Dimethylcarbamoyl chloride | *12*, 77 (1976); *Suppl. 7*, 199 (1987) |
| Dimethylformamide | *47*, 171 (1989) |
| 1,1-Dimethylhydrazine | *4*, 137 (1974); *Suppl.7*, 62 (1987) |
| 1,2-Dimethylhydrazine | *4*, 145 (1974) (*corr. 42*, 253); *Suppl. 7*, 62 (1987) |
| Dimethyl hydrogen phosphite | *48*, 85 (1990) |
| 1,4-Dimethylphenanthrene | *32*, 349 (1983); *Suppl. 7*, 62 (1987) |
| Dimethyl sulphate | *4*, 271 (1974); *Suppl. 7*, 200 (1987) |
| 3,7-Dinitrofluoranthene | *46*, 189 (1989) |
| 3,9-Dinitrofluoranthene | *46*, 195 (1989) |
| 1,3-Dinitropyrene | *46*, 201 (1989) |
| 1,6-Dinitropyrene | *46*, 215 (1989) |
| 1,8-Dinitropyrene | *33*, 171 (1984); *Suppl. 7*, 63 (1987); *46*, 231 (1989) |
| Dinitrosopentamethylenetetramine | *11*, 241 (1976); *Suppl. 7*, 63 (1987) |
| 1,4-Dioxane | *11*, 247 (1976); *Suppl. 7*, 201 (1987) |
| 2,4'-Diphenyldiamine | *16*, 313 (1978); *Suppl. 7*, 63 (1987) |
| Direct Black 38 (*see also* Benzidine-based dyes) | *29*, 295 (1982) (*corr. 42*, 261) |
| Direct Blue 6 (*see also* Benzidine-based dyes) | *29*, 311 (1982) |
| Direct Brown 95 (*see also* Benzidine-based dyes) | *29*, 321 (1982) |
| Disperse Blue 1 | *48*, 139 (1990) |
| Disperse Yellow 3 | *48*, 149 (1990) |
| Disulfiram | *12*, 85 (1976); *Suppl. 7*, 63 (1987) |
| Dithranol | *13*, 75 (1977); *Suppl. 7*, 63 (1987) |
| Divinyl ether (*see* Anaesthetics, volatile) | |

| | |
|---|---|
| Dulcin | 12, 97 (1976); Suppl. 7, 63 (1987) |

## E

| | |
|---|---|
| Endrin | 5, 157 (1974); Suppl. 7, 63 (1987) |
| Enflurane (see Anaesthetics, volatile) | |
| Eosin | 15, 183 (1977); Suppl. 7, 63 (1987) |
| Epichlorohydrin | 11, 131 (1976) (corr. 42, 256); Suppl. 7, 202 (1987) |
| 1,2-Epoxybutane | 47, 217 (1989) |
| 1-Epoxyethyl-3,4-epoxycyclohexane | 11, 141 (1976); Suppl. 7, 63 (1987) |
| 3,4-Epoxy-6-methylcyclohexylmethyl-3,4-epoxy-6-methyl-cyclohexane carboxylate | 11, 147 (1976); Suppl. 7, 63 (1987) |
| cis-9,10-Epoxystearic acid | 11, 153 (1976); Suppl. 7, 63 (1987) |
| Erionite | 42, 225 (1987); Suppl. 7, 203 (1987) |
| Ethinyloestradiol (see also Steroidal oestrogens) | 6, 77 (1974); 21, 233 (1979) |
| Ethionamide | 13, 83 (1977); Suppl. 7, 63 (1987) |
| Ethyl acrylate | 19, 57 (1979); 39, 81 (1986); Suppl. 7, 63 (1987) |
| Ethylene | 19, 157 (1979); Suppl. 7, 63 (1987) |
| Ethylene dibromide | 15, 195 (1977); Suppl. 7, 204 (1987) |
| Ethylene oxide | 11, 157 (1976); 36, 189 (1985) (corr. 42, 263); Suppl. 7, 205 (1987) |
| Ethylene sulphide | 11, 257 (1976); Suppl. 7, 63 (1987) |
| Ethylene thiourea | 7, 45 (1974); Suppl. 7, 207 (1987) |
| Ethyl methanesulphonate | 7, 245 (1974); Suppl. 7, 63 (1987) |
| N-Ethyl-N-nitrosourea | 1, 135 (1972); 17, 191 (1978); Suppl. 7, 63 (1987) |
| Ethyl selenac (see also Selenium and selenium compounds) | 12, 107 (1976); Suppl. 7, 63 (1987) |
| Ethyl tellurac | 12, 115 (1976); Suppl. 7, 63 (1987) |
| Ethynodiol diacetate (see also Progestins; Combined oral contraceptives) | 6, 173 (1974); 21, 387 (1979) |
| Eugenol | 36, 75 (1985); Suppl. 7, 63 (1987) |
| Evans blue | 8, 151 (1975); Suppl. 7, 63 (1987) |

## F

| | |
|---|---|
| Fast Green FCF | 16, 187 (1978); Suppl. 7, 63 (1987) |
| Ferbam | 12, 121 (1976) (corr. 42, 256); Suppl. 7, 63 (1987) |
| Ferric oxide | 1, 29 (1972); Suppl. 7, 216 (1987) |
| Ferrochromium (see Chromium and chromium compounds) | |
| Fluometuron | 30, 245 (1983); Suppl. 7, 63 (1987) |
| Fluoranthene | 32, 355 (1983); Suppl. 7, 63 (1987) |

| | |
|---|---|
| Fluorene | *32*, 365 (1983); *Suppl. 7*, 63 (1987) |
| Fluorides (inorganic, used in drinking-water) | *27*, 237 (1982); *Suppl. 7*, 208 (1987) |
| 5-Fluorouracil | *26*, 217 (1981); *Suppl. 7*, 210 (1987) |
| Fluorspar (*see* Fluorides) | |
| Fluosilicic acid (*see* Fluorides) | |
| Fluroxene (*see* Anaesthetics, volatile) | |
| Formaldehyde | *29*, 345 (1982); *Suppl. 7*, 211 (1987) |
| 2-(2-Formylhydrazino)-4-(5-nitro-2-furyl)thiazole | *7*, 151 (1974) (*corr. 42*, 253); *Suppl. 7*, 63 (1987) |
| Fuel oils (heating oils) | *45*, 239 (1989) (*corr. 47*, 505) |
| Furazolidone | *31*, 141 (1983); *Suppl. 7*, 63 (1987) |
| Furniture and cabinet-making | *25*, 99 (1981); *Suppl. 7*, 380 (1987) |
| 2-(2-Furyl)-3-(5-nitro-2-furyl)acrylamide (*see* AF-2) | |
| Fusarenon-X | *11*, 169 (1976); *31*, 153 (1983); *Suppl. 7*, 64 (1987) |

## G

| | |
|---|---|
| Gasoline | *45*, 159 (1989) (*corr. 47*, 505) |
| Gasoline engine exhaust (*see* Diesel and gasoline engine exhausts) | |
| Glass fibres (*see* Man-made mineral fibres) | |
| Glasswool (*see* Man-made mineral fibres) | |
| Glass filaments (*see* Man-made mineral fibres) | |
| Glu-P-1 | *40*, 223 (1986); *Suppl. 7*, 64 (1987) |
| Glu-P-2 | *40*, 235 (1986); *Suppl. 7*, 64 (1987) |
| L-Glutamic acid, 5-[2-(4-hydroxymethyl)phenylhydrazide] (*see* Agaratine) | |
| Glycidaldehyde | *11*, 175 (1976); *Suppl. 7*, 64 (1987) |
| Some glycidyl ethers | *47*, 237 (1989) |
| Glycidyl oleate | *11*, 183 (1976); *Suppl. 7*, 64 (1987) |
| Glycidyl stearate | *11*, 187 (1976); *Suppl. 7*, 64 (1987) |
| Griseofulvin | *10*, 153 (1976); *Suppl. 7*, 391 (1987) |
| Guinea Green B | *16*, 199 (1978); *Suppl. 7*, 64 (1987) |
| Gyromitrin | *31*, 163 (1983); *Suppl. 7*, 391 (1987) |

## H

| | |
|---|---|
| Haematite | *1*, 29 (1972); *Suppl. 7*, 216 (1987) |
| Haematite and ferric oxide | *Suppl. 7*, 216 (1987) |
| Haematite mining, underground, with exposure to radon | *1*, 29 (1972); *Suppl. 7*, 216 (1987) |
| Hair dyes, epidemiology of | *16*, 29 (1978); *27*, 307 (1982) |
| Halothane (*see* Anaesthetics, volatile) | |
| α-HCH (*see* Hexachlorocyclohexanes) | |
| β-HCH (*see* Hexachlorocyclohexanes) | |

γ-HCH (see Hexachlorocyclohexanes)
Heating oils (see Fuel oils)
Heptachlor (see also Chlordane/Heptachlor)  5, 173 (1974); 20, 129 (1979)
Hexachlorobenzene  20, 155 (1979); Suppl. 7, 219 (1987)
Hexachlorobutadiene  20, 179 (1979); Suppl. 7, 64 (1987)
Hexachlorocyclohexanes  5, 47 (1974); 20, 195 (1979)
 (corr. 42, 258); Suppl. 7, 220 (1987)
Hexachlorocyclohexane, technical-grade (see Hexachlorocyclohexanes)
Hexachloroethane  20, 467 (1979); Suppl. 7, 64 (1987)
Hexachlorophene  20, 241 (1979); Suppl. 7, 64 (1987)
Hexamethylphosphoramide  15, 211 (1977); Suppl. 7, 64 (1987)
Hexoestrol (see Nonsteroidal oestrogens)
Hycanthone mesylate  13, 91 (1977); Suppl. 7, 64 (1987)
Hydralazine  24, 85 (1980); Suppl. 7, 222 (1987)
Hydrazine  4, 127 (1974); Suppl. 7, 223 (1987)
Hydrogen peroxide  36, 285 (1985); Suppl. 7, 64 (1987)
Hydroquinone  15, 155 (1977); Suppl. 7, 64 (1987)
4-Hydroxyazobenzene  8, 157 (1975); Suppl. 7, 64 (1987)
17α-Hydroxyprogesterone caproate (see also Progestins)  21, 399 (1979) (corr. 42, 259)
8-Hydroxyquinoline  13, 101 (1977); Suppl. 7, 64 (1987)
8-Hydroxysenkirkine  10, 265 (1976); Suppl. 7, 64 (1987)

# I

Indeno[1,2,3-cd]pyrene  3, 229 (1973); 32, 373 (1983);
 Suppl. 7, 64 (1987)
IQ  40, 261 (1986); Suppl. 7, 64 (1987)
Iron and steel founding  34, 133 (1984); Suppl. 7, 224 (1987)
Iron-dextran complex  2, 161 (1973); Suppl. 7, 226 (1987)
Iron-dextrin complex  2, 161 (1973) (corr. 42, 252);
 Suppl. 7, 64 (1987)
Iron oxide (see Ferric oxide)
Iron oxide, saccharated (see Saccharated iron oxide)
Iron sorbitol-citric acid complex  2, 161 (1973); Suppl. 7, 64 (1987)
Isatidine  10, 269 (1976); Suppl. 7, 65 (1987)
Isoflurane (see Anaesthetics, volatile)
Isoniazid (see Isonicotinic acid hydrazide)
Isonicotinic acid hydrazide  4, 159 (1974); Suppl. 7, 227 (1987)
Isophosphamide  26, 237 (1981); Suppl. 7, 65 (1987)
Isopropyl alcohol  15, 223 (1977); Suppl. 7, 229 (1987)
Isopropyl alcohol manufacture (strong-acid process)  Suppl. 7, 229 (1987)
 (see also Isopropyl alcohol)
Isopropyl oils  15, 223 (1977); Suppl. 7, 229 (1987)
Isosafrole  1, 169 (1972); 10, 232 (1976);
 Suppl. 7, 65 (1987)

## J

Jacobine　　　　　　　　　　　　　　　　　　　　　　　*10*, 275 (1976); *Suppl. 7*, 65 (1987)
Jet fuel　　　　　　　　　　　　　　　　　　　　　　　*45*, 203 (1989)
Joinery (*see* Carpentry and joinery)

## K

Kaempferol　　　　　　　　　　　　　　　　　　　　　31, 171 (1983); *Suppl. 7*, 65 (1987)
Kepone (*see* Chlordecone)

## L

Lasiocarpine　　　　　　　　　　　　　　　　　　　　*10*, 281 (1976); *Suppl. 7*, 65 (1987)
Lauroyl peroxide　　　　　　　　　　　　　　　　　　*36*, 315 (1985); Suppl. 7, 65 (1987)
Lead acetate (*see* Lead and lead compounds)
Lead and lead compounds　　　　　　　　　　　　　　*1*, 40 (1972) (*corr. 42*, 251); 2, 52,
　　　　　　　　　　　　　　　　　　　　　　　　　　150 (1973); *12*, 131 (1976);
　　　　　　　　　　　　　　　　　　　　　　　　　　23, 40, 208, 209, 325 (1980);
　　　　　　　　　　　　　　　　　　　　　　　　　　*Suppl. 7*, 230 (1987)

Lead arsenate (*see* Arsenic and arsenic compounds)
Lead carbonate (*see* Lead and lead compounds)
Lead chloride (*see* Lead and lead compounds)
Lead chromate (*see* Chromium and chromium compounds)
Lead chromate oxide (*see* Chromium and chromium compounds)
Lead naphthenate (*see* Lead and lead compounds)
Lead nitrate (*see* Lead and lead compounds)
Lead oxide (*see* Lead and lead compounds)
Lead phosphate (*see* Lead and lead compounds)
Lead subacetate (*see* Lead and lead compounds)
Lead tetroxide (*see* Lead and lead compounds)
Leather goods manufacture　　　　　　　　　　　　　　*25*, 279 (1981); *Suppl. 7*, 235 (1987)
Leather industries　　　　　　　　　　　　　　　　　　*25*, 199 (1981); *Suppl. 7*, 232 (1987)
Leather tanning and processing　　　　　　　　　　　　*25*, 201 (1981); *Suppl. 7*, 236 (1987)
Ledate (*see also* Lead and lead compounds)　　　　　　*12*, 131 (1976)
Light Green SF　　　　　　　　　　　　　　　　　　　*16*, 209 (1978); *Suppl. 7*, 65 (1987)
Lindane (*see* Hexachlorocyclohexanes)
The lumber and sawmill industries (including logging)　　*25*, 49 (1981); *Suppl. 7*, 383 (1987)
Luteoskyrin　　　　　　　　　　　　　　　　　　　　　*10*, 163 (1976); *Suppl. 7*, 65 (1987)
Lynoestrenol (*see also* Progestins; Combined oral contraceptives)　*21*, 407 (1979)

## M

Magenta　　　　　　　　　　　　　　　　　　　　　　*4*, 57 (1974) (*corr. 42*, 252);
　　　　　　　　　　　　　　　　　　　　　　　　　　*Suppl. 7*, 238 (1987)

| | |
|---|---|
| Magenta, manufacture of (*see also* Magenta) | *Suppl. 7*, 238 (1987) |
| Malathion | *30*, 103 (1983); *Suppl. 7*, 65 (1987) |
| Maleic hydrazide | *4*, 173 (1974) (*corr. 42*, 253); *Suppl. 7*, 65 (1987) |
| Malonaldehyde | *36*, 163 (1985); *Suppl. 7*, 65 (1987) |
| Maneb | *12*, 137 (1976); *Suppl. 7*, 65 (1987) |
| Man-made mineral fibres | *43*, 39 (1988) |
| Mannomustine | *9*, 157 (1975); *Suppl. 7*, 65 (1987) |
| MCPA (*see also* Chlorophenoxy herbicides; Chlorophenoxy herbicides, occupational exposures to) | *30*, 255 (1983) |
| MeA-α-C | *40*, 253 (1986); *Suppl. 7*, 65 (1987) |
| Medphalan | *9*, 168 (1975); *Suppl. 7*, 65 (1987) |
| Medroxyprogesterone acetate | *6*, 157 (1974); *21*, 417 (1979) (*corr. 42*, 259); *Suppl. 7*, 289 (1987) |
| Megestrol acetate (*see also* Progestins; Combined oral contraceptives) | |
| MeIQ | *40*, 275 (1986); *Suppl. 7*, 65 (1987) |
| MeIQx | *40*, 283 (1986); *Suppl. 7*, 65 (1987) |
| Melamine | *39*, 333 (1986); *Suppl. 7*, 65 (1987) |
| Melphalan | *9*, 167 (1975); *Suppl. 7*, 239 (1987) |
| 6-Mercaptopurine | *26*, 249 (1981); *Suppl. 7*, 240 (1987) |
| Merphalan | *9*, 169 (1975); *Suppl. 7*, 65 (1987) |
| Mestranol (*see also* Steroidal oestrogens) | *6*, 87 (1974); *21*, 257 (1979) (*corr. 42*, 259) |
| Methanearsonic acid, disodium salt (*see* Arsenic and arsenic compounds) | |
| Methanearsonic acid, monosodium salt (*see* Arsenic and arsenic compounds | |
| Methotrexate | *26*, 267 (1981); *Suppl. 7*, 241 (1987) |
| Methoxsalen (*see* 8-Methoxypsoralen) | |
| Methoxychlor | *5*, 193 (1974); *20*, 259 (1979); *Suppl. 7*, 66 (1987) |
| Methoxyflurane (*see* Anaesthetics, volatile) | |
| 5-Methoxypsoralen | *40*, 327 (1986); *Suppl. 7*, 242 (1987) |
| 8-Methoxypsoralen (*see also* 8-Methoxypsoralen plus ultraviolet radiation) | *24*, 101 (1980) |
| 8-Methoxypsoralen plus ultraviolet radiation | *Suppl. 7*, 243 (1987) |
| Methyl acrylate | *19*, 52 (1979); *39*, 99 (1986); *Suppl. 7*, 66 (1987) |
| 5-Methylangelicin plus ultraviolet radiation (*see also* Angelicin and some synthetic derivatives) | *Suppl. 7*, 57 (1987) |
| 2-Methylaziridine | *9*, 61 (1975); *Suppl. 7*, 66 (1987) |
| Methylazoxymethanol acetate | *1*, 164 (1972); *10*, 131 (1976); *Suppl. 7*, 66 (1987) |

| | |
|---|---|
| Methyl bromide | *41*, 187 (1986) (*corr. 45*, 283); *Suppl. 7*, 245 (1987) |
| Methyl carbamate | *12*, 151 (1976); *Suppl. 7*, 66 (1987) |
| Methyl-CCNU [*see* 1-(2-Chloroethyl)-3-(4-methylcyclohexyl)-1-nitrosourea] | |
| Methyl chloride | *41*, 161 (1986); *Suppl. 7*, 246 (1987) |
| 1-, 2-, 3-, 4-, 5- and 6-Methylchrysenes | *32*, 379 (1983); *Suppl. 7*, 66 (1987) |
| *N*-Methyl-*N*,4-dinitrosoaniline | *1*, 141 (1972); *Suppl. 7*, 66 (1987) |
| 4,4'-Methylene bis(2-chloroaniline) | *4*, 65 (1974) (*corr. 42*, 252); *Suppl. 7*, 246 (1987) |
| 4,4'-Methylene bis(*N*,*N*-dimethyl)benzenamine | *27*, 119 (1982); *Suppl. 7*, 66 (1987) |
| 4,4'-Methylene bis(2-methylaniline) | *4*, 73 (1974); *Suppl. 7*, 248 (1987) |
| 4,4'-Methylenedianiline | *4*, 79 (1974) (*corr. 42*, 252); *39*, 347 (1986); *Suppl. 7*, 66 (1987) |
| 4,4'-Methylenediphenyl diisocyanate | *19*, 314 (1979); *Suppl. 7*, 66 (1987) |
| 2-Methylfluoranthene | *32*, 399 (1983); *Suppl. 7*, 66 (1987) |
| 3-Methylfluoranthene | *32*, 399 (1983); *Suppl. 7*, 66 (1987) |
| Methyl iodide | *15*, 245 (1977); *41*, 213 (1986); *Suppl. 7*, 66 (1987) |
| Methyl methacrylate | *19*, 187 (1979); *Suppl. 7*, 66 (1987) |
| Methyl methanesulphonate | *7*, 253 (1974); *Suppl. 7*, 66 (1987) |
| 2-Methyl-1-nitroanthraquinone | *27*, 205 (1982); *Suppl. 7*, 66 (1987) |
| *N*-Methyl-*N'*-nitro-*N*-nitrosoguanidine | *4*, 183 (1974); *Suppl. 7*, 248 (1987) |
| 3-Methylnitrosaminopropionaldehyde (*see* 3-(*N*-Nitrosomethylamino)propionaldehyde) | |
| 3-Methylnitrosaminopropionitrile (*see* 3-(*N*-Nitrosomethylamino)propionitrile) | |
| 4-(Methylnitrosamino)-4-(3-pyridyl)-1-butanal (*see* 4-(*N*-Nitrosomethylamino)-4-(3-pyridyl)-1-butanal) | |
| 4-(Methylnitrosamino)-1-(3-pyridyl)-1-butanone (*see* 4-(*N*-Nitrosomethylamino)-1-(3-pyridyl)-1-butanone) | |
| *N*-Methyl-*N*-nitrosourea | *1*, 125 (1972); *17*, 227 (1978); *Suppl. 7*, 66 (1987) |
| *N*-Methyl-*N*-nitrosourethane | *4*, 211 (1974); *Suppl. 7*, 66 (1987) |
| Methyl parathion | *30*, 131 (1983); *Suppl. 7*, 392 (1987) |
| 1-Methylphenanthrene | *32*, 405 (1983); *Suppl. 7*, 66 (1987) |
| 7-Methylpyrido[3,4-*c*]psoralen | *40*, 349 (1986); *Suppl. 7*, 71 (1987) |
| Methyl red | *8*, 161 (1975); *Suppl. 7*, 66 (1987) |
| Methyl selenac (*see also* Selenium and selenium compounds) | *12*, 161 (1976); *Suppl. 7*, 66 (1987) |
| Methylthiouracil | *7*, 53 (1974); *Suppl. 7*, 66 (1987) |
| Metronidazole | *13*, 113 (1977); *Suppl. 7*, 250 (1987) |
| Mineral oils | *3*, 30 (1973); *33*, 87 (1984) (*corr. 42*, 262); *Suppl. 7*, 252 (1987) |

| | |
|---|---|
| Mirex | 5, 203 (1974); 20, 283 (1979) (corr. 42, 258); Suppl. 7, 66 (1987) |
| Mitomycin C | 10, 171 (1976); Suppl. 7, 67 (1987) |
| MNNG (see N-Methyl-N'-nitro-N-nitrosoguanidine) | |
| MOCA (see 4,4'-Methylene bis(2-chloroaniline)) | |
| Modacrylic fibres | 19, 86 (1979); Suppl. 7, 67 (1987) |
| Monocrotaline | 10, 291 (1976); Suppl. 7, 67 (1987) |
| Monuron | 12, 167 (1976); Suppl. 7, 67 (1987) |
| MOPP and other combined chemotherapy including alkylating agents | Suppl. 7, 254 (1987) |
| Morpholine | 47, 199 (1989) |
| 5-(Morpholinomethyl)-3-[(5-nitrofurfurylidene)amino]-2-oxazolidinone | 7, 161 (1974); Suppl. 7, 67 (1987) |
| Mustard gas | 9, 181 (1975) (corr. 42, 254); Suppl. 7, 259 (1987) |
| Myleran (see 1,4-Butanediol dimethanesulphonate) | |

# N

| | |
|---|---|
| Nafenopin | 24, 125 (1980); Suppl. 7, 67 (1987) |
| 1,5-Naphthalenediamine | 27, 127 (1982); Suppl. 7, 67 (1987) |
| 1,5-Naphthalene diisocyanate | 19, 311 (1979); Suppl. 7, 67 (1987) |
| 1-Naphthylamine | 4, 87 (1974) (corr. 42, 253); Suppl. 7, 260 (1987) |
| 2-Naphthylamine | 4, 97 (1974); Suppl. 7, 261 (1987) |
| 1-Naphthylthiourea | 30, 347 (1983); Suppl. 7, 263 (1987) |
| Nickel acetate (see Nickel and nickel compounds) | |
| Nickel ammonium sulphate (see Nickel and nickel compounds) | |
| Nickel and nickel compounds | 2, 126 (1973) (corr. 42, 252); 11, 75 (1976); Suppl. 7, 264 (1987) (corr. 45, 283) |
| Nickel carbonate (see Nickel and nickel compounds) | |
| Nickel carbonyl (see Nickel and nickel compounds) | |
| Nickel chloride (see Nickel and nickel compounds) | |
| Nickel-gallium alloy (see Nickel and nickel compounds) | |
| Nickel hydroxide (see Nickel and nickel compounds) | |
| Nickelocene (see Nickel and nickel compounds) | |
| Nickel oxide (see Nickel and nickel compounds) | |
| Nickel subsulphide (see Nickel and nickel compounds) | |
| Nickel sulphate (see Nickel and nickel compounds) | |
| Niridazole | 13, 123 (1977); Suppl. 7, 67 (1987) |
| Nithiazide | 31, 179 (1983); Suppl. 7, 67 (1987) |
| Nitrilotriacetic acid and its salts | 48, 181 (1990) |
| 5-Nitroacenaphthene | 16, 319 (1978); Suppl. 7, 67 (1987) |
| 5-Nitro-ortho-anisidine | 27, 133 (1982); Suppl. 7, 67 (1987) |

| | |
|---|---|
| 9-Nitroanthracene | *33*, 179 (1984); *Suppl. 7*, 67 (1987) |
| 7-Nitrobenz[*a*]anthracene | *46*, 247 (1989) |
| 6-Nitrobenzo[*a*]pyrene | *33*, 187 (1984); *Suppl. 7*, 67 (1987); *46*, 255 (1989) |
| 4-Nitrobiphenyl | *4*, 113 (1974); *Suppl. 7*, 67 (1987) |
| 6-Nitrochrysene | *33*, 195 (1984); *Suppl. 7*, 67 (1987); *46*, 267 (1989) |
| Nitrofen (technical-grade) | *30*, 271 (1983); *Suppl. 7*, 67 (1987) |
| 3-Nitrofluoranthene | *33*, 201 (1984); *Suppl. 7*, 67 (1987) |
| 2-Nitrofluorene | *46*, 277 (1989) |
| 5-Nitro-2-furaldehyde semicarbazone | *7*, 171 (1974); *Suppl. 7*, 67 (1987) |
| 1-[(5-Nitrofurfurylidene)amino]-2-imidazolidinone | *7*, 181 (1974); *Suppl. 7*, 67 (1987) |
| N-[4-(5-Nitro-2-furyl)-2-thiazolyl]acetamide | *1*, 181 (1972); *7*, 185 (1974); *Suppl. 7*, 67 (1987) |
| Nitrogen mustard | *9*, 193 (1975); *Suppl. 7*, 269 (1987) |
| Nitrogen mustard *N*-oxide | *9*, 209 (1975); *Suppl. 7*, 67 (1987) |
| 1-Nitronaphthalene | *46*, 291 (1989) |
| 2-Nitronaphthalene | *46*, 303 (1989) |
| 3-Nitroperylene | *46*, 313 (1989) |
| 2-Nitropropane | *29*, 331 (1982); *Suppl. 7*, 67 (1987) |
| 1-Nitropyrene | *33*, 209 (1984); *Suppl. 7*, 67 (1987); *46*, 321 (1989) |
| 2-Nitropyrene | *46*, 359 (1989) |
| 4-Nitropyrene | *46*, 367 (1989) |
| *N*-Nitrosatable drugs | *24*, 297 (1980) *(corr. 42, 260)* |
| *N*-Nitrosatable pesticides | *30*, 359 (1983) |
| *N'*-Nitrosoanabasine | *37*, 225 (1985); *Suppl. 7*, 67 (1987) |
| *N'*-Nitrosoanatabine | *37*, 233 (1985); *Suppl. 7*, 67 (1987) |
| *N*-Nitrosodi-*n*-butylamine | *4*, 197 (1974); *17*, 51 (1978); *Suppl. 7*, 67 (1987) |
| *N*-Nitrosodiethanolamine | *17*, 77 (1978); *Suppl. 7*, 67 (1987) |
| *N*-Nitrosodiethylamine | *1*, 107 (1972) *(corr. 42, 251)*; *17*, 83 (1978) *(corr. 42, 257)*; *Suppl. 7*, 67 (1987) |
| *N*-Nitrosodimethylamine | *1*, 95 (1972); *17*, 125 (1978) *(corr. 42, 257)*; *Suppl. 7*, 67 (1987) |
| *N*-Nitrosodiphenylamine | *27*, 213 (1982); *Suppl. 7*, 67 (1987) |
| *para*-Nitrosodiphenylamine | *27*, 227 (1982) *(corr. 42, 261)*; *Suppl. 7*, 68 (1987) |
| *N*-Nitrosodi-*n*-propylamine | *17*, 177 (1978); *Suppl. 7*, 68 (1987) |
| *N*-Nitroso-*N*-ethylurea (*see N*-Ethyl-*N*-nitrosourea) | |
| *N*-Nitrosofolic acid | *17*, 217 (1978); *Suppl. 7*, 68 (1987) |
| *N*-Nitrosoguvacine | *37*, 263 (1985); *Suppl. 7*, 68 (1987) |
| *N*-Nitrosoguvacoline | *37*, 263 (1985); *Suppl. 7*, 68 (1987) |
| *N*-Nitrosohydroxyproline | *17*, 304 (1978); *Suppl. 7*, 68 (1987) |

| | |
|---|---|
| 3-(*N*-Nitrosomethylamino)propionaldehyde | *37*, 263 (1985); *Suppl. 7*, 68 (1987) |
| 3-(*N*-Nitrosomethylamino)propionitrile | *37*, 263 (1985); *Suppl. 7*, 68 (1987) |
| 4-(*N*-Nitrosomethylamino)-4-(3-pyridyl)-1-butanal | *37*, 205 (1985); *Suppl. 7*, 68 (1987) |
| 4-(*N*-Nitrosomethylamino)-1-(3-pyridyl)-1-butanone | *37*, 209 (1985); *Suppl. 7*, 68 (1987) |
| *N*-Nitrosomethylethylamine | *17*, 221 (1978); *Suppl. 7*, 68 (1987) |
| *N*-Nitroso-*N*-methylurea (*see N*-Methyl-*N*-nitrosourea) | |
| *N*-Nitroso-*N*-methylurethane (*see N*-Methyl-*N*-methylurethane) | |
| *N*-Nitrosomethylvinylamine | *17*, 257 (1978); *Suppl. 7*, 68 (1987) |
| *N*-Nitrosomorpholine | *17*, 263 (1978); *Suppl. 7*, 68 (1987) |
| *N'*-Nitrosonornicotine | *17*, 281 (1978); *37*, 241 (1985); *Suppl. 7*, 68 (1987) |
| *N*-Nitrosopiperidine | *17*, 287 (1978); *Suppl. 7*, 68 (1987) |
| *N*-Nitrosoproline | *17*, 303 (1978); *Suppl. 7*, 68 (1987) |
| *N*-Nitrosopyrrolidine | *17*, 313 (1978); *Suppl. 7*, 68 (1987) |
| *N*-Nitrososarcosine | *17*, 327 (1978); *Suppl. 7*, 68 (1987) |
| Nitrosoureas, chloroethyl (*see* Chloroethyl nitrosoureas) | |
| 5-Nitro-*ortho*-toluidine | *48*, 169 (1990) |
| Nitrous oxide (*see* Anaesthetics, volatile) | |
| Nitrovin | *31*, 185 (1983); *Suppl. 7*, 68 (1987) |
| NNA (*see* 4-(*N*-Nitrosomethylamino)-4-(3-pyridyl)-1-butanal) | |
| NNK (*see* 4-(*N*-Nitrosomethylamino)-1-(3-pyridyl)-1-butanone) | |
| Nonsteroidal oestrogens (*see also* Oestrogens, progestins and combinations) | *Suppl. 7*, 272 (1987) |
| Norethisterone (*see also* Progestins; Combined oral contraceptives) | *6*, 179 (1974); *21*, 461 (1979) |
| Norethynodrel (*see also* Progestins; Combined oral contraceptives | *6*, 191 (1974); *21*, 461 (1979) (*corr. 42*, 259) |
| Norgestrel (*see also* Progestins, Combined oral contraceptives) | *6*, 201 (1974); *21*, 479 (1979) |
| Nylon 6 | *19*, 120 (1979); *Suppl. 7*, 68 (1987) |

# O

| | |
|---|---|
| Ochratoxin A | *10*, 191 (1976); *31*, 191 (1983) (*corr. 42*, 262); *Suppl. 7*, 271 (1987) |
| Oestradiol-17β (*see also* Steroidal oestrogens) | *6*, 99 (1974); *21*, 279 (1979) |
| Oestradiol 3-benzoate (*see* Oestradiol-17β) | |
| Oestradiol dipropionate (*see* Oestradiol-17β) | |
| Oestradiol mustard | *9*, 217 (1975) |
| Oestradiol-17β-valerate (*see* Oestradiol-17β) | |
| Oestriol (*see also* Steroidal oestrogens) | *6*, 117 (1974); *21*, 327 (1979) |
| Oestrogen-progestin combinations (*see* Oestrogens, progestins and combinations) | |
| Oestrogen-progestin replacement therapy (*see also* Oestrogens, progestins and combinations) | *Suppl. 7*, 308 (1987) |

| | |
|---|---|
| Oestrogen replacement therapy (see also Oestrogens, progestins and combinations) | Suppl. 7, 280 (1987) |
| Oestrogens (see Oestrogens, progestins and combinations) | |
| Oestrogens, conjugated (see Conjugated oestrogens) | |
| Oestrogens, nonsteroidal (see Nonsteroidal oestrogens) | |
| Oestrogens, progestins and combinations | 6 (1974); 21 (1979); Suppl. 7, 272 (1987) |
| Oestrogens, steroidal (see Steroidal oestrogens) | |
| Oestrone (see also Steroidal oestrogens) | 6, 123 (1974); 21, 343 (1979) (corr. 42, 259) |
| Oestrone benzoate (see Oestrone) | |
| Oil Orange SS | 8, 165 (1975); Suppl. 7, 69 (1987) |
| Oral contraceptives, combined (see Combined oral contraceptives) | |
| Oral contraceptives, investigational (see Combined oral contraceptives) | |
| Oral contraceptives, sequential (see Sequential oral contraceptives) | |
| Orange I | 8, 173 (1975); Suppl. 7, 69 (1987) |
| Orange G | 8, 181 (1975); Suppl. 7, 69 (1987) |
| Organolead compounds (see also Lead and lead compounds) | Suppl. 7, 230 (1987) |
| Oxazepam | 13, 58 (1977); Suppl. 7, 69 (1987) |
| Oxymetholone (see also Androgenic (anabolic) steroids) | 13, 131 (1977) |
| Oxyphenbutazone | 13, 185 (1977); Suppl. 7, 69 (1987) |

## P

| | |
|---|---|
| Paint manufacture and painting (occupational exposures in) | 47, 329 (1989) |
| Panfuran S (see also Dihydroxymethylfuratrizine) | 24, 77 (1980); Suppl. 7, 69 (1987) |
| Paper manufacture (see Pulp and paper manufacture) | |
| Parasorbic acid | 10, 199 (1976) (corr. 42, 255); Suppl. 7, 69 (1987) |
| Parathion | 30, 153 (1983); Suppl. 7, 69 (1987) |
| Patulin | 10, 205 (1976); 40, 83 (1986); Suppl. 7, 69 (1987) |
| Penicillic acid | 10, 211 (1976); Suppl. 7, 69 (1987) |
| Pentachloroethane | 41, 99 (1986); Suppl. 7, 69 (1987) |
| Pentachloronitrobenzene (see Quintozene) | |
| Pentachlorophenol (see also Chlorophenols; Chlorophenols, occupational exposures to) | 20, 303 (1979) |
| Perylene | 32, 411 (1983); Suppl. 7, 69 (1987) |
| Petasitenine | 31, 207 (1983); Suppl. 7, 69 (1987) |
| *Petasites japonicus* (see Pyrrolizidine alkaloids) | |
| Petroleum refining (occupational exposures in) | 45, 39 (1989) |
| Some petroleum solvents | 47, 43 (1989) |
| Phenacetin | 3, 141 (1973); 24, 135 (1980); Suppl. 7, 310 (1987) |

| | |
|---|---|
| Phenanthrene | *32*, 419 (1983); *Suppl. 7*, 69 (1987) |
| Phenazopyridine hydrochloride | *8*, 117 (1975); *24*, 163 (1980) (*corr.* *42*, 260); *Suppl. 7*, 312 (1987) |
| Phenelzine sulphate | *24*, 175 (1980); *Suppl. 7*, 312 (1987) |
| Phenicarbazide | *12*, 177 (1976); *Suppl. 7*, 70 (1987) |
| Phenobarbital | *13*, 157 (1977); *Suppl. 7*, 313 (1987) |
| Phenol | *47*, 263 (1989) |
| Phenoxyacetic acid herbicides (*see* Chlorophenoxy herbicides) | |
| Phenoxybenzamine hydrochloride | *9*, 223 (1975); *24*, 185 (1980); *Suppl. 7*, 70 (1987) |
| Phenylbutazone | *13*, 183 (1977); *Suppl. 7*, 316 (1987) |
| *meta*-Phenylenediamine | *16*, 111 (1978); *Suppl. 7*, 70 (1987) |
| *para*-Phenylenediamine | *16*, 125 (1978); *Suppl. 7*, 70 (1987) |
| *N*-Phenyl-2-naphthylamine | *16*, 325 (1978) (*corr.* *42*, 257); *Suppl. 7*, 318 (1987) |
| *ortho*-Phenylphenol | *30*, 329 (1983); *Suppl. 7*, 70 (1987) |
| Phenytoin | *13*, 201 (1977); *Suppl. 7*, 319 (1987) |
| Piperazine oestrone sulphate (*see* Conjugated oestrogens) | |
| Piperonyl butoxide | *30*, 183 (1983); *Suppl. 7*, 70 (1987) |
| Pitches, coal-tar (*see* Coal-tar pitches) | |
| Polyacrylic acid | *19*, 62 (1979); *Suppl. 7*, 70 (1987) |
| Polybrominated biphenyls | *18*, 107 (1978); *41*, 261 (1986); *Suppl. 7*, 321 (1987) |
| Polychlorinated biphenyls | *7*, 261 (1974); *18*, 43 (1978) (*corr.* *42*, 258); *Suppl. 7*, 322 (1987) |
| Polychlorinated camphenes (*see* Toxaphene) | |
| Polychloroprene | *19*, 141 (1979); *Suppl. 7*, 70 (1987) |
| Polyethylene | *19*, 164 (1979); *Suppl. 7*, 70 (1987) |
| Polymethylene polyphenyl isocyanate | *19*, 314 (1979); *Suppl. 7*, 70 (1987) |
| Polymethyl methacrylate | *19*, 195 (1979); *Suppl. 7*, 70 (1987) |
| Polyoestradiol phosphate (*see* Oestradiol-17β) | |
| Polypropylene | *19*, 218 (1979); *Suppl. 7*, 70 (1987) |
| Polystyrene | *19*, 245 (1979); *Suppl. 7*, 70 (1987) |
| Polytetrafluoroethylene | *19*, 288 (1979); *Suppl. 7*, 70 (1987) |
| Polyurethane foams | *19*, 320 (1979); *Suppl. 7*, 70 (1987) |
| Polyvinyl acetate | *19*, 346 (1979); *Suppl. 7*, 70 (1987) |
| Polyvinyl alcohol | *19*, 351 (1979); *Suppl. 7*, 70 (1987) |
| Polyvinyl chloride | *7*, 306 (1974); *19*, 402 (1979); *Suppl. 7*, 70 (1987) |
| Polyvinyl pyrrolidone | *19*, 463 (1979); *Suppl. 7*, 70 (1987) |
| Ponceau MX | *8*, 189 (1975); *Suppl. 7*, 70 (1987) |
| Ponceau 3R | *8*, 199 (1975); *Suppl. 7*, 70 (1987) |
| Ponceau SX | *8*, 207 (1975); *Suppl. 7*, 70 (1987) |
| Potassium arsenate (*see* Arsenic and arsenic compounds) | |

| | |
|---|---|
| Potassium arsenite (*see* Arsenic and arsenic compounds) | |
| Potassium bis(2-hydroxyethyl)dithiocarbamate | *12*, 183 (1976); *Suppl. 7*, 70 (1987) |
| Potassium bromate | *40*, 207 (1986); *Suppl. 7*, 70 (1987) |
| Potassium chromate (*see* Chromium and chromium compounds) | |
| Potassium dichromate (*see* Chromium and chromium compounds) | |
| Prednisone | *26*, 293 (1981); *Suppl. 7*, 326 (1987) |
| Procarbazine hydrochloride | *26*, 311 (1981); *Suppl. 7*, 327 (1987) |
| Proflavine salts | *24*, 195 (1980); *Suppl. 7*, 70 (1987) |
| Progesterone (*see also* Progestins; Combined oral contraceptives) | *6*, 135 (1974); *21*, 491 (1979) (*corr. 42*, 259) |
| Progestins (*see also* Oestrogens, progestins and combinations) | *Suppl. 7*, 289 (1987) |
| Pronetalol hydrochloride | *13*, 227 (1977) (*corr. 42*, 256); *Suppl. 7*, 70 (1987) |
| 1,3-Propane sultone | *4*, 253 (1974) (*corr. 42*, 253); *Suppl. 7*, 70 (1987) |
| Propham | *12*, 189 (1976); *Suppl. 7*, 70 (1987) |
| β-Propiolactone | *4*, 259 (1974) (*corr. 42*, 253); *Suppl. 7*, 70 (1987) |
| *n*-Propyl carbamate | *12*, 201 (1976); *Suppl. 7*, 70 (1987) |
| Propylene | *19*, 213 (1979); *Suppl. 7*, 71 (1987) |
| Propylene oxide | *11*, 191 (1976); *36*, 227 (1985) (*corr. 42*, 263); *Suppl. 7*, 328 (1987) |
| Propylthiouracil | *7*, 67 (1974); *Suppl. 7*, 329 (1987) |
| Ptaquiloside (*see also* Bracken fern) | *40*, 55 (1986); *Suppl. 7*, 71 (1987) |
| Pulp and paper manufacture | *25*, 157 (1981); *Suppl. 7*, 385 (1987) |
| Pyrene | *32*, 431 (1983); *Suppl. 7*, 71 (1987) |
| Pyrido[3,4-*c*]psoralen | *40*, 349 (1986); *Suppl. 7*, 71 (1987) |
| Pyrimethamine | *13*, 233 (1977); *Suppl. 7*, 71 (1987) |
| Pyrrolizidine alkaloids (*see also* Hydroxysenkirkine; Isatidine; Jacobine; Lasiocarpine; Monocrotaline; Retrorsine; Riddelliine; Seneciphylline; Senkirkine) | |

# Q

| | |
|---|---|
| Quercetin (*see also* Bracken fern) | *31*, 213 (1983); *Suppl. 7*, 71 (1987) |
| *para*-Quinone | *15*, 255 (1977); *Suppl. 7*, 71 (1987) |
| Quintozene | *5*, 211 (1974); *Suppl. 7*, 71 (1987) |

# R

| | |
|---|---|
| Radon | *43*, 173 (1988) (*corr. 45*, 283) |
| Reserpine | *10*, 217 (1976); *24*, 211 (1980) (*corr. 42*, 260); *Suppl. 7*, 330 (1987) |
| Resorcinol | *15*, 155 (1977); *Suppl. 7*, 71 (1987) |

| | |
|---|---|
| Retrorsine | *10*, 303 (1976); *Suppl. 7*, 71 (1987) |
| Rhodamine B | *16*, 221 (1978); *Suppl. 7*, 71 (1987) |
| Rhodamine 6G | *16*, 233 (1978); *Suppl. 7*, 71 (1987) |
| Riddelliine | *10*, 313 (1976); *Suppl. 7*, 71 (1987) |
| Rifampicin | *24*, 243 (1980); *Suppl. 7*, 71 (1987) |
| Rockwool (*see* Man-made mineral fibres) | |
| The rubber industry | 28 (1982) (*corr.* 42, 261); *Suppl. 7*, 332 (1987) |
| Rugulosin | *40*, 99 (1986); *Suppl. 7*, 71 (1987) |

## S

| | |
|---|---|
| Saccharated iron oxide | *2*, 161 (1973); *Suppl. 7*, 71 (1987) |
| Saccharin | *22*, 111 (1980) (*corr.* 42, 259); *Suppl. 7*, 334 (1987) |
| Safrole | *1*, 169 (1972); *10*, 231 (1976); *Suppl. 7*, 71 (1987) |
| The sawmill industry (including logging) (*see* The lumber and sawmill industry (including logging)) | |
| Scarlet Red | *8*, 217 (1975); *Suppl. 7*, 71 (1987) |
| Selenium and selenium compounds | *9*, 245 (1975) (*corr.* 42, 255); *Suppl. 7*, 71 (1987) |
| Selenium dioxide (*see* Selenium and selenium compounds) | |
| Selenium oxide (*see* Selenium and selenium compounds) | |
| Semicarbazide hydrochloride | *12*, 209 (1976) (*corr.* 42, 256); *Suppl. 7*, 71 (1987) |
| *Senecio jacobaea* L. (*see* Pyrrolizidine alkaloids) | |
| *Senecio longilobus* (*see* Pyrrolizidine alkaloids) | |
| Seneciphylline | *10*, 319, 335 (1976); *Suppl. 7*, 71 (1987) |
| Senkirkine | *10*, 327 (1976); *31*, 231 (1983); *Suppl. 7*, 71 (1987) |
| Sepiolite | *42*, 175 (1987); *Suppl. 7*, 71 (1987) |
| Sequential oral contraceptives (*see also* Oestrogens, progestins and combinations) | *Suppl. 7*, 296 (1987) |
| Shale-oils | *35*, 161 (1985); *Suppl. 7*, 339 (1987) |
| Shikimic acid (*see also* Bracken fern) | *40*, 55 (1986); *Suppl. 7*, 71 (1987) |
| Shoe manufacture and repair (*see* Boot and shoe manufacture and repair) | |
| Silica (*see also* Amorphous silica; Crystalline silica) | *42*, 39 (1987) |
| Slagwool (*see* Man-made mineral fibres) | |
| Sodium arsenate (*see* Arsenic and arsenic compounds) | |
| Sodium arsenite (*see* Arsenic and arsenic compounds) | |
| Sodium cacodylate (*see* Arsenic and arsenic compounds) | |
| Sodium chromate (*see* Chromium and chromium compounds) | |

| | |
|---|---|
| Sodium cyclamate (*see* Cyclamates) | |
| Sodium dichromate (*see* Chromium and chromium compounds) | |
| Sodium diethyldithiocarbamate | *12*, 217 (1976); *Suppl. 7*, 71 (1987) |
| Sodium equilin sulphate (*see* Conjugated oestrogens) | |
| Sodium fluoride (*see* Fluorides) | |
| Sodium monofluorophosphate (*see* Fluorides) | |
| Sodium oestrone sulphate (*see* Conjugated oestrogens) | |
| Sodium *ortho*-phenylphenate (*see also ortho*-Phenylphenol) | *30*, 329 (1983); *Suppl. 7*, 392 (1987) |
| Sodium saccharin (*see* Saccharin) | |
| Sodium selenate (*see* Selenium and selenium compounds) | |
| Sodium selenite (*see* Selenium and selenium compounds) | |
| Sodium silicofluoride (*see* Fluorides) | |
| Soots | *3*, 22 (1973); *35*, 219 (1985); *Suppl. 7*, 343 (1987) |
| Spironolactone | *24*, 259 (1980); *Suppl. 7*, 344 (1987) |
| Stannous fluoride (*see* Fluorides) | |
| Steel founding (*see* Iron and steel founding) | |
| Sterigmatocystin | *1*, 175 (1972); *10*, 245 (1976); *Suppl. 7*, 72 (1987) |
| Steroidal oestrogens (*see also* Oestrogens, progestins and combinations) | *Suppl. 7*, 280 (1987) |
| Streptozotocin | *4*, 221 (1974); *17*, 337 (1978); *Suppl. 7*, 72 (1987) |
| Strobane® (*see* Terpene polychlorinates) | |
| Strontium chromate (*see* Chromium and chromium compounds) | |
| Styrene | *19*, 231 (1979) (*corr. 42*, 258); *Suppl. 7*, 345 (1987) |
| Styrene-acrylonitrile copolymers | *19*, 97 (1979); *Suppl. 7*, 72 (1987) |
| Styrene-butadiene copolymers | *19*, 252 (1979); *Suppl. 7*, 72 (1987) |
| Styrene oxide | *11*, 201 (1976); *19*, 275 (1979); *36*, 245 (1985); *Suppl. 7*, 72 (1987) |
| Succinic anhydride | *15*, 265 (1977); *Suppl. 7*, 72 (1987) |
| Sudan I | *8*, 225 (1975); *Suppl. 7*, 72 (1987) |
| Sudan II | *8*, 233 (1975); *Suppl. 7*, 72 (1987) |
| Sudan III | *8*, 241 (1975); *Suppl. 7*, 72 (1987) |
| Sudan Brown RR | *8*, 249 (1975); *Suppl. 7*, 72 (1987) |
| Sudan Red 7B | *8*, 253 (1975); *Suppl. 7*, 72 (1987) |
| Sulfafurazole | *24*, 275 (1980); *Suppl. 7*, 347 (1987) |
| Sulfallate | *30*, 283 (1983); *Suppl. 7*, 72 (1987) |
| Sulfamethoxazole | *24*, 285 (1980); *Suppl. 7*, 348 (1987) |
| Sulphisoxazole (*see* Sulfafurazole) | |
| Sulphur mustard (*see* Mustard gas) | |
| Sunset Yellow FCF | *8*, 257 (1975); *Suppl. 7*, 72 (1987) |
| Symphytine | *31*, 239 (1983); *Suppl. 7*, 72 (1987) |

## T

| | |
|---|---|
| 2,4,5-T (*see also* Chlorophenoxy herbicides; Chlorophenoxy herbicides, occupational exposures to) | *15*, 273 (1977) |
| Talc | *42*, 185 (1987); *Suppl. 7*, 349 (1987) |
| Tannic acid | *10*, 253 (1976) (*corr. 42*, 255); *Suppl. 7*, 72 (1987) |
| Tannins (*see also* Tannic acid) | *10*, 254 (1976); *Suppl. 7*, 72 (1987) |
| TCDD (*see* 2,3,7,8-Tetrachlorodibenzo-*para*-dioxin) | |
| TDE (*see* DDT) | |
| Terpene polychlorinates | *5*, 219 (1974); *Suppl. 7*, 72 (1987) |
| Testosterone (*see also* Androgenic (anabolic) steroids) | *6*, 209 (1974); *21*, 519 (1979) |
| Testosterone oenanthate (*see* Testosterone) | |
| Testosterone propionate (*see* Testosterone) | |
| 2,2',5,5'-Tetrachlorobenzidine | *27*, 141 (1982); *Suppl. 7*, 72 (1987) |
| 2,3,7,8-Tetrachlorodibenzo-*para*-dioxin | *15*, 41 (1977); *Suppl. 7*, 350 (1987) |
| 1,1,1,2-Tetrachloroethane | *41*, 87 (1986); *Suppl. 7*, 72 (1987) |
| 1,1,2,2-Tetrachloroethane | *20*, 477 (1979); *Suppl. 7*, 354 (1987) |
| Tetrachloroethylene | *20*, 491 (1979); *Suppl. 7*, 355 (1987) |
| 2,3,4,6-Tetrachlorophenol (*see* Chlorophenols; Chlorophenols, occupational exposures to) | |
| Tetrachlorvinphos | *30*, 197 (1983); *Suppl. 7*, 72 (1987) |
| Tetraethyllead (*see* Lead and lead compounds) | |
| Tetrafluoroethylene | *19*, 285 (1979); *Suppl. 7*, 72 (1987) |
| Tetrakis(hydroxymethyl) phosphonium salts | *48*, 95 (1990) |
| Tetramethyllead (*see* Lead and lead compounds) | |
| Textile manufacturing industry, exposures in | *48*, 215 (1990) |
| Thioacetamide | *7*, 77 (1974); *Suppl. 7*, 72 (1987) |
| 4,4'-Thiodianiline | *16*, 343 (1978); *27*, 147 (1982); *Suppl. 7*, 72 (1987) |
| Thiotepa (*see* Tris(1-aziridinyl)phosphine sulphide) | |
| Thiouracil | *7*, 85 (1974); *Suppl. 7*, 72 (1987) |
| Thiourea | *7*, 95 (1974); *Suppl. 7*, 72 (1987) |
| Thiram | *12*, 225 (1976); *Suppl. 7*, 72 (1987) |
| Titanium dioxide | *47*, 307 (1989) |
| Tobacco habits other than smoking (*see* Tobacco products, smokeless) | |
| Tobacco products, smokeless | *37* (1985) (*corr. 42*, 263); *Suppl. 7*, 357 (1987) |
| Tobacco smoke | *38* (1986) (*corr. 42*, 263); *Suppl. 7*, 357 (1987) |
| Tobacco smoking (*see* Tobacco smoke) | |
| *ortho*-Tolidine (*see* 3,3'-Dimethylbenzidine) | |
| 2,4-Toluene diisocyanate (*see also* Toluene diisocyanates) | *19*, 303 (1979); *39*, 287 (1986) |
| 2,6-Toluene diisocyanate (*see also* Toluene diisocyanates) | *19*, 303 (1979); *39*, 289 (1986) |

| | |
|---|---|
| Toluene | *47*, 79 (1989) |
| Toluene diisocyanates | *39*, 287 (1986) (*corr. 42*, 264); Suppl. 7, 72 (1987) |
| Toluenes, α-chlorinated (*see* α-Chlorinated toluenes) | |
| *ortho*-Toluenesulphonamide (*see* Saccharin) | |
| *ortho*-Toluidine | *16*, 349 (1978); *27*, 155 (1982); Suppl. 7, 362 (1987) |
| Toxaphene | *20*, 327 (1979); Suppl. 7, 72 (1987) |
| Tremolite (*see* Asbestos) | |
| Treosulphan | *26*, 341 (1981); Suppl. 7, 363 (1987) |
| Triaziquone (*see* Tris(aziridinyl)-*para*-benzoquinone) | |
| Trichlorfon | *30*, 207 (1983); Suppl. 7, 73 (1987) |
| 1,1,1-Trichloroethane | *20*, 515 (1979); Suppl. 7, 73 (1987) |
| 1,1,2-Trichloroethane | *20*, 533 (1979); Suppl. 7, 73 (1987) |
| Trichloroethylene | *11*, 263 (1976); *20*, 545 (1979); Suppl. 7, 364 (1987) |
| 2,4,5-Trichlorophenol (*see also* Chlorophenols; Chlorophenols occupational exposures to) | *20*, 349 (1979) |
| 2,4,6-Trichlorophenol (*see also* Chlorophenols; Chlorophenols, occupational exposures to) | *20*, 349 (1979) |
| (2,4,5-Trichlorophenoxy)acetic acid (*see* 2,4,5-T) | |
| Trichlorotriethylamine hydrochloride | *9*, 229 (1975); Suppl. 7, 73 (1987) |
| T$_2$-Trichothecene | *31*, 265 (1983); Suppl. 7, 73 (1987) |
| Triethylene glycol diglycidyl ether | *11*, 209 (1976); Suppl. 7, 73 (1987) |
| 4,4',6-Trimethylangelicin plus ultraviolet radiation (*see also* Angelicin and some synthetic derivatives) | Suppl. 7, 57 (1987) |
| 2,4,5-Trimethylaniline | *27*, 177 (1982); Suppl. 7, 73 (1987) |
| 2,4,6-Trimethylaniline | *27*, 178 (1982); Suppl. 7, 73 (1'987) |
| 4,5',8-Trimethylpsoralen | *40*, 357 (1986); Suppl. 7, 366 (1987) |
| Triphenylene | *32*, 447 (1983); Suppl. 7, 73 (1987) |
| Tris(aziridinyl)-*para*-benzoquinone | *9*, 67 (1975); Suppl. 7, 367 (1987) |
| Tris(1-aziridinyl)phosphine oxide | *9*, 75 (1975); Suppl. 7, 73 (1987) |
| Tris(1-aziridinyl)phosphine sulphide | *9*, 85 (1975); Suppl. 7, 368 (1987) |
| 2,4,6-Tris(1-aziridinyl)-*s*-triazine | *9*, 95 (1975); Suppl. 7, 73 (1987) |
| Tris(2-chloroethyl) phosphate | *48*, 109 (1990) |
| 1,2,3-Tris(chloromethoxy)propane | *15*, 301 (1977); Suppl. 7, 73 (1987) |
| Tris(2,3-dibromopropyl)phosphate | *20*, 575 (1979); Suppl. 7, 369 (1987) |
| Tris(2-methyl-1-aziridinyl)phosphine oxide | *9*, 107 (1975); Suppl. 7, 73 (1987) |
| Trp-P-1 | *31*, 247 (1983); Suppl. 7, 73 (1987) |
| Trp-P-2 | *31*, 255 (1983); Suppl. 7, 73 (1987) |
| Trypan blue | *8*, 267 (1975); Suppl. 7, 73 (1987) |
| *Tussilago farfara* L. (*see* Pyrrolizidine alkaloids) | |

## U

| | |
|---|---|
| Ultraviolet radiation | *40*, 379 (1986) |
| Underground haematite mining with exposure to radon | *1*, 29 (1972); *Suppl. 7*, 216 (1987) |
| Uracil mustard | *9*, 235 (1975); *Suppl. 7*, 370 (1987) |
| Urethane | *7*, 111 (1974); *Suppl. 7*, 73 (1987) |

## V

| | |
|---|---|
| Vat Yellow 4 | *48*, 161 (1990) |
| Vinblastine sulphate | *26*, 349 (1981) (*corr. 42*, 261); *Suppl. 7*, 371 (1987) |
| Vincristine sulphate | *26*, 365 (1981); *Suppl. 7*, 372 (1987) |
| Vinyl acetate | *19*, 341 (1979); *39*, 113 (1986); *Suppl. 7*, 73 (1987) |
| Vinyl bromide | *19*, 367 (1979); *39*, 133 (1986); *Suppl. 7*, 73 (1987) |
| Vinyl chloride | *7*, 291 (1974); *19*, 377 (1979) (*corr. 42*, 258); *Suppl. 7*, 373 (1987) |
| Vinyl chloride-vinyl acetate copolymers | *7*, 311 (1976); *19*, 412 (1979) (*corr. 42*, 258); *Suppl. 7*, 73 (1987) |
| 4-Vinylcyclohexene | *11*, 277 (1976); *39*, 181 (1986); *Suppl. 7*, 73 (1987) |
| Vinyl fluoride | *39*, 147 (1986); *Suppl. 7*, 73 (1987) |
| Vinylidene chloride | *19*, 439 (1979); *39*, 195 (1986); *Suppl. 7*, 376 (1987) |
| Vinylidene chloride-vinyl chloride copolymers | *19*, 448 (1979) (*corr. 42*, 258); *Suppl. 7*, 73 (1987) |
| Vinylidene fluoride | *39*, 227 (1986); *Suppl. 7*, 73 (1987) |
| N-Vinyl-2-pyrrolidone | *19*, 461 (1979); *Suppl. 7*, 73 (1987) |

## W

| | |
|---|---|
| Wollastonite | *42*, 145 (1987); *Suppl. 7*, 377 (1987) |
| Wood industries | *25* (1981); *Suppl. 7*, 378 (1987) |

## X

| | |
|---|---|
| Xylene | *47*, 125 (1989) |
| 2,4-Xylidine | *16*, 367 (1978); *Suppl. 7*, 74 (1987) |
| 2,5-Xylidine | *16*, 377 (1978); *Suppl. 7*, 74 (1987) |

## Y

| | |
|---|---|
| Yellow AB | *8*, 279 (1975); *Suppl. 7*, 74 (1987) |

Yellow OB					8, 287 (1975); *Suppl.* 7, 74 (1987)

# Z

Zearalenone					*31*, 279 (1983); *Suppl.* 7, 74 (1987)
Zectran					*12*, 237 (1976); *Suppl.* 7, 74 (1987)
Zinc beryllium silicate (*see* Beryllium and beryllium compounds)
Zinc chromate (*see* Chromium and chromium compounds)
Zinc chromate hydroxide (*see* Chromium and chromium compounds)
Zinc potassium chromate (*see* Chromium and chromium compounds)
Zinc yellow (*see* Chromium and chromium compounds)
Zineb					*12*, 245 (1976); *Suppl.* 7, 74 (1987)
Ziram					*12*, 259 (1976); *Suppl.* 7, 74 (1987)

www.ingramcontent.com/pod-product-compliance
Ingram Content Group UK Ltd.
Pitfield, Milton Keynes, MK11 3LW, UK
UKHW051258180426
11947UKWH00020B/1785